# Spine Surgery

## Tricks of the Trade

### Second Edition

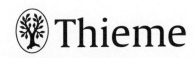

# Spine Surgery
## Tricks of the Trade
### Second Edition

**Alexander R. Vaccaro, MD, PhD**
Vice Chairman of Orthopaedic Surgery
Professor of Orthopaedics and Neurosurgery
Co-Director of the Delaware Valley Spinal Cord Injury Center
Co-Chief of Spine Surgery and of the Spine Fellowship Program
Thomas Jefferson University Hospital
Philadelphia, Pennsylvania

**Todd J. Albert, MD**
Richard H. Rothman Professor and Chairman of Orthopaedic Surgery
Professor of Neurosurgery
Co-Chief of Spine Surgery and of the Spine Fellowship Program
Thomas Jefferson University Hospital
Philadelphia, Pennsylvania

**Medical Illustrator**
Birck Cox

Thieme
New York • Stuttgart

Thieme Medical Publishers, Inc.
333 Seventh Avenue
New York, NY 10001

Executive Editor: Kalan Conerly
Managing Editor: J. Owen Zurhellen IV
Editorial Assistants: Adriana di Giorgio, Jacquelyn DeSanti, Chad Hollingsworth
Vice President, Production and Electronic Publishing: Anne T. Vinnicombe
Production Editor: Martha Wetherill
Vice President, International Marketing and Sales: Cornelia Schulze
Sales Director: Ross Lumpkin
Chief Financial Officer: Peter van Woerden
President: Brian D. Scanlan
Compositor: Macmillan Solutions
Printer: The Maple-Vail Book Manufacturing Group
Medical Illustrator: Birck Cox
Cover Photographer: Robert Neroni

**Library of Congress Cataloging-in-Publication Data**

Spine surgery : tricks of the trade / [edited by] Alexander R. Vaccaro, Todd J. Albert. — 2nd ed.
   p. ; cm.
   Includes index.
   ISBN-13: 978-1-58890-519-2
   1. Spine—Surgery.   I. Vaccaro, Alexander R.    II. Albert, Todd J.
   [DNLM: 1. Spinal Diseases—surgery.   2. Spine—surgery.   WE 725 S75992 2009]
   RD768.S685 2009
   617.4'71059—dc22

                                              2008035607

   **Important note:** Medical knowledge is ever-changing. As new research and clinical experience broaden our knowledge, changes in treatment and drug therapy may be required. The authors and editors of the material herein have consulted sources believed to be reliable in their efforts to provide information that is complete and in accord with the standards accepted at the time of publication. However, in view of the possibility of human error by the authors, editors, or publisher of the work herein, or changes in medical knowledge, neither the authors, editors, or publisher, nor any other party who has been involved in the preparation of this work, warrants that the information contained herein is in every respect accurate or complete, and they are not responsible for any errors or omissions or for the results obtained from use of such information. Readers are encouraged to confirm the information contained herein with other sources. For example, readers are advised to check the product information sheet included in the package of each drug they plan to administer to be certain that the information contained in this publication is accurate and that changes have not been made in the recommended dose or in the contraindications for administration. This recommendation is of particular importance in connection with new or infrequently used drugs.

   Some of the product names, patents, and registered designs referred to in this book are in fact registered trademarks or proprietary names even though specific reference to this fact is not always made in the text. Therefore, the appearance of a name without designation as proprietary is not to be construed as a representation by the publisher that it is in the public domain.

Printed in the United States of America

5 4 3 2

ISBN 978-1-58890-519-2

# Dedications

I dedicate this book to my children, Max, Alex, and Juliana, and to my parents, Alexander and Sue, all of whom have supported the efforts put forward in bringing this book to fruition.

*—Alexander R. Vaccaro, MD, PhD*

I dedicate this book to the memory of Herman Merinoff, who taught me so much about the "trade" of life.

*—Todd J. Albert, MD*

# Contents

# Foreword

Over the past twenty-five years, significant changes in the management of spinal disorders have taken place. We have moved from managing deformities and fractures with straight rods and single point fixation to complex three-dimensional reconstruction using multi-segmental pedicular instrumentation. We have moved from maximally invasive surgical exposures to minimally invasive techniques that allow patients to rapidly regain their normal activities and work status while minimizing their downtime. We are now beginning to embrace the idea of maintaining motion with arthroplasty rather automatically proceeding with arthrodesis. As these transitions have occurred, the technical expertise required for the procedures has become more demanding. Due to the imperfect nature of the human biologic system, not all of these procedures will be successful, so options for salvage techniques must be devised.

Alexander Vaccaro and Todd Albert are to be congratulated for the publication of this second edition of the book that provides the answers to many of the "how to, when to, and how do I get out of this" questions related to spine surgery. This revised edition has eighty-one chapters written by internationally recognized giants in the spine surgery arena. These contributors have compiled their experiences into a very concise, organized presentation of each topic, allowing rapid overview but also providing strict attention to detail. The format is consistent throughout the textbook, with each chapter providing an initial description of the technique or problem, key principles and expectations, indications, contraindications, and special considerations. Next, specific instructions, positioning, and anesthesia requirements are discussed. This is followed by tips, pearls and lessons learned, difficulties encountered, key procedural steps and pitfalls that may occur. The last section of each chapter includes what many texts fail to provide: recommendations regarding bailout, rescue, and salvage procedures. When all of these sections are combined as a complete chapter, one has at their fingertips the most concise, contemporary, authoritative "How To" manual of spinal surgery.

*Spine Surgery: Tricks of the Trade, Second Edition,* is a must for all orthopaedic and neurosurgical residents and fellows managing spine patients in their training. It is useful for the practicing spinal surgeon who has been in the community for a number of years and needs an up-to-date reference for his or her library.

*Robert A. McGuire, Jr., MD*
Professor and Chairman
Department of Orthopaedics and Rehabilitation
University of Mississippi Medical Center
Jackson, Mississippi

# Preface

Beginning in 1964 with Lyman Smith's work of injecting chymopapain into the intervertebral disk for the purpose of hydrolyzing a herniated nucleus pulposus, spine physicians have been developing techniques to minimize the morbidity of spine surgery procedures. This is a noble effort, as minimizing soft tissue or bone surgical invasion theoretically reduces operative time with less potential blood loss while avoiding unnecessary soft tissue trauma. If successful, patients may experience less need for postoperative pain medication, shorter hospital stays, and an expedited return to normal activities.

To keep current with these changing times, the authors of *Spine Surgery: Tricks of the Trade* have decided to write this second edition to incorporate contemporary surgical procedures while preserving topics that emphasize the basic tenets of spinal surgical care. For a second time, we have sought out the most qualified masters of the field for this undertaking. This book has brought together over 80 internationally renowned physicians to provide the most up-to-date guidance on commonly and not so commonly performed spinal procedures.

This second edition has been fully revised and updated. There are 81 chapters divided into eighteen sections. Each chapter follows a standard format: (1) a concise description of the procedure and key principles; (2) the expectations of what the surgeon is able to achieve with the procedure; (3) the indications and contraindications for the surgical technique; (4) special considerations and instructions when performing the described surgical procedure; (5) tips, pearls, and lessons learned in order to help minimize any complications or difficulties encountered; (6) key procedural steps; (7) pitfalls associated with the described technique; and (8) available bailout, rescue, and salvage procedures, should they become necessary.

This format has been created for ease of use by interested medical students, residents, spine fellows, pain management specialists, and spine surgeons from orthopedic and neurosurgical backgrounds. Each chapter is concise and rich in content, to provide readers interested in spinal care the most important aspects of a specific procedure.

*Peter M. Fleischut, MD*
New York-Presbyterian Hospital/Cornell
New York, New York

# Acknowledgments

This second edition of *Spine Surgery: Tricks of the Trade* was brought to publication with great efforts put forth by many individuals. We would especially like to thank Peter M. Fleischut, MD, without whose relentless work this edition would not have been possible. We will be forever grateful for Dr. Fleischut's selfless service to this project. The authors and Thieme also thank Medtronic Sofamor Danek, Inc., for its kind support of the art program for this book.

# Contributors

Kuniyoshi Abumi
Department of Orthopaedic Surgery
Hokkaido University Hospital
Sapporo, Japan

Todd J. Albert, MD
Rothman Institute
Philadelphia, Pennsylvania

D. Greg Anderson, MD
Rothman Institute
Philadelphia, Pennsylvania

Paul A. Anderson, MD
Department of Orthopedic Surgery and
  Rehabilitation
University Hospital
Madison, Wisconsin

Alexios Apazidis, MD
Department of Orthopedics
University of Medicine and Dentistry of New Jersey
Newark, New Jersey

Paul M. Arnold, MD
Spinal Cord Injury Center
University of Kansas
Kansas City, Kansas

JahanGir Asghar, MD
Shriners' Hospitals for Children
Philadelphia, Pennsylvania

Geoffrey N. Askin, MD
Mater Medical Centre
South Brisbane, Queensland, Australia

Joshua D. Auerbach, MD
Spine Surgery Service
Department of Orthopaedic Surgery
University of Pennsylvania
Philadelphia, Pennsylvania

Hyun Bae, MD
Spine Institute at Saint John's Health Center
Santa Monica, California

Eli M. Baron, MD
Private Practice
Philadelphia, Pennsylvania

John M. Beiner, MD
Connecticut Orthopaedic Specialists
Hamden, Connecticut

Edward C. Benzel, MD
Cleveland Clinic Spine Institute
Cleveland, Ohio

Randal R. Betz, MD
Shriners' Hospital for Children
Philadelphia, Pennsylvania

Scott L. Blumenthal, MD
Texas Back Institute
Plano, Texas

Christopher M. Bono, MD
Department of Orthopaedic Surgery
Boston University Medical Center
Boston, Massachusetts

Jared F. Brandoff, MD
Private Practice
Plainview, New York

Salvador A. Brau, MD
Spine Access Surgery Associates
Los Angeles, California

Keith H. Bridwell, MD
Department of Orthopaedic Surgery
Washington University School of Medicine
St. Louis, Missouri

Darrel S. Brodke, MD
University of Utah Orthopaedic Center
Salt Lake City, Utah

Douglas C. Burton, MD
Department of Orthopedic Surgery
University of Kansas Medical Center
Kansas City, Kansas

Frank P. Cammisa, Jr., MD
Hospital for Special Surgery
New York, New York

Robert M. Campbell, Jr., MD
Thoracic Institute
Christus Santa Rosa Children's Hospital
San Antonio, Texas

Kazuhiro Chiba MD, PhD
Section of Spine and Spinal Cord Surgery
School of Medicine
Keio University
Tokyo, Japan

Kingsley R. Chin, MD
Spine Surgery Service
University of Pennsylvania Medical School
Philadelphia, Pennsylvania

Norman B. Chutkan, MD
Medical College of Georgia
Augusta, Georgia

**Bradford L. Currier, MD**
Department of Orthopaedics
Mayo Clinic
Rochester, Minnesota

**Linda P. D'Andrea, MD**
Shriners' Hospital for Children
Philadelphia, Pennsylvania

**Jason C. Datta, MD**
Spine Education and Research Institute
Thornton, Colorado

**Rick B. Delamarter, MD**
Spine Institute at Saint John's Health Center
Santa Monica, California

**Vincent J. Devlin, MD**
Private Practice
Gilbert, Arizona

**Carrie A. Diulus, MD**
Department of Orthopaedic Surgery
Cleveland Clinic Foundation
Cleveland, Ohio

**Marcel F. S. Dvorak, MD**
Department of Orthopaedics
University of British Columbia
Vancouver, British Columbia, Canada

**Robert K. Eastlack, MD**
Private Practice
San Diego, California

**Charles C. Edwards, MD**
Maryland Spine Center
Baltimore, Maryland

**Charles C. Edwards II, MD**
Maryland Spine Center
Baltimore, Maryland

**James C. Farmer, MD**
Hospital for Special Surgery
New York, New York

**Jeffrey S. Fischgrund, MD**
Private Practice
Southfield, Mississippi

**Charles G. Fisher, MD**
Department of Orthopaedics
University of British Columbia
Vancouver, British Columbia, Canada

**Peter M. Fleischut, MD**
Private Practice
New York, New York

**Kevin T. Foley, MD**
Department of Neurosurgery
University of Tennessee
Memphis, Tennessee

**Steven R. Garfin, MD**
Department of Orthopedic Surgery
University of California–San Diego
San Diego, California

**Ben J. Garrido, MD**
Department of Orthopaedic Surgery
Indiana University School of Medicine
Indianapolis, Indiana

**Daniel E. Gelb, MD**
Department of Orthopaedics
University of Maryland School of Medicine
Timonium, Maryland

**Federico P. Girardi, MD**
Hospital for Special Surgery
New York, New York

**Ziya L. Gokaslan, MD**
Department of Neurology
Johns Hopkins Hospital
Baltimore, Maryland

**John T. Gorczyca, MD**
University of Rochester
Rochester, New York

**M. Sean Grady, MD**
Department of Neurosurgery
Hospital of the University of Pennsylvania
Philadelphia, Pennsylvania

**James T. Guille, MD**
Brandywine Institute of Orthopaedics
Pottstown, Pennsylvania

**Troy D. Gust, MD**
Department of Neurosurgery
University of Kansas Medical Center
Kansas City, Kansas

**Amgad Hanna, MD**
Private Practice
Philadelphia, Pennsylvania

**James S. Harrop, MD**
Department of Neurological Surgery
Thomas Jefferson University Hospital
Philadelphia, Pennsylvania

**Neal G. Haynes, MD**
Department of Neurosurgery
University of Kansas Medical Center
Kansas City, Kansas

**Langston T. Holly, MD**
Division of Neurosurgery
University of California–Los Angeles
Los Angeles, California

**Russel C. Huang, MD**
Hospital for Special Surgery
New York, New York

**R. John Hurlbert, MD**
Department of Clinical Neurosciences
University of Calgary Spine Program
Foothills Hospital and Medical Centre
Calgary, Alberta, Canada

**Roger P. Jackson, MD**
Private Practice
North Kansas City, Kansas

**Jack I. Jallo, MD**
Department of Neurosurgery
Temple University
Philadelphia, Pennsylvania

**Michael E. Janssen, DO**
Center for Spinal Disorders
Denver, Colorado

**Wade K. Jensen, MD**
Private Practice
Madison, Wisconsin

**Shiveindra Jeyamohan, MD**
Department of Neurological and Orthopedic
    Surgery
Thomas Jefferson University
Philadelphia, Pennsylvania

**G. Alexander Jones, MD**
Hudson Valley Neurosurgical Associates
Goshen, New York

**Iain H. Kalfas, MD**
Department of Neurosurgery
Cleveland Clinic Foundation
Cleveland, Ohio

**James D. Kang, MD**
Department of Orthopedic Surgery
University of Pittsburgh
Pittsburgh, Pennsylvania

**Mustafa H. Khan, MD**
Private Practice
Chicago, Illinois

**Choll W. Kim, MD**
Private Practice
La Jolla, California

**Daniel H. Kim, MD**
Private Practice
Houston, Texas

**David H. Kim, MD**
Boston Spine Group
Boston, Massachusetts

**Mark A. Knaub, MD**
Department of Orthopaedics and Rehabilitation
Penn State Milton S. Hershey College of
    Medicine
Hershey, Pennsylvania

**Timothy R. Kuklo, MD**
Washington University School of
    Medicine
St. Louis, Missouri

**Brian Kwon, MD**
Boston Spine Group
New England Baptist Hospital
Boston, Massachusetts

**Joon Yung Lee, MD**
Department of Orthopaedic Surgery
University of Pittsburgh
Pittsburgh, Pennsylvania

**Max C. Lee, MD**
Private Practice
Fox Point, Wisconsin

**Yu-Po Lee, MD**
Department of Orthopaedic Surgery
University of California–San Diego
San Diego, California

**Lawrence G. Lenke, MD**
Washington University Medical Center
Saint Louis, Missouri

**Howard B. Levene, MD**
Department of Neurosurgery
Temple University
Philadelphia, Pennsylvania

**Paul Licina, MD**
Brisbane Orthopaedic Specialist Services
Holy Spirit Northside Hospital
Chermside, Queensland, Australia

**Isador H. Lieberman, MD**
Cleveland Clinic Foundation
Cleveland, Ohio

**Moe R. Lim, MD**
Department of Orthopaedics
University of North Carolina
Chapel Hill, North Carolina

**Steven C. Ludwig, MD**
Private Practice
Baltimore, Maryland

**Neil R. Malhotra, MD**
Department of Neurosurgery
University of Pennsylvania
Philadelphia, Pennsylvania

**Linda Mascolo, RN**
Norwalk Hospital
Norwalk, Connecticut

**Sameer Mathur, MD**
Department of Orthopaedics
University of North Carolina
Chapel Hill, North Carolina

**Ralph J. Mobbs**
Prince of Wales Private Hospital
Barker Street, Randwick, Australia

**Milan G. Mody, MD**
WK Orthopedic and Sports Medicine Center
Shreveport, Louisiana

**Kenneth C. Moghadam, CO**
University of Calgary Spine Program
Foothills Hospital and Medical Centre
Calgary, Alberta, Canada

**Robert W. Molinari, MD**
University of Rochester Spine Center
Rochester, New York

**Seamus Morris, MD**
Private Practice
New York, New York

**Patrick F. O'Leary, MD**
Private Practice
New York, New York

**Stephen L. Ondra, MD**
Department of Neurological Surgery
Northwestern University
Chicago, Illinois

**Brian A. O'Shaughnessy, MD**
Department of Neurosurgery
Northwestern University
McGraw Medical Center
Chicago, Illinois

**John H. Peloza, MD**
Center for Spine Care
Dallas, Texas

**Matías G. Petracchi, MD**
Department of Orthopaedic Surgery
Hospital for Special Surgery
New York-Presbyterian Hospital
New York, New York

**Frank M. Phillips, MD**
Department of Orthopaedic Surgery
Rush University Medical Center
Chicago, Illinois

**Luiz Pimenta, MD, PhD**
Department of Spine Surgery
Santa Rita Hospital
São Paulo, Brazil

**Ben B. Pradhan, MD, MSE**
Spine Institute at Saint John's Health
   Center
Santa Monica, California

**Gregory J. Przybylski, MD**
Department of Neurosurgery
JFK Medical Center/Seton Hall University
Edison, New Jersey

**Y. Raja Rampersaud, MD**
University of Toronto
Toronto Western Hospital
University Health Network
Toronto, Ontario, Canada

**Bernard A. Rawlins, MD**
Hospital for Special Surgery
New York, New York

**Daniel K. Resnick, MD**
Department of Neurosurgery
University of Wisconsin
Madison, Wisconsin

**Laurence D. Rhines, MD**
University of Texas M.D. Anderson Cancer Center
Houston, Texas

**Paul T. Rubery, MD**
Division of Spinal Surgery
University of Rochester Medical Center
Rochester, New York

**Sanjeev Sabharwal**
University Hospital
Newark, New Jersey

**Harvinder S. Sandhu, MD**
Hospital for Special Surgery
New York, New York

**Rick C. Sasso, MD**
Indiana Spine Group
Indianapolis, Indiana

**Kristina M. Schmidt, MD**
Private Practice
Enid, Oklahoma

**James D. Schwender, MD**
Twin Cities Spine Center
Minneapolis, Minnesota

**Thomas N. Scioscia, MD**
West End Orthopaedic Clinic
Richmond, Virginia

**Arya Nick Shamie, MD**
Department of Orthopaedic Surgery
University of California–Los Angeles
Santa Monica, California

**Ashwini D. Sharan, MD**
Private Practice
Philadelphia, Pennsylvania

**Jeff S. Silber, MD**
Department of Orthopedic Surgery
North Shore-Long Island Jewish Health System
Great Neck, New York

**Fernando E. Silva, MD**
Private Practice
Irvine, California

**Kern Singh, MD**
Department of Orthopaedic Surgery
Rush University Medical Center
Chicago, Illinois

**Laura Snyder, BS**
Thomas Jefferson University
Philadelphia, Pennsylvania

**Erik Spayde**
Spine Institute at Saint John's Health Center
Santa Monica, California

**Jeffrey M. Spivak, MD**
Spine Center
Hospital for Joint Diseases
New York, New York

**John T. Street, MB**
Private Practice
Vancouver, British Columbia, Canada

**Chadi Tannoury, MD**
Private Practice

**Raja Taunk, BS**
Private Practice
Newark, New Jersey

**Brett A. Taylor, MD**
Orthopedic Center of St. Louis
Chesterfield, Missouri

**John E. Tis, MD**
Department of Pediatric Orthopaedics
Walter Reed Army Medical Center
Washington, DC

**Eeric Truumees, MD**
Private Practice
Royal Oak, Mississippi

**Alexander R. Vaccaro, MD, PhD**
Rothman Institute
Philadelphia, Pennsylvania

**Gianluca Vadalà, MD**
Department of Orthopedic Surgery
University Campus Bio-Medico of Rome
Rome, Italy

**Michael J. Vives, MD**
UMDNJ Medical School
Newark, New Jersey

**Jeffrey C. Wang, MD**
Department of Orthopaedic Surgery
University of California–Los Angeles
Los Angeles, California

**Timothy F. Witham, MD**
Department of Neurosurgery
Johns Hopkins University
Baltimore, Maryland

**David A. Wong, MD**
Denver Spine Center
Denver, Colorado

**Kirkham B. Wood, MD**
Massachusetts General Hospital
Wang Ambulatory Care Center
Boston, Massachusetts

**Michael A. Woods, MD**
Department of Radiology
University of Wisconsin Hospital
Madison, Wisconsin

# 1

# Foramen Magnum Decompression

*Ashwini D. Sharan, Laura Snyder, and Gregory J. Przybylski*

## Description
To achieve adequate decompression of the posterior cranial fossa without injury to the neurovascular structures at the craniocervical junction.

## Key Principles
Bony removal should include sufficient occipital bone and upper cervical lamina to incorporate both the rostral-caudal as well as the lateral extent of pathology while protecting the transverse sinus and vertebral arteries. Dural expansion may be an additional component of decompression of the upper cervical spinal cord and lower medulla.

## Expectations
Although spinal instability after foramen magnum decompression is not common, excessive lateral decompression in conjunction with disruption of posterior craniocervical ligaments may result in hypermobility of the craniocervical junction. One must be prepared to encounter a vestigial venous sinus within the dural leaves at the foramen magnum.

## Indications
Chiari malformation, achondroplasia, syringobulbia, basilar invagination, complex C1, C2 fractures.

## Contraindications
Adequate treatment of associated hydrocephalus should be achieved prior to foramen magnum decompression. Similarly, supratentorial masses should be excluded before opening the dura in the infratentorial posterior fossa.

## Special Considerations
Magnetic resonance imaging (MRI) of the brain and craniocervical junction preoperatively is imperative to define the extent of compression. The extent of caudal cerebellar displacement (for Chiari malformation), hydrocephalus, or other supratentorial mass lesions can be detected on MRI. Additionally, the venous sinuses and vertebral artery are visualized on MRI. A computed tomography (CT) scan may be beneficial in gauging the thickness of the keel and bony anatomy when considering instrumentation of the craniocervical junction.

## Special Instructions, Position, and Anesthesia
The patient is positioned prone with a Mayfield pin head holder. Maintaining the head in a flexed posture facilitates decompression, but may not be appropriate during stabilization procedures. Neurophysiologic monitoring may be used to monitor spinal cord and brainstem function, and arterial monitoring is beneficial in detecting blood pressure lability and bradycardia from brainstem compression.

## Tips, Pearls, and Lessons Learned
Flexion of the neck so that the mandible is two fingerbreadths away from the sternum facilitates separation of the inferior occipital margin of the foramen magnum and the posterior atlas, thereby improving ease of craniocervical ligament dissection from the dura. Extensive flexion of the neck may exacerbate postoperative swallowing or respiratory problems.

   Although the tentorium cerebelli and the transverse sinus are typically in the same axial plane as the upper third of the ear lobe, patients with hindbrain malformations may have a small posterior fossa and therefore a low-lying transverse sinus. A gross way to identify the transverse sinus is to connect a curved line from the mastoid process to the external occipital protuberance (EOP, or inion). Bony removal should be initiated inferior to these points to avoid sinus injury. Venous sinus bleeding can be controlled by pinching the inner and outer dural leaves together or sometimes by using vascular clips.

   Subperiosteal dissection along the atlas should be limited to 1.5 cm from the midline of the posterior tubercle of the atlas in adults and 1 cm in children. Dissection beyond this must be performed with extreme caution to avoid injury to the vertebral artery. A large venous plexus is typically encountered at the lateral margin of decompression at the craniocervical junction, signifying proximity to the vertebral arteries.

### Difficulties Encountered

The midline bony keel is thicker than the paramedian occipital bone. Burr holes on either side of the midline keel at the rostral extent of the craniectomy can facilitate separation of the dura from the inner skull table. Rapid bleeding from the occipital or marginal sinus during dural opening may occur, but can be avoided by surgical clip placement on both sides of the dural opening in advance of the incision. Bleeding from emissary veins during subperiosteal dissection of the occiput may also occur, but can be controlled with bone wax.

### Key Procedural Steps

Shave and preparation of the skin should extend from above the EOP to the lower cervical spine. A midline incision with subperiosteal dissection provides exposure from the EOP to the predetermined caudal cervical lamina chosen for removal (**Fig. 1.1**). A Y-shaped incision of the fascia provides for a fascial flap attached to the superior nuchal line, aiding closure. Exposure is maintained with cerebellar retractors. Margins of the foramen magnum are defined with a curette. Preservation of muscular and ligamentous attachments of C2 are recommended if the axis is not removed in the decompression.

Typically, a $3 \times 3$ cm section of occipital bone with the posterior rim of the foramen magnum is removed. A high-speed drill is used to create a craniectomy on either side of the midline bony keel. The dura is dissected from the inner skull table as needed as the bone is gradually lifted away (**Fig. 1.2**). Additionally, it will be beneficial to thin the midline keel and the foramen magnum with the drill until a thin remnant of bone remains. This thinned bone easily cracks as a curette is then used to lift the isolated occipital bone starting at the foramen magnum away from the posterior fossa. Extreme care should be exercised when placing instruments between the bone and the dura in a compressed foramen magnum. Similarly, narrow troughs can be drilled at the lateral borders of each lamina to be removed until a thin remnant of bone remains. The detached lamina can be lifted away from the spinal canal with a rongeur while a curette is used to separate the underlying dura from the inner laminar surface. Rongeurs can be used to enlarge the lateral extent of decompression if needed.

The dura may contain a thickened band at the craniocervical junction that can be released with a curette. Dural expansion can be performed with a midline incision over the cervical region extending bilaterally and diagonally over the posterior fossa dura up to the transverse sinus, forming a Y-shaped opening. Cerebrospinal fluid egress can be prevented by maintaining the integrity of the arachnoid layer. Bleeding from within the dural leaves may be encountered, but can be controlled either with surgical clips or by using bipolar cautery across the inner and outer dural leaves. A dural patch or fascia lata graft can

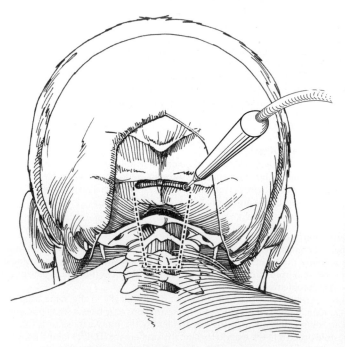

**Fig. 1.1** *Posterior exposure from the inion to the rostral margin of the C2 spinous process, showing an outline of the occipital and atlas bone removed.*

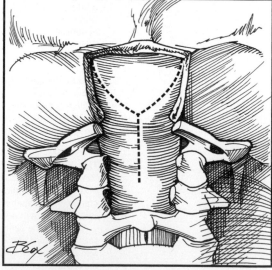

**Fig. 1.2** *Posterior exposure of the dura after bony removal, showing an outline of the Y-shaped dural incision.*

## PITFALLS

- Inadequate decompression, typically laterally or caudally, can result in failure of the surgery to ameliorate neurologic symptoms of craniocervical junction compression. Failure to incise a constricting dural band at the craniocervical junction may also result in inadequate decompression. Rapid substantial bleeding can be encountered if dural venous sinuses are not identified and controlled.

be sewn to the dural margins with 4–0 suture. Recently, greater success has been noted in dural repair with 6-0 Gore-Tex suture. Additional procedures in treatment of Chiari malformations including resecting the cerebellar tonsils, opening the foramen of Magendie, placing a stent, and plugging the obex remain controversial.

### Bailout, Rescue, Salvage Procedures

Copious bleeding from a low-pressure dural venous sinus can be controlled with compression of the inner and outer dural leaves against each other. Laceration of the transverse sinus can be managed by packing the site with a hemostatic agent and tamponade, being careful not to occlude the sinus completely with the packing material. Bleeding from injury to the vertebral artery can be managed with tamponade. If repair cannot be performed, subsequent angiography should be done to determine whether additional future treatment is necessary. Persistent compression at the foramen magnum might necessitate either a lateral transcondylar approach or even an anterior transoral decompression.

# 2

# Cervical Laminectomy and Foraminotomy

*Brian Kwon and David H. Kim*

## Description

The removal of compressive bone and soft tissue structures surrounding the cervical spinal cord (laminectomy) or its nerve roots (foraminotomy).

## Key Principles

Laminectomy is used for expansion of the cervical canal in individuals with symptomatic cervical stenosis. This is typically found in individuals with spondylotic degeneration overlying developmentally narrow canals. Multilevel decompression can be easily accomplished through a simple posterior surgical approach. Foraminotomy can be performed as an independent procedure or in conjunction with laminectomy to address unilateral or bilateral single-level or multilevel foraminal stenosis caused by spondylotic osteophyte formation or soft disk herniations.

## Expectations

Laminectomy performed for cervical myelopathy typically involves multilevel decompression. Recently laminectomy performed as a stand-alone procedure has fallen out of favor due to the incidence of postoperative kyphosis and recurrent symptoms. In current practice, laminectomy is more commonly performed with concomitant instrumented fusion. Clinical results in patients who are ambulatory preoperatively are generally favorable with most patients experiencing at least partial neurologic recovery.

Foraminotomy yields good to excellent relief of arm pain in the majority of patients. Best results have been observed in single-level disease associated with lateral soft disk herniation.

## Indications

### Laminectomy

- Multilevel cervical stenosis in a patient with neutral or lordotic sagittal alignment
- Cervical spondylotic myelopathy
- Previous anterior cervical spine decompression with recurrent myelopathy
- Diffuse ossification of the posterior longitudinal ligament (OPLL)
- Patient anatomy interfering with anterior surgery (e.g., previous anterior neck dissection, obesity, short neck, barrel chest)

### Foraminotomy

- Cervical radiculopathy caused by radiologically identified foraminal stenosis associated with lateral osteophytes or soft disk herniation
- Single-level or multilevel disease
- Failure of nonsurgical management
- Previous anterior cervical decompression with inadequate relief of radiculopathy due to insufficient foraminal decompression

## Contraindications

### Laminectomy

Kyphotic sagittal alignment.

### Foraminotomy

Medial pathology, i.e., disk herniation or compressive osteophyte, where surgical access may be associated with increased risk of neurological injury.

## Special Considerations

Laminectomy requires lordotic or neutral alignment, measured from the superior end plate of C3 to the inferior end plate of C7 on upright cervical spine films. The number of levels included should be determined by the anatomic distribution of compressive pathology noted on magnetic resonance imaging (MRI) or computed tomography (CT) after myelography. Facet resection in excess of 50% during foraminotomy can lead to segmental instability. Preoperative lateral flexion/extension films are recommended to assess for the presence of instability.

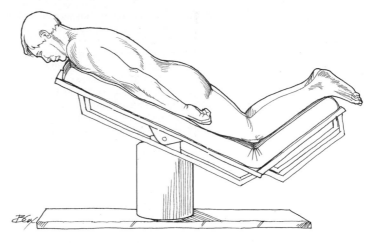

**Fig. 2.1** *Patient position on operating bed. Bed position should be in 30-degree reverse Trendelenburg, with the foot of the bed flexed 30 degrees to prevent migration of the patient toward the foot of the bed.*

### Special Instructions, Position, and Anesthesia

For both procedures, patients can be positioned prone or seated. The seated position can facilitate surgery by decreasing blood loss, but may risk air embolism. Familiarity with this position is crucial for both surgical and anesthesia staff. The prone position on chest rolls is more widely utilized. The patient's head can be secured with Mayfield tongs. While the patient is in the prone position, the eyes and nose should be protected and periodically checked. If possible, the head and neck should be placed in the "military position" without flexion or extension and slight posterior translation of the head. The use of neurophysiologic spinal cord monitoring is recommended in the setting of myelopathy. Baseline evoked potential signals should be obtained prior to patient positioning and then rechecked shortly after the patient has been placed in the final operative position. Arms are tucked at the sides. Gentle caudal traction can be placed on the shoulders with tape to help with radiographic visualization of the lower cervical levels, especially in individuals with broad or thick shoulders. Bed position should be in 30-degree reverse Trendelenburg, with the foot of the bed flexed 30 degrees to prevent migration of the patient toward the foot of the bed (**Fig. 2.1**). Hypotension should be avoided in myelopathic patients.

### Tips, Pearls, and Lessons Learned

In patients with myeloradiculopathy and significant radicular symptoms, the presence of significant foraminal stenosis should be sought on preoperative imaging studies and appropriate concomitant foraminotomies planned. In preoperative positioning, excessive flexion or extension should be avoided in myelopathic patients. For foraminotomies, slight kyphosis opens the interspaces and foramina, but care must be taken during dissection as the dural sac is more susceptible to injury.

The surgical exposure for laminectomy proceeds caudal to rostral; this facilitates subperiosteal detachment of paraspinal muscles, which attach in the same direction and reduce bleeding. A clamp is placed on an exposed spinous process and a lateral radiograph is obtained to confirm levels. Dissection should proceed to the lateral margin of the facet joints. This extent of exposure establishes landmarks needed for safe placement of lateral mass screws and ensures that more than half of the facet joint is not removed during any associated foraminotomy. Dissection beyond the lateral margin risks significant bleeding from the soft tissue in this area. Care must be taken not to injure the facet capsules at any level where fusion is not planned.

### Difficulties Encountered

The epidural venous plexus surrounding the cervical cord can be severely compressed in myelopathic patients. Brisk bleeding can occur from the epidural plexus as well as the venous plexus surrounding the cervical nerve root within the neuroforamen following decompression. Careful bipolar coagulation or use of Surgicel can provide adequate hemostasis. Blind compression or coagulation can lead to serious nerve root or spinal cord injury and should be avoided.

### Key Procedural Steps

With the neck in neutral position, the ligamentum nuchae is relatively lax and tends to meander from the midline. Maintaining dorsal traction using hooks or retractors can facilitate midline dissection and reduce bleeding. Avoid detaching the muscular insertions from the cephalad border of the C2 spinous process. The cephalad and caudad border of each lamina should be carefully freed of soft tissue. Preparation of screw holes for implant placement should be performed prior to the actual laminectomy to minimize the risk of spinal cord injury. Laminectomy margins should be created 2 mm medial to the junction of the lamina and lateral mass using a 2-mm high-speed burr. This reduces bleeding from epidural vessels localized directly anterior to the junction of the laminae and lateral masses. In the setting of severe stenosis, sublaminar placement of instruments risks injury to the spinal cord and should be avoided. The angle of approach with the burr should be 30 to 45 degrees in the horizontal plane to avoid burring into the lateral mass (**Fig. 2.2A,B**). A gentle sweeping motion with the burr should be performed to gradually and evenly deepen the laminectomy trough. Once all laminae have been divided they can be removed en bloc by detaching the interspinous ligament and ligamentum flavum with a Kerrison rongeur or knife (**Fig. 2.2C**). Gentle dorsal traction is maintained on the detached laminae using towel clips on the individual spinous processes. To reduce the risk of postoperative C5 and C6 root palsy, a concomitant C5 and C6 foraminotomy is routinely performed. Once laminectomy has been completed, prior to rod placement, additional restoration of anatomic lordosis can be accomplished by loosening the Mayfield attachment and gently extending the patient's neck.

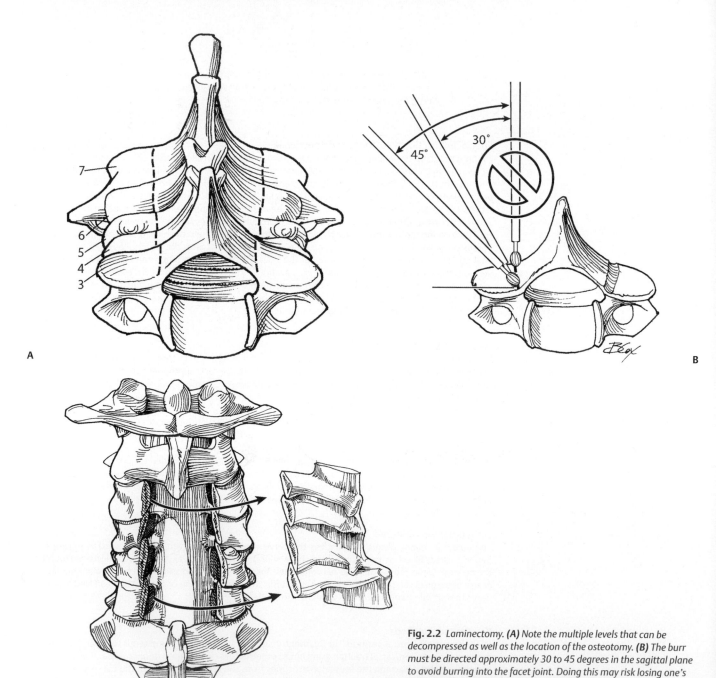

**Fig. 2.2** *Laminectomy. **(A)** Note the multiple levels that can be decompressed as well as the location of the osteotomy. **(B)** The burr must be directed approximately 30 to 45 degrees in the sagittal plane to avoid burring into the facet joint. Doing this may risk losing one's orientation and burring too deeply, endangering the dural sac or spinal cord. **(C)** En bloc removal of laminae.*

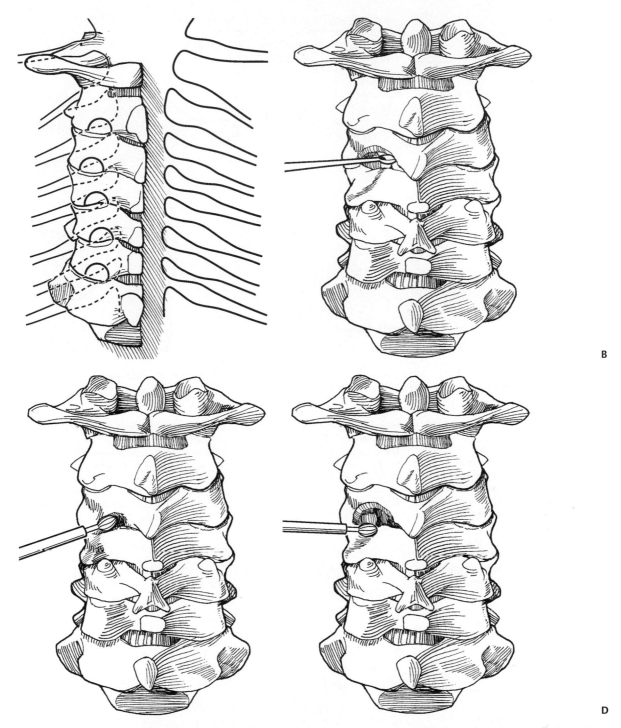

**Fig. 2.3** *Foraminotomy. (A) The entire facet joint should be visualized, and the capsule protected. Note the relationship of the nerve root to the superior and inferior articular processes. (B) The medial half of the inferior articular process is removed with a burr. (C) The ligamentum can be dissected free from superior, lateral, and inferior margins using a small curette or nerve hook. (D) The remaining superior articular process can then be removed by using a burr to thin it and a 1-mm Kerrison rongeur to remove remaining articular process, leaving the nerve root decompressed.*

For foraminotomy a unilateral exposure can be performed. An operating microscope or loupe magnification is recommended. Once the level has been confirmed and the facet joint visualized, a 2-mm high-speed burr is used to remove a portion of the laminae and the medial half of the inferior articular process of the cephalad vertebra (**Fig. 2.3**) initially. The ligamentum is then removed using a fine curette. This leaves a "triangle" of bone representing the superior articular process of the caudal vertebra with any associated

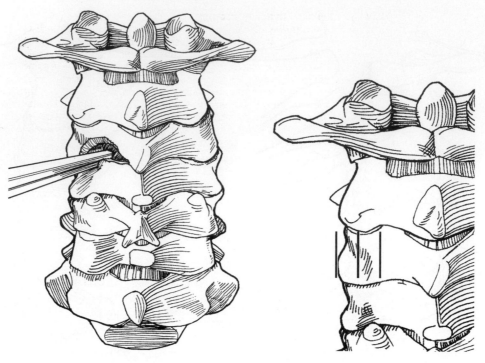

A                                                                                                      B

**Fig. 2.4** *(A)* A Kerrison rongeur removing the thinned superior articular process. *(B)* Final image showing decompressed foramen, highlighting removal of 50% of the facet joint.

**PITFALLS**

- Laminectomy accomplishes indirect decompression of the spinal cord by allowing posterior translation of the cord away from anterior compressive pathology. Typically a minimum of three or four levels is required to allow adequate cord translation. When performing laminectomy for cervical stenosis, to minimize the risk of iatrogenic cord injury, instruments with taller profiles than the footplate of a 2-mm Kerrison rongeur should not be placed underneath the lamina near the central canal. Postsurgical C5 radiculopathy occurs in 10 to 15% of patients and typically appears between the second and fifth postoperative day. Most spontaneously resolve over 6 to 12 months.

- Foraminal decompression risks nerve root injury, especially if high-profile Kerrison rongeurs are placed into the foramen. Air embolus is a rare complication associated with posterior cervical surgery with the patient in the seated position. Occurrence can be monitored using end tidal $CO_2$ sensors. If a significant air embolism is suspected, the patient should undergo immediate electrocauterization of any readily accessible bleeding veins, and the wound should be quickly covered. If a central venous catheter was placed preoperatively, the line can be advanced into the right atrium to attempt evacuation of the air. If this fails, the patient can be placed in the left lateral decubitus position to trap the air in the right atrium.

osteophytes. A diamond-coated burr (with constant saline irrigation) is then used to thin or remove entirely the medial half of the superior articular process. A fine curette or a 1-mm Kerrison can be used to complete the foraminotomy by removing remaining bone and soft tissue overlying the neuroforamen (**Fig. 2.4**). With severe stenosis resulting from spondylosis, unroofing the neuroforamen with a fine curette is preferable to minimize the risk of iatrogenic nerve root injury. If removal of a soft disk herniation is necessary, a fine nerve hook is used to gently retract the nerve root in the *cephalad* direction to expose the disk. Care must be taken to retract both rami of the nerve root when present, as the smaller, more anterior and caudally located motor branch can be mistaken for a fragment of disk material (**Fig. 2.5**).

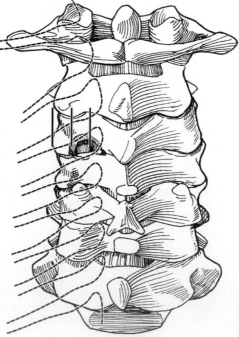

**Fig. 2.5** *Relationship between cervical nerve roots and articular processes. Note also the proximity between the superior articular process and nerve root.*

**Bailout, Rescue, Salvage Procedures**

If compression remains at C2 after C3 is removed, the ventral portion of C2 can be removed with a burr and Kerrison rongeur while protecting the cervical cord—the dome osteotomy. Progressive postoperative kyphosis can be associated with neck pain and recurrent myelopathy. Typically, this complication occurs when laminectomy is performed without concomitant fusion. Sagittal alignment can be restored by performing multilevel anterior cervical diskectomy and interbody structural graft reconstruction followed by posterior cervical instrumented fusion. Adjacent segment degeneration is a theoretical concern following fusion. To minimize the risk of recurrent symptomatology from adjacent segment disease, fusion should be extended to include adjacent levels when preoperative subluxation or instability is identified. Occasionally, progressive cervicothoracic kyphosis occurs below a previous laminectomy and fusion. This risk may be increased in the setting of preoperative cervicothoracic kyphosis or when the posterior midline tethering ligaments are disrupted. Extension of the fusion to the upper thoracic spine with appropriate instrumentation typically allows restoration of sagittal alignment.

# 3

# Laminoplasty

*Kazuhiro Chiba*

## Description
To achieve adequate decompression of the spinal cord and the nerve roots by shifting the laminae posteriorly, yet preserving cervical stability by retaining the posterior bone–ligamentous complex.

## Key Principles
In addition to the local decompression effect by the posterior shift of the laminae, the total or indirect decompression effect by the posterior migration of the spinal cord away from anterior pathologic structures, such as disk herniation, osteophyte, and ossified ligament, can be expected in this procedure, unless the patient's cervical alignment is kyphotic. Preserved laminae provide protection to the spinal cord and serve as an attachment to the stripped muscles and preserved ligaments, including the supraspinous, interspinous, and yellow ligaments.

## Expectations
Relief of myelopathy caused by multilevel compression due to cervical degenerative diseases and ossification of the posterior longitudinal ligament. Long-term outcomes of expansive laminoplasty are satisfactory, for example, neurologic improvement assessed by the Japanese Orthopaedic Association (JOA) scoring system is approximately 50 to 60%. Adjacent segment disease and nonunion, which are noted after anterior fusions, can be avoided. No postoperative external support is necessary.

## Indications
Patients with multilevel spinal cord compression due to cervical spondylosis, or ossification of the posterior longitudinal ligament. Patients who have developmental spinal stenosis are also good candidates for laminoplasty even if they have single-level disease, such as a disk herniation.

## Contraindications
Preoperatively established severe kyphosis (C2–C7 kyphotic angle over 10 degrees); severely unstable cervical spine, for example, athetoid cerebral palsy, rheumatoid arthritis, and destructive spondyloarthropathy.

## Special Considerations
Careful evaluation of the lateral radiographs to assess for developmental spinal canal stenosis (anteroposterior diameter of the spinal canal <13 mm), which, if symptomatic, is an indication for this procedure. Computed tomography (CT) is used to measure the thickness of the laminae and to decide the optimal positions of the gutters. Magnetic resonance imaging (MRI) is used to assess the laterality of spinal cord compression, thereby deciding the side of laminar opening. Laminae are usually opened at the side of predominant compression.

## Special Instructions, Position, and Anesthesia
A prone position with a Mayfield pin headrest. Flex the neck slightly to open up the space between the occiput and cervical spine to obtain adequate exposure. Tilt the surgical table about 30 degrees to bring the flexed neck parallel to the horizontal plane. Use endotracheal general anesthesia.

## Tips, Pearls, and Lessons Learned
Incise the nuchal ligament and paracervical muscles at the exact midline, and strip the muscles subperiosteally to avoid bleeding. Complete the hinge side gutter last, after completion of the open side gutter and the resection of the ligamentum flava at both ends of the laminar door. Check the stability of the hinge frequently while making the hinge gutter. Preserve the spinous process of C7 whenever possible, to reduce postoperative axial symptoms. Encourage early active neck exercise.

## Difficulties Encountered
Uncontrollable epidural bleeding is sometimes encountered during the laminar opening procedure, especially in ossification of the posterior longitudinal ligament (OPLL) procedures. In some cases, the laminar door cannot be opened readily, due to remaining bony continuity on the open gutter side, inadequate resection of the ligamenta flava, and inadequate drilling of the hinge gutter.

## Key Procedural Steps
The laminae, in most cases, from C3 to C6 or C7, are exposed through a midline incision followed by dissection of bilateral paracervical muscles. At the junction of the lamina and the facet joint, the open side gutter is made using a high-speed drill. The ventral cortex of the laminae is perforated

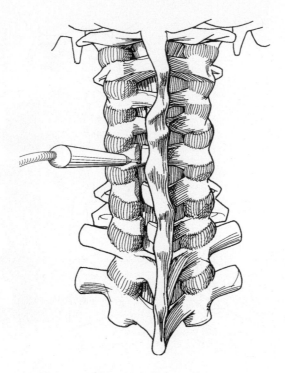

**Fig. 3.1** *Starting the gutter on the open side.*

using a diamond burr (**Fig. 3.1**). Ligamenta flava at the cranial and caudal ends of the intended laminar expansion, usually at the C2-3, C6-7, or C7-T1 interspaces, are resected using a thin-bladed Kerrison rongeur, while opening the interspace with a small laminar spreader. Another gutter in the contralateral side is made, while preserving the ventral cortex. This side now functions as a hinge. Make the hinge gutter slightly wider and more lateral than the open gutter side to avoid abutting of the cut edges of the lamina and facet joint and to allow adequate opening (**Fig. 3.2**). To prevent

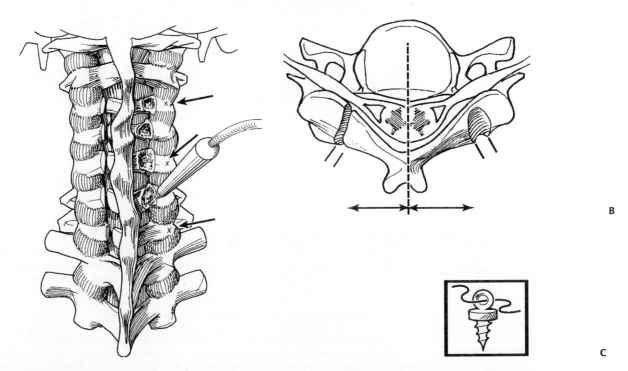

A

B

C

**Fig. 3.2** *Make the hinge gutter last. (A) Note that the hinge gutter is made wider and more lateral than the one in the open side. (B) Both gutters completed. (C) Suture anchor.*

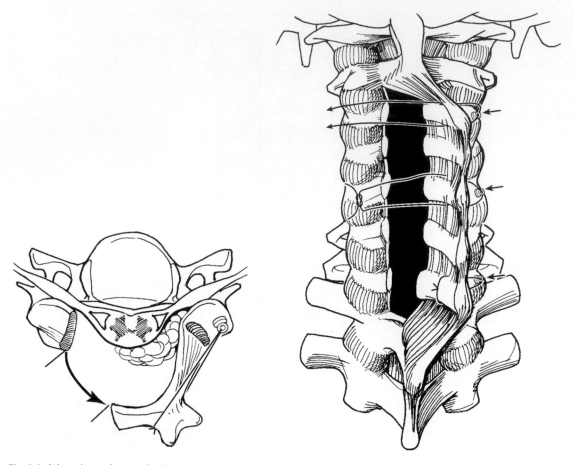

A
B

**Fig. 3.3** **(A)** *Axial view showing the hinge in operation. The lamina is held securely with threads of the anchor screw inserted into the corresponding lateral mass.* **(B)** *Passage of the threads prior to laminar opening.*

hinge problems, the stability of the hinge is checked frequently while deepening the hinge gutter by applying a gentle bending force to the spinous processes.

After the completion of the hinge gutter, anchor sutures (PeBA Anchor Screw®, Smith & Nephew, Orthopaedic Biosystem, Andover, MA) may be placed in the lateral mass and the threads are passed through interspinous ligaments around the base of the corresponding spinous process at each level (**Fig. 3.3**). Each lamina is lifted one by one using a large Kerrison rongeur placed under the open edge. This is repeated until the open side laminae become almost horizontal. Dural pulsation can usually be observed at this stage. To maintain the expanded position and to prevent the closure of the laminar door, threads previously placed at the base of the spinous processes are securely tied (**Fig. 3.3**). A suction drain is placed and the wound is closed in layers. Patients are mobilized 1 to 3 days after the surgery without external supports. Early active neck exercise are encouraged.

**Bailout, Rescue, Salvage Procedures**

- If the laminar door cannot be opened readily, check, in the following order, if (1) the ventral cortex of the laminae in the open side gutter has been removed completely, (2) the ligamentum flava at the both ends are completely resected, or (3) the hinge side gutter is deep enough. Then remove the remaining bone and ligaments, or drill further. If only one lamina is detached, a secure tightening of the adjacent laminae will hold the broken lamina, preventing its migration into the spinal canal. If more than two consecutive laminae are detached, the whole laminar door should be removed.
- Do not try to coagulate the massive bleeding from the epidural venous plexus. A gentle pack of hemostatic materials (e.g., collagen fibrils) for 5 minutes should work in most cases.
- The exact mechanism of segmental paralysis is unknown, but mainly attributed to radiculopathy due to tethering of the nerve roots after posterior migration of the spinal cord; however, involvement of spinal cord pathology has also been implied. This paralysis usually resolves spontaneously within several weeks to 6 months.

PITFALLS

- Detachment of the hinge due to excessive drilling or fracture of the hinge due to inadequate drilling
- Segmental motor paralysis, particularly at the C5 and C6 segments, which occurs in about 5 to 10% of patients
- Postoperative axial pain and limited cervical range of motion
- Closure of the opened laminae
- Cerebrospinal fluid leakage due to a dural tear
- Neurologic complications due to postoperative epidural hematoma

- Preservation of the C7 spinous process and early active exercise reduces postoperative axial pain and preserves cervical range of motion.
- Using lateral mass anchor screw fixation minimizes the potential for laminar closure.
- Use a diamond burr to perforate the ventral cortex to avoid dural injury.
- Place two suction drains especially if the patient is at high risk for bleeding, such as in the setting of hypertension, hemorrhagic tendency due to liver dysfunction, severe myelopathy, and absence of dural pulsation after decompression.

# 4

# Surgical Removal of Intradural Spinal Cord Tumors

*Timothy F. Witham and Ziya L. Gokaslan*

## Description

Resection of intradural tumors is performed almost exclusively through a posterior approach. Laminectomies performed rostral and caudal to the level of the lesion are critical to provide adequate exposure for tumor resection. Coronal exposure is also important with wide, but facet-sparing, laminectomies that allow for gentle manipulation of the tumor and spinal cord if necessary. Even ventrally situated tumors can most often be approached in this fashion.

A dural opening rostral and caudal to the level of the lesion is critical. The arachnoid should initially be preserved to prevent spinal cord herniation. Opening the dura rostral to the lesion first also helps to prevent herniation of the spinal cord if the arachnoid is not preserved. Techniques to allow for gentle manipulation of the spinal cord include wide laminectomies, a lengthy dural opening, sectioning of the dentate ligaments, and, in some cases, nerve root sectioning.

## Expectations

Intradural spinal tumors are classified as extramedullary or intramedullary. In most cases, the extramedullary tumors are benign, and the surgical goal is complete resection. In some cases with lesions such as neurofibromas, complete resection is not possible without complete or partial transection of the nerve root of origin. If the root is one that subserves a critical function (i.e., C5 root) then consideration is given to subtotal resection. The majority of extramedullary tumors may be cured with complete surgical excision. Intramedullary tumors are less likely to be cured by surgery alone. Ependymomas, hemangioblastomas, angiolipomas, and pilocytic tumors are usually amenable to complete resection, whereas malignant astrocytic tumors require subtotal resection or biopsy followed by adjuvant therapy.

## Indications

A contrast-enhancing intradural spinal lesion in a symptomatic patient is usually approached surgically for diagnostic and therapeutic purposes. Symptoms include motor or sensory deficits, sphincter dysfunction, and pain localized to the area of the lesion. Pain that is not mechanical and tends to be exacerbated by recumbency is common with intradural spinal tumors.

## Contraindications

Transverse myelitis and multiple sclerosis are two disease entities that may be confused with intramedullary spinal cord tumors. Clinical history and imaging can differentiate these diseases from intradural tumors. However, if the clinical picture is not clear, then neurologic workup for demyelinating disease should be initiated. Drop metastases are typically not approached surgically. Elderly patients who are asymptomatic may be initially followed with serial imaging. Tumors with highly aggressive behavior may be considered for biopsy and adjuvant therapy.

## Special Considerations

Perioperative administration of corticosteroids is not supported by scientific evidence. However, many surgeons routinely administer up to 100 mg of Decadron prior to resection of intramedullary tumors and continue high-dose steroids postoperatively. A subsequent slow taper is performed over 2 to 4 weeks.

For intradural meningiomas that require dural resection and for intramedullary cases in which spinal cord swelling is a potential issue, a dural patch graft may be necessary. Meticulous dural closure is paramount in the prevention of a cerebrospinal fluid (CSF) fistula or pseudomeningocele. A dural sealant is routinely placed along the suture line as well.

## Special Instructions, Position, and Anesthesia

Patients are placed in the prone position, and the chest is well padded. A Mayfield cranial clamp is used for cervical and upper thoracic lesions. Perioperative corticosteroids and broad-spectrum antibiotics are routinely administered to all patients. The horseshoe adapter to the Mayfield is avoided to prevent skin breakdown on the face or ocular pressure leading to ocular ischemia that can be observed during prolonged cases in the prone position with this device.

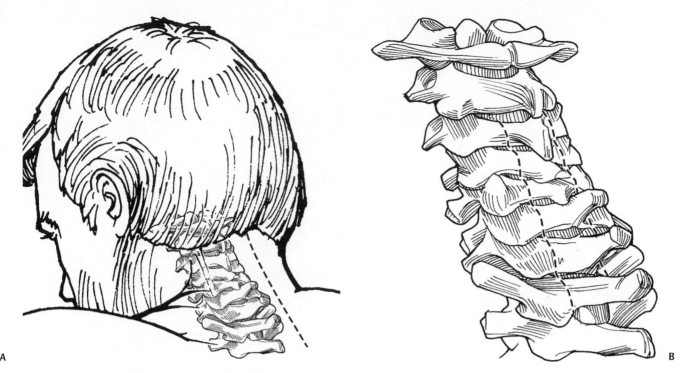

**Fig. 4.1** *(A)* *Intraoperative illustration of a patient with a C4–C7 ependymoma. The skin incision is marked.* *(B)* *The laminectomy is extended one level above and below the tumor zone.*

### Tips, Pearls, and Lessons Learned

For intramedullary spinal cord tumors, the dissection is usually begun at the middle portion of the neoplasm where the lesion is the bulkiest. Dissection in this location is least likely to result in injury to the surrounding neural tissues.

For lesions with tumor-associated cysts, laminectomies to provide exposure of the cyst outside the area of the solid tumor component are not necessary. The cyst walls are typically nonneoplastic, and complete tumor resection results in the disappearance of the cyst. Intraoperative monitoring with epidural motor evoked potential (MEPs) leads may be helpful as a way to avoid rather than merely detect irreversible neurologic injury. With experienced electrophysiologists, spinal epidural MEPs are a reliable predictor of postoperative outcome. All patients should be followed with plain radiographs for the development of postlaminectomy kyphosis. Children less than 3 years of age, those with preoperative deformity, and those with preoperative neurologic deficits are at greatest risk. Although there is no scientific evidence to support the use of laminoplasty, this technique is used in all children and in those patients at high risk for the development of postlaminectomy kyphosis. Titanium miniplates can be used to reconstruct and stabilize the lamina.

### Key Procedural Steps

Continuous somatosensory evoked potentials (SSEPs) are monitored in all patients. MEPs are monitored as described above when a good baseline may be followed. Although SSEPs and MEPs are thought to be predictive of postoperative outcome at centers with extensive experience, this finding remains controversial.

A standard midline skin incision is fashioned with subsequent subperiosteal dissection of the paraspinal muscles (**Fig. 4.1A**). Laminectomies or osteoplastic laminotomies are performed one level above and below the superior and inferior poles of the tumor (**Fig. 4.1B**). Large moist cottonoids are placed along the edges of the paraspinal muscles. Intraoperative ultrasonography is commonly helpful prior to dural opening for intramedullary tumors to determine if the tumor is sufficiently exposed rostrocaudally.

A midline durotomy is performed rostral to the superior pole of the tumor and carried inferiorly. Dural tack-up sutures are placed to tent the dural edges laterally to the muscles. The arachnoid is preserved and opened separately under microscopic guidance (**Fig. 4.2**). The edges of the arachnoid are clipped to the dura with small vascular clips.

Finding the midline is important for minimizing neurologic morbidity, but may be difficult secondary to spinal cord rotation or distortion from the tumor. The posterior median sulcus may be estimated by inspection of the dorsal root entry zones bilaterally or by identifying the convergence of very small vessels in the midline. A midline myelotomy is started at the area of maximum cord enlargement and is extended to expose the tumor in its entirety. We have recently started using dorsal column mapping by stimulating the cord directly and recording SSEPs from the scalp to identify the midline in cases in which the spinal cord is distorted.

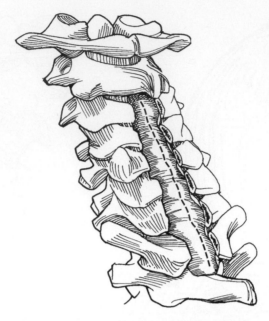

**Fig. 4.2** *The durotomy is completed and the arachnoid is incised.*

The dissection is initiated in the midportion of the tumor (**Fig. 4.3**). This region is the safest with respect to risk of neurologic injury. Microdissectors are used to gently spread the posterior columns. Pial traction sutures are used to maintain gentle traction on the myelotomy. With a portion of the tumor exposed, a frozen section or touch prep is obtained. The results of the biopsy may change the goals of the subsequent resection. High-grade lesions may be biopsied or debulked with the notion that adjuvant therapies will be required postoperatively. Low-grade glial tumors and ependymomas are more aggressively approached. Ependymomas are usually well circumscribed, and smaller lesions can be resected *en bloc*. Larger lesions are more challenging with regard to *en bloc* resection, particularly at the poles of the tumor.

We recommend *en bloc* resection when possible for several reasons (**Fig. 4.4**). *En bloc* resection reduces the potential for tumor spillage while avoiding intralesional bleeding. With reduced bleeding, a better surgical plane is maintained. With some larger tumors, *en bloc* resection is not possible and piecemeal resection is performed.

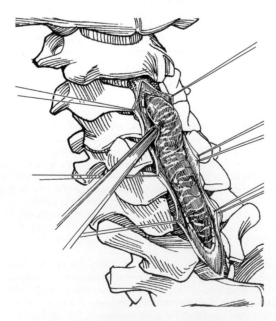

**Fig. 4.3** *Tumor dissection is initiated in the middle portion of the tumor, which is the bulkiest.*

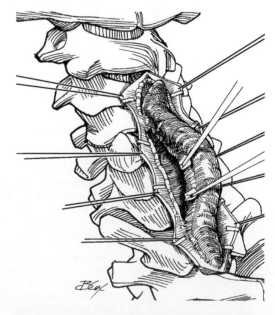

**Fig. 4.4** *The rostral pole of the tumor is being dissected in an* en bloc *fashion.*

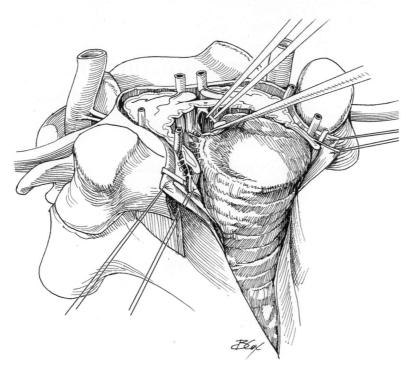

**Fig. 4.5** *Great caution must be exerted while coagulating branches of the anterior spinal artery supplying the neoplasm along the anterior aspect of the cord.*

Tumor resection or dissection along the anterior median raphe is often difficult because of tumor adherence to this thinned-out portion of the spinal cord (**Fig. 4.5**). Great caution must be taken in coagulating vessels in this location that frequently represent small branches of the anterior spinal artery that penetrate the tumor. Following tumor resection, intraoperative ultrasonography is utilized to assess the extent of resection.

### Bailout, Rescue, Salvage Procedures

Spinal deformity may progress to result in neurologic compression and deficit. Therefore, frequent postoperative plain film imaging is important to recognize spinal deformity early in its course. Spinal deformity should be treated aggressively with reduction and fixation. Limiting the laminectomy and avoiding denervation or disruption of the facet joints may reduce the likelihood of this complication.

**PITFALLS**

- Paralysis following resection of an intramedullary spinal cord tumor is most commonly associated with the degree of preoperative deficit and less commonly a function of tumor histology or extent of surgical resection. A dense preoperative motor deficit has the highest likelihood of becoming a permanent deficit postoperatively. It follows that it is imperative for patients with a known intramedullary spinal cord tumor to undergo surgical resection prior to the progression of motor deficit.
- Impaired joint position sense is a potential complication that can be functionally debilitating. Careful placement of the myelotomy in the posterior median raphe with limited dissection/traction of the posterior columns may help prevent this problem.
- Spinal deformity represents a significant postoperative complication particularly in children. Recognition of postoperative deformity and differentiation from tumor recurrence has subsequent treatment implications. In children, osteoplastic laminotomy may minimize the incidence of postoperative kyphoscoliosis. Tumor resection in conjunction with instrumented stabilization is sometimes performed in patients who are felt to be a high risk for postoperative kyphosis. Spinal instrumentation, however, may limit postoperative magnetic resonance imaging capabilities.

# 5

# Open Reduction of Unilateral and Bilateral Facet Dislocations

*Moe R. Lim, Sameer Mathur, and Alexander R. Vaccaro*

## Description
Open posterior reduction of unilateral or bilateral facet dislocations or fracture/dislocations.

## Key Principles
The key principle for achieving reduction is the gentle re-creation of the injury mechanism followed by manipulation of the affected segments into normal alignment.

## Expectations
Avoidance of neurologic injury with the reduction maneuver.

## Indications
- Unilateral or bilateral facet dislocations or fracture/dislocations that have failed attempted closed reduction
- Unilateral or bilateral facet dislocations or fracture/dislocations that have failed attempted open anterior reduction
- Unilateral or bilateral facet dislocations or fracture/dislocations with no evidence of a disk herniation on preoperative magnetic resonance imaging (MRI)

## Contraindications
- Hemodynamic instability
- Aborted closed reduction in a patient with worsening sensory or motor function who is subsequently noted to have a significant disk herniation on MRI; such a patient requires an anterior diskectomy prior to open posterior reduction

## Special Considerations
After a failed attempt at closed reduction, a cervical spine MRI is mandatory to search for a disk herniation. A significant disk herniation may be dragged into the canal and cause spinal cord compression during open reduction under general anesthesia. In the presence of a disk herniation, an anterior diskectomy is required prior to open posterior reduction.

## Special Instructions, Position, and Anesthesia
Neurophysiologic spinal cord monitoring during the reduction maneuver is extremely helpful. If an alert is detected, the reduction maneuver can readily be reversed, potentially avoiding neurologic injury. Multimodality monitoring is preferred with motor evoked potentials, somatosensory evoked potentials, and spontaneous electromyogram (EMG) recordings. For anesthesia, awake fiberoptic intubation avoids excessive cervical extension and allows a neurologic exam after intubation. Neurophysiologic baselines are recorded after the administration of general anesthesia, prone positioning, shoulder taping, and other closed cervical manipulation. The patient is placed in traction with Gardner-Wells tongs on a Stryker frame to allow for the preservation of cervical stability while turning the patient prone.

## Tips, Pearls, and Lessons Learned
The reduction should be achievable with only gentle manipulation. Greater amounts of force may cause a spinous process fracture or neurologic injury. If difficulty in reduction is encountered, additional muscle relaxation from anesthesia may be helpful. If additional relaxation does not allow safe reduction, the superior articular facet(s) of the caudal vertebra can be trimmed with a burr. This decreases the barrier to posterior translation of the inferior facet of the cephalad level. The amount of bone resected, however, should be minimized to allow native bony stability following the reduction. A nerve hook placed along the medial edge of the inferior cephalad facet can also provide addition leverage.

## Difficulties Encountered
If significant neurophysiologic signal changes are encountered during the reduction maneuver, the procedure should be halted. Once other potential causes of the signal changes (such as hypotension) are ruled out, the patient should be carefully turned supine and a diskectomy performed. Because reduction should afford an indirect decompression of the spinal cord, neurophysiologic changes with attempted reduction likely indicate anterior cord compression by a herniated disk.

Traumatic dural lacerations may also occur in facet dislocations with a concomitant lamina fracture. When encountered, a watertight repair should be performed. If repair is not possible, a lumbar drain can be used to divert cerebrospinal fluid (CSF) flow.

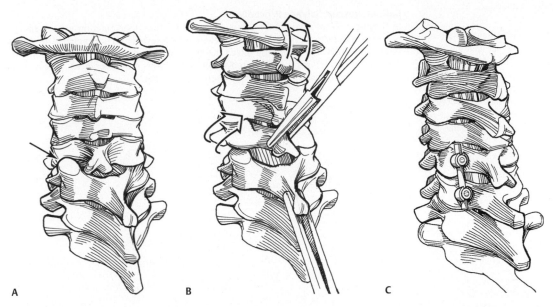

**Fig. 5.1** *(A) The open reduction technique for a unilateral facet dislocation (arrow). (B) A gentle distraction and kyphotic moment is applied to the cephalad tenaculum to re-create the injury mechanism. (C) Posterior compression is applied using spinous process wiring or lateral mass screws.*

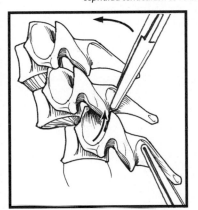

**Fig. 5.2** *Lateral view of the reduction of the facet joint (arrows indicate traction).*

## Key Procedural Steps

After prone positioning and establishment of neurophysiology baseline recordings, a standard subperiosteal dissection of the posterior cervical spine is performed. Care should be taken to avoid violating the facet capsules and interspinous ligaments of levels not involved in the intended fusion. The dislocated level can often be detected by a step-off in the spinous processes or the associated soft tissue injuries. Once the dislocated levels are identified, the lateral masses are exposed completely. The dislocation can be reduced by grasping the involved cephalad and caudal spinous process with a tenaculum at the spinolaminar junction. The neurophysiologist should be warned of the possibility of an acute signal change. If any significant neurophysiologic changes are detected, the procedure should be halted.

Axial caudal traction is applied to the caudal tenaculum. A gentle distraction and kyphotic moment is applied to the cephalad tenaculum to re-create the injury mechanism. A rotational force may also be additionally required for unilateral facet dislocations. The maneuver is applied until the inferior articular processes of the cephalad vertebra are freed from underneath the superior articular processes of the caudal vertebra. Once the inferior facets of the cephalad vertebra clear and become posterior to the superior facets of the caudal vertebra, the difficult portion of the reduction is complete. To achieve anatomic alignment, posterior compression is applied using spinous process wiring or lateral mass screws (**Fig. 5.1, Fig. 5.2, and Fig. 5.3**).

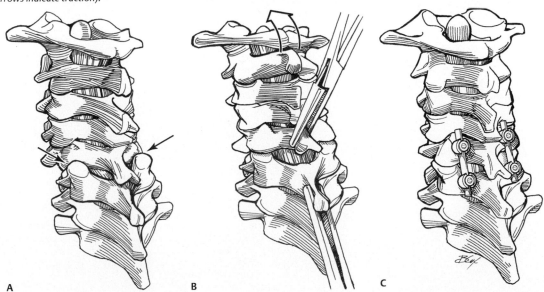

**Fig. 5.3.** *(A) The open reduction technique for a bilateral facet dislocation (arrows). (B) A gentle distraction and kyphotic moment is applied to the cephalad tenaculum to re-create the injury mechanism. (C) Posterior compression is applied using spinous process wiring or lateral mass screws.*

**PITFALLS**

- In a severe injury, concomitant lateral mass or facet fractures may limit the degree of inherent stability following reduction of the dislocation. In addition, the use of lateral mass fixation at that site may be prohibited. Should this occur, extension of the stabilization construct or other forms of instrumentation may be warranted.

**Bailout, Rescue, Salvage Procedures**

In the presence of a lamina or spinous process fracture, manipulation via the spinous process is not possible. In this situation, lateral mass screws can be inserted into the cephalad levels bilaterally. With the screwdrivers still attached to the screws in a fixed angle, the screw–screwdriver construct can be used to manipulate and reduce the dislocated vertebra. With this maneuver, great care must be taken to avoid destruction of the bony purchase of the lateral mass screws.

# 6

# Occipital Wiring and Plating Techniques

*Neal G. Haynes, Troy D. Gust, and Paul M. Arnold*

### Description

The safe fixation of the occipital cervical junction with both plates and screws, or wires, cables, and rods, without durotomy, neural, or vascular injury. Internal occipital-cervical stabilization has proven over time to be advantageous to external fixation for complication-free immobilization of the unstable occipital cervical junction.

### Expectations

Occipital screws and plates are more stable under axial loads and should be considered for severe instability or when needed to counterbalance additional force vectors such as odontoid migration or multiple fractures.

Wires secured to the inner surface of the occipital bone can provide a solid point of purchase to secure cervical rods. This avoids potential screw pullout and can be used when bone is less than optimal. Additionally, this provides flexibility to the surgeon in choosing cervical wire purchase location.

### Indications

Occipitocervical instability or dislocation from trauma, rheumatoid arthritis or other inflammatory process, basilar impression, neoplasm, congenital anomalies, osteomyelitis, or iatrogenic causes.

### Contraindications

Active infection, irreducible odontoid migration greater than 15 mm above the foramen magnum, or presence of a sequestrum.

### Special Considerations

Preoperative planning should include computed tomography (CT) scanning to locate the transverse sinus as well as any anomalous vasculature to prevent inadvertent vascular injury. Preoperative positioning with lateral x-ray or fluoroscopic guidance is crucial to establish optimal alignment of the basiocciput and cervical spine to prevent postoperative occipitocervical kyphosis. The patient is placed in the prone position secured in a Mayfield head holder. In cases of spinal cord compression, somatosensory or motor evoked potential monitoring should be used.

### Tips, Pearls, and Lessons Learned

For dual plating, occipital screws should be placed three to a side on either side of the midline just below the superior nuchal line and as close to the external occipital protuberance as possible (**Fig. 6.1**). An independent occipital plate may only require two or three screws, usually oriented in a vertical or transverse orientation. Cerebrospinal fluid (CSF) leaks at this stage can usually be stopped by placing a screw into the hole. Bone wax may also be helpful to prevent CSF leak.

For wire placement, intraoperative fluoroscopy is useful in that it helps to match the malleable rod template to the profile of the occipitocervical junction. The rod implant is then bent to match the template. Patience is required during this step to ensure that the rods rest on the occiput and that no space exists between the rods and the cervical lamina, as this can result in the wire cutting through the bone. A small suboccipital craniotomy surrounded by four burr holes can make wire passage easier and safer. Bending the tip of the wire 180 degrees over a distance of less than 10 mm such that the bend is being advanced between the bone and dura rather than the blunt end can help prevent inadvertent durotomy and neural injury.

### Key Procedural Steps

Occipital screw placement immediately lateral to the external occipital protuberance and up to 20 mm laterally along the superior nuchal line can accommodate screws from 14 mm in length medially to 5 mm in length at 20 mm. This optimal screw placement zone tapers downward to the foramen magnum in a triangular fashion. Bicortical occipital fixation provides the strongest construct. To do this, both the inner and outer table must be drilled and tapped prior to screw placement. Before drilling, the drill stop should be set to 10 mm.

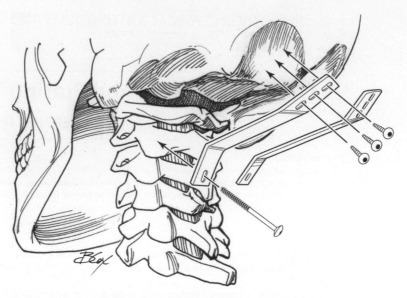

**Fig. 6.1** *Upper cervical spine and occiput. Note there are three holes on each side for the cranial fixation.*

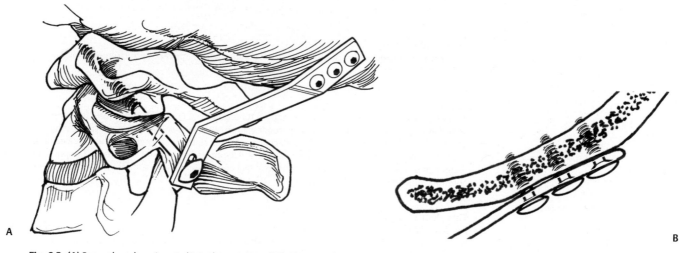

**Fig. 6.2 (A)** *Screws have been inserted into the occiput and C2. The cranial screws are below the superior nuchal line.* **(B)** *Detail of bicortical occipital screws.*

C2 pedicle screws should be placed first, followed by subaxial lateral mass screws. Occipital screws may be placed after cervical fixation, as there is more room for variability at the occiput than in the spine (**Fig. 6.2**).

Rods or plates should be bent to shape prior to drilling occipital holes. If the rods or plate extends above the superior nuchal line, a reverse bend is required at this level to ensure that it will lie flat on the occiput. When rods are used, the pivot point should be at the occipitocervical junction with the cephalad portion angling medially. In plating, a coronal plane bend should be applied to angle the occipital portion medially.

For wire placement a small suboccipital craniectomy can be performed (**Fig. 6.3**). Once the final rod position is determined, four burr holes are drilled around the craniectomy (**Fig. 6.4**). The dura is then dissected away from the inner table using a curette or dental instrument so that the bent wire tip can be passed without risk of injury (**Fig. 6.5**).

The use of a cranial bolt, the so-called inside-outside technique, can be used in patients with poor quality bone. This technique allows for a bolt to be attached to the skull via a small burr hole and trough. A plate or rod connector is placed over the bolt and secured with a nut.

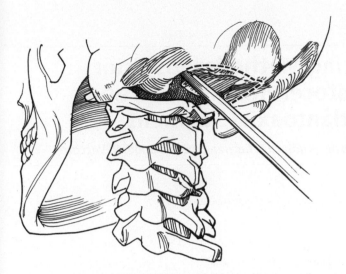

**Fig. 6.3** *Suboccipital craniectomy performed with a Kerrison rongeur to facilitate wire placement.*

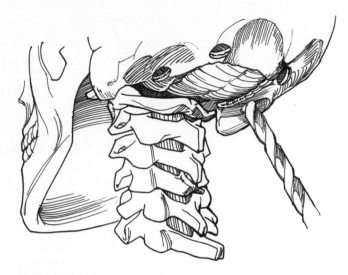

**Fig. 6.4** *Burr holes placed laterally to the craniectomy.*

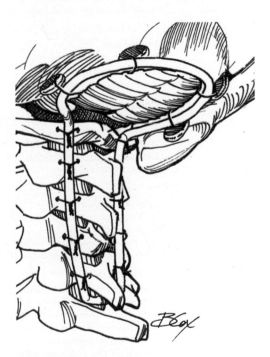

**Fig. 6.5** *Rod has been contoured and wired in place from the occiput to C5.*

PITFALLS

• Perpendicular screw placement can be especially difficult due to the steep angle required close to the foramen magnum. Unusually thin occipital bone close to the foramen magnum or in certain pathologic states can make adequate screw purchase difficult or even impossible. Cervical screw placement at the desired level can be compromised by diseased bone such as in osteomyelitis or neoplasm. Avoid these problems by placing screws closer to the superior nuchal line, but no more than 20 mm lateral to the midline, and as far superior to the foramen magnum as feasible. If the desired cervical fusion levels are too diseased for adequate screw placement, extend the construct inferiorly as many levels as necessary. Stabilization must be performed in the neutral position as rigid flexion or extension can be extremely distressing to the patient. Durotomy and neural or vascular injury can occur during drilling, screw placement, wire passage, or suboccipital craniotomy. A poor fit of the plates or rods can lead to bony erosion of the lamina or pressure ulcers of the overlying skin with subsequent hardware exposure and infection.

Independent plates are becoming popular. Fewer screws are often needed and their diameters range from 4.5 to 5 mm with a smaller screw pitch than standard cortical screws. This allows shorter screws to be used when necessary.

**Bailout, Rescue, Salvage Procedures**

If screws cannot be placed below the superior nuchal line, they may with caution be placed cephalad to it. Bear in mind that the transverse sinus typically runs deep to this landmark. If the sinus is encountered during drilling, immediately place a screw and do not attempt a repair. With a foreign body in the sinus, the patient should be placed on antiplatelet therapy postoperatively to prevent thrombosis. Screw placement can also fix most cranial CSF leaks.

# 7

# Grafting Methods: Posterior Occipitocervical Junction and Atlantoaxial Segment

*Robert K. Eastlack, Bradford L. Currier, and Alexander R. Vaccaro*

## Description

To facilitate arthrodesis of the occipitocervical or atlantoaxial segments.

## Key Principles

- Prepare the donor sites or bony bed adequately.
- Autograft bone is the gold standard choice in graft material.
- Adequate internal fixation plays an important role in maximizing fusion success.

## Expectations

Thorough preparation of the grafting site and use of autograft bone with adequate stabilization should result in a healthy fusion mass.

## Indications

- Occipitocervical instability
- Atlantoaxial instability

## Contraindications

Grossly infected sites should be debrided and treated with appropriate surgical/medical management before application of metal instrumentation and bone grafting in some cases. The timing of the graft placement and instrumentation must be addressed on an individual basis. Shortened life expectancy (less than 3 to 6 months) may obviate the usefulness of bone grafting, but it is prudent to err on the side of overtreatment.

## Special Considerations

- Occipitocervical fusions require careful intraoperative positioning to leave patients in an optimized functional alignment.
- Preserve the subaxial muscular and ligamentous attachments to the spinous process of C2 (semispinalis cervicis muscles, interspinalis muscles, interspinous ligament) when not planning for subaxial fusion.

## Special Instructions, Position, and Anesthesia

- Be sure that anesthesiology is aware of the need for neuromonitoring, as the choice of anesthetic may change when motor evoked potentials are employed.
- Position the patient prone with the head held with a pinion or halo secured to the operating table with a Mayfield attachment.
- Position the occipitocervical junction intraoperatively using fluoroscopy. The intersection of lines drawn parallel with the opening of the foramen magnum and the superior end plate of C3 should approximate 45 degrees. Ensure that neutral rotation has been obtained before fusing the atlantoaxial junction as well.

## Tips, Pearls, and Lessons Learned

Autograft bone may be harvested from the posterior-superior iliac spine or ribs. Bicortical specimens should be obtained when the graft is providing structural support in the area of fusion. If there is inadequate structural or morselized autograft bone specimen available, allograft bone may be used or autograft bone can be supplemented with demineralized bone matrix adjuncts. Do not place bone graft directly on neural elements, including the C2 exiting nerve root or ganglion.

Remove the cortex on the occipital bone below the external occipital protuberance to expose bleeding cancellous bone. This can be done with a high-speed burr following placement of occipital hardware, which may include a plate and screws. Analyze the preoperative computed tomography (CT) images for bone dimensions and the location of neurovascular structures. There is considerable anatomic variability. The occiput is thickest in the region of the external occipital protuberance (EOP), but the adjacent venous sinuses must be avoided. A thick midline keel of bone runs from the EOP to the foramen magnum and may be used for rigid fixation. Do not stray greater than 2 cm laterally from midline, as the bone thickness diminishes considerably.

Prepare the atlas and axis similarly prior to graft placement. It is very important to adequately expose and decorticate the C1 arch and laminae of C2. Using a Kerrison rongeur to decorticate the caudal portion of C1 and cranial portion of C2 will avoid a dural tear from the burr.

**Difficulties Encountered**

Absence of the C1 posterior arch, or the need for laminectomy at C1 or C2, may necessitate placement of bone graft into the atlantoaxial joints. Carefully elevate the C2 ganglion to expose the atlantoaxial joint on each side. Remove cartilage joints with a curette or burr and pack morselized cancellous graft into the joints. Corticocancellous strut grafts can be applied laterally and held in place with wires or cables secured to the bone or the instrumentation. This bone graft can be carried up to a prepared occipital bony surface when occipitocervical fusion is desired. The occipital bone should be prepared sufficiently laterally from midline to accommodate the graft placement over the C1–2 articulation.

**Key Procedural Steps**

*Occipitocervical Grafting*

This step can be accomplished in a variety of ways, depending on the extent of fusion required below the axis, as well as the accompanying instrumentation. Corticocancellous strips placed parasagittally in a longitudinal fashion can be employed (**Fig. 7.1**). Alternatively, a large unicortical piece of iliac crest autograft can be placed over the occiput–C2 region, using a midline caudal notch to help with its positioning on the cephalad aspect of the C2 spinous process (**Fig. 7.2**). Prepare the dorsal aspect of the posterior elements and occiput by decorticating them, and ensure that the cancellous surface of the graft abuts those areas well. The graft can be secured to the occiput by a midline screw or wire, or held in place by the overlying soft tissues. With newer rod/screw fixation techniques, morselized cancellous autograft bone appears to be sufficient if applied liberally to well-decorticated surfaces. Bilateral instrumentation in combination with secure occipital fixation obviates the apparent need for structural bone graft material. Because of the small surface area comprising the posterior arch of C1, we typically use a supplemental interlaminar bicortical bone graft (via one of the methods described below) at the atlantoaxial site.

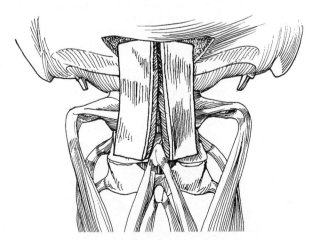

**Fig. 7.1** *Posterior perspective of the occipitocervical spine bony elements. Note the corticocancellous strips laid longitudinally on either side of the spinous processes parasagittally. The cancellous surface should be facing the decorticated surfaces of the occiput and laminae.*

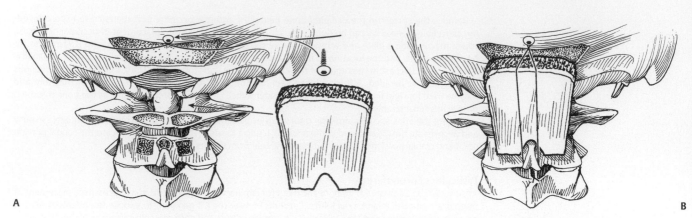

**Fig. 7.2** *(A) A large unicortical piece of iliac crest bone is applied to the occipitocervical junction, using a notch in the caudal edge that engages the cephalad margin of the C2 spinous process. (B) The inset of this unicortical iliac crest graft demonstrates the cancellous surface that should be placed in contact with the decorticated surfaces of the occiput and laminae.*

### Atlantoaxial Grafting

#### Brooks Technique (Fig. 7.3)

Two individual bicortical corticocancellous grafts (iliac crest or rib) are fashioned to fit snugly between the C1 and C2 laminae. The cephalad and caudal edges can be shaped concavely to accept the convex laminar edges they approximate. Once sublaminar wires are passed below both C1 and C2, the bony surfaces of the host bone are decorticated with careful attention given to preparing the caudal and cephalad aspects of the C1 and C2 laminae, respectively. This can be accomplished with a Kerrison rongeur or a high-speed burr. Gently use a midline laminar spreader to obtain mild distraction of the atlantoaxial interlaminar space, and place the grafts between the lamina parasagittally.

#### Dickman-Sonntag Hybrid Technique (Fig. 7.4)

A 4-cm tricortical corticocancellous graft from the iliac crest or rib is converted to a bicortical graft with a saw. Harvest the graft from the posterolateral aspect of the crest starting approximately 2 cm lateral to the posterior-superior iliac spine to obtain a graft of ideal proportions. Trim the graft to match the length between medial edges of the right and left atlantoaxial articulations. The long edges can be contoured to key into the convex surfaces of the cephalad and caudal laminae. Sublaminar wires are placed only under C1, and bone graft sites are denuded as in the Brooks technique, prior to placement of the graft. The graft is placed horizontally between the C1 and C2 laminae, with the concave surface of the graft placed toward the dura. A midline notch in the caudal surface of the graft typically aids in positioning of the graft, so that it conforms to the cranial surface of the C2 spinous process. The notch should be deeper anteriorly than posteriorly to match the upward slope of the C2 spinous process.

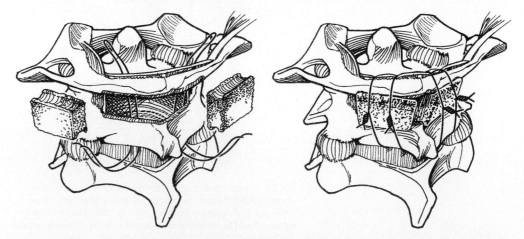

**Fig. 7.3** *Brooks technique for C1-C2 posterior arthrodesis. (A) Note the concave preparation of the cancellous mantle that mates with the lamina at both C1 and C2, and provides an extra measure of graft stability. Two pieces of bicortical iliac crest graft are placed between the C1 and C2 lamina on each side of the (B) C2 spinous process, and they are typically wired in place.*

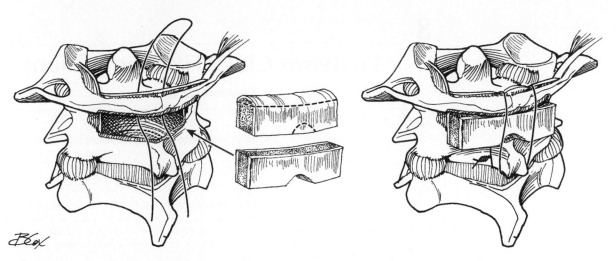

**Fig. 7.4 (A)** *Dickman-Sonntag hybrid graft for C1-C2 posterior arthrodesis. This 4-cm piece of tricortical graft is excised from the iliac crest, and converted to bicortical via resection of the longitudinal section delineated by the dashed line. The curvilinear dashed line* *demonstrates the area of notch preparation that will engage the C2 spinous process. **(B)** After application of the hybrid graft between C1 and C2, wiring is typically employed to capture and stabilize the graft between the laminae.*

## PITFALLS

- The course of the vertebral artery varies as it passes from lateral to medial just posterior to the lateral mass of C1. Limit exposure of the posterior arch beyond 8 mm from the midline to prevent injury to the vertebral artery in this area.
- When only atlantoaxial arthrodesis is desired, be careful to limit exposure of the occipital bone in children. Younger patients have a heightened propensity to autofuse the occipitocervical junction following exposure alone.

## Bailout, Rescue, Salvage Procedures

When inadequate laminar bone stock remains due to congenital anomaly or laminectomy, central placement of the bone graft must be accomplished with extreme caution. If the bone graft does not have secure fixation to the occipital and axial surfaces, the corticocancellous graft should be morselized and placed lateral to the cord.

If the posterior arch of C1 fractures during atlantoaxial graft placement or fixation, grafting should be applied laterally as well. A small amount of cancellous graft can be packed into the atlantoaxial joints, or corticocancellous strips may be placed dorsally to span the atlantoaxial articular recess. Avoid impingement of the C2 nerve or the spinal cord with the graft. Immobilize the region postoperatively with a cervical orthosis or halo vest depending on the degree of instability, type of internal fixation, and the quality of the bone.

# 8

# Posterior C1, C2 Fixation Options

*Norman B. Chutkan*

## Description

Review of fixation options for C1-C2 posterior fusion including posterior wiring, transarticular screws, lateral mass screws, and translaminar screws. The relevant anatomy and structures at risk are reviewed.

## Key Principles

Although posterior wiring is an accepted method of atlantoaxial fixation, newer techniques have been developed that provide rigid fixation. These include transarticular screw fixation, C1-C2 lateral mass screw fixation, and C2 translaminar screws. Although these techniques do allow for more rigid fixation, they are technically more demanding and are associated with an increased risk of complications.

## Expectations

In cases of C1-C2 instability, there are several options for secure fixation of the atlantoaxial complex. The suitability of each technique depends on the specific anatomy and the presence or absence of intact posterior elements.

## Indications

- C1, C2 instability
- Nonunion or delayed union of odontoid fractures
- Pseudarthrosis of previous atlantoaxial fusion

## Contraindications

Related to specific techniques, as follows.

### Posterior Wiring

- Absent or fractured C1 or C2 lamina; marked C1 canal encroachment by bone, pannus, or other tissue; congenital occipital–C1 fusion

### Transarticular Screws

- Aberrant vertebral artery anatomy
- Inability to reduce the atlantoaxial complex
- Relative contraindication: previous injury or known unilateral vertebral artery occlusion

### C1-C2 Lateral Mass Screws

- Aberrant vertebral artery passage
- Destruction or fracture of C1 lateral mass or C2 pedicle

### C2 Translaminar Screws

- Fractured or absent C2 lamina

## Special Considerations

Detailed preoperative evaluation of the bone morphology and neurovascular anatomy is critical to maximize surgical success and minimize the risk of complications. Computed tomography (CT) and magnetic resonance imaging (MRI) facilitate determining the location of the vertebral arteries, assessing the reduction of the atlantoaxial complex, assessing the integrity of the posterior elements, and evaluating the pars of the axis. CT angiography provides better visualization of the vertebral arteries than does standard CT. Stereotactic image guidance systems may be beneficial in demonstrating the proposed screw trajectory. In cases where posterior wiring is being considered, care should be taken if there is significant anterior canal encroachment by hypertrophied bone (odontoid), pannus, infected tissue, or large tissue mass, as this may increase the risk of neurologic injury.

### Special Instructions, Position, and Anesthesia
- With gross instability, consider awake intubation and a rotational table such as an OSI Jackson (Orthopedic Systems, Inc., Union City, CA).
- Prone position with rolls or spine frame
- Head fixed with Mayfield pin holder or graphite halo ring
- Neurophysiologic monitoring may be helpful.
- Lateral intraoperative fluoroscopy is mandatory. Anteroposterior (AP) fluoroscopy is optional, as is stereotactic guidance.

### Tips, Pearls, and Lessons Learned
For cases of posterior wiring, flexing the head on C1 can facilitate wire passage. Anatomic reduction should be achieved prior to passing wires. Large curved blunt needles can be used to pass sutures under the lamina. Wires or cables can then be pulled through. Unicortical grafts with a thick cancellous component should fit snugly against the decorticated posterior and inferior ring of C1 and the lamina of C2. In cases where screw fixation is being considered, it is important to remember that there is significant variation in bony morphology and vascular anatomy among individuals. Careful preoperative assessment facilitates determining the best options for screw fixation. The use of intraoperative tactile and visual landmarks as well as fluoroscopy is critical. Although not mandatory, stereotactic imaging may be of benefit. Direct palpation of the medial border of the C2 isthmus is most important, as it serves as a guide for correct medial-lateral screw placement.

### Difficulties Encountered
Increased thoracic kyphosis may present a challenge for percutaneous placement of transarticular screws. The venous plexus overlying the C1-C2 facet joint can lead to significant bleeding. This can be minimized with careful dissection and packing with hemostatic agents. Appropriate positioning prior to beginning the case is critical. The neck should be positioned with lower cervical flexion and midcervical protraction while maintaining reduction of the atlantoaxial complex. With posterior wiring, if wires or cables cannot be passed safely or easily under the lamina of C2, passing it through or around the spinous process should be considered.

### Key Procedural Steps
Exposure should be limited to the C1-C2 posterior elements. Care should be taken to avoid injury to the C2-C3 facet capsule. For posterior wiring, limit the exposure of C1 to 1.5 to 2 cm laterally from the midline to avoid injuring the vertebral artery. Free the edges of the lamina of C1 and C2. The interspinous ligament between C2 and C3 is maintained. A small, central soft tissue window is created between C2 and C3. A large blunt needle is used to pass a looped suture under C1 and C2. If a Gallie-type fusion is planned, a single suture is sufficient; however, a Gallie construct provides little rotational stability, and a Brooks-type construct is preferred. This requires the passage of two separate sutures. Wire or cables can then be pulled through. For a Gallie fusion a looped wire or cable is pulled under C1 and wrapped around the spinous process of C2. For a Brooks fusion two looped wires or cables are pulled under the lamina of C1 and C2. With a Gallie fusion a single large unicortical autograft is placed between the lamina of C1 and C2 and secured in place by tightening the wires or cables. In a Brooks fusion two corticocancellous autograft rectangular wedges are used (**Fig. 8.1**). The grafts should fit snugly once the wires or cables are tightened. Gaps between the graft and lamina can be filled with cancellous bone.

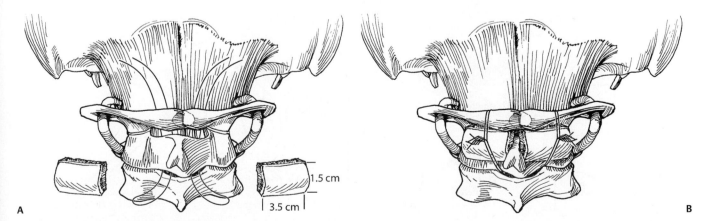

**A**                                                                                    **B**

**Fig. 8.1** *(A,B) Brooks wiring with corticocancellous struts.*

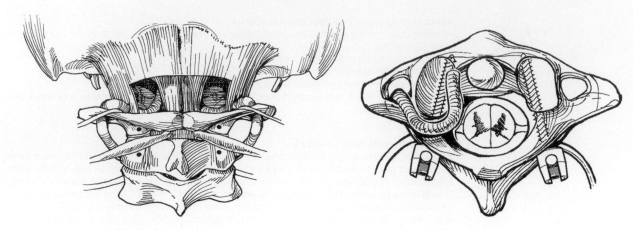

**Fig. 8.2** *(A,B) C1 lateral mass screws.*

Placement of C1 lateral mass screws as originally described requires exposure of the C1 lateral mass, which can be associated with significant bleeding from the venous plexus. Careful dissection and packing with hemostatic agents can minimize this risk. Alternating from side to side until adequate exposure is achieved is a useful technique. A modification of the original technique involves starting the screws on the posterior ring of C1 to avoid having to dissect out the lateral mass. With this technique it is necessary to ensure that the posterior ring is thick enough to accommodate a screw and that there is not an aberrant interosseous vertebral artery. A starting hole is created using a 2-mm high-speed burr and the lateral mass is then drilled under fluoroscopic control (**Fig. 8.2**). Bicortical fixation is recommended.

Placement of C2 pedicle screws and transarticular screws is similar. In both cases palpation of the medial wall of the C2 isthmus serves as a critical landmark in lateral to medial angulation. For transarticular screws the starting point is more inferior (2 mm cephalad to the C2-C3 facet joint) with a steeper angulation (**Fig. 8.3** and **Fig. 8.4**). This usually requires percutaneous placement at the cervicothoracic junction to achieve the appropriate angulation. The ability to achieve this angulation should be verified preoperatively by using a long guidewire external to the body. A small high-speed burr is used to create a starting hole. Multiple lateral fluoroscopic images are used to ensure correct screw trajectory. For C2 pedicle screws the starting point is usually higher, in the superior medial portion of the lateral mass, angulated approximately 15 degrees toward midline (**Fig. 8.5**). Direct exposure of the C1-C2 facet carries the potential of significant bleeding, but does allow for curettage and bone grafting of the joint.

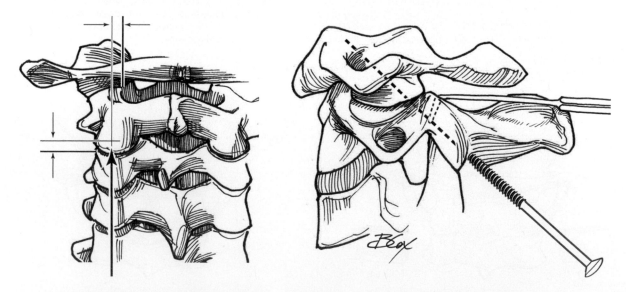

**Fig. 8.3** *Starting point and trajectory in the coronal plane.*    **Fig. 8.4** *Screw trajectory through the C1-C2 articulation.*

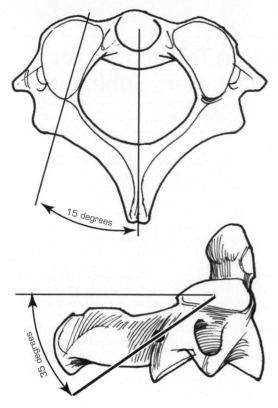

**Fig. 8.5** *Placement of C2 pedicle screw in the transverse and sagittal planes.*

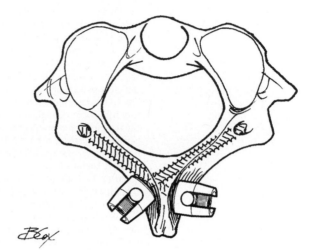

**Fig. 8.6** *C2 translaminar screws.*

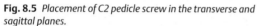

**PITFALLS**

- With posterior wiring, care should be taken to use thin flexible wire or cables to avoid indenting the dura. Undersized grafts may cause loss of reduction or a posteriorly directed vector. Posterior wiring is not as rigid as screw fixation, and in patients with gross instability additional external immobilization such as a halo may be necessary. In cases of screw fixation the vertebral artery is the structure most at risk. Inadvertent inferior or lateral placement of transarticular or C2 pedicle screws may place the artery at risk. Cannulated systems are not recommended to prevent accidental advancement of the guidewire into the neck.

Recently, C2 translaminar screw placement has been described with possibly less risk to the vertebral arteries. This involves creating a starting hole at the junction of the C2 spinous process and lamina (**Fig. 8.6**). A drill is then used to create a screw hole between the inner and outer cortical tables. Using a hand drill may reduce the risk of cortical breach. Although the technique is relatively simple it is important to plan screw placement carefully, as placement of the first screw in its most optimal position may block placement of the second screw. The use of polyaxial screws facilitates combining this technique with C1 lateral mass screws or subaxial lateral mass screw fixation.

**Bailout, Rescue, Salvage Procedures**

Injury to the vertebral artery requires that the procedure be aborted. Bone wax, hemostatic agents, and tamponade may control bleeding; however, further exposure and ligation may be necessary. Repair of the vertebral artery is technically very demanding. Placement of a short screw to control bleeding followed by emergent angiography with neurovascular assistance should be considered. Unilateral vertebral artery injury is often well tolerated. Repair should not be attempted unless there is evidence of neurologic disturbance. With transarticular fixation, placement of sublaminar wires or cables prior to screw hole preparation is recommended to allow for some provisional fixation in the event of a vertebral artery injury. Anterior transarticular fixation is an option if posterior wiring or screw fixation is not possible. Alternatively extending the fusion to an occipitocervical fusion may be necessary in extreme cases.

# 9

# Reduction Techniques for Atlantoaxial Rotary Subluxation

*Rick C. Sasso*

## Description

Atlantoaxial rotatory subluxation is an anterior displacement of one C1-C2 joint with a concomitant posterior migration of the contralateral articulation. The pivot point is usually an intact anterior arch of C1–odontoid articulation with a preserved transverse atlantal ligament (TAL). This type of C1-C2 subluxation is different from the more common anterior subluxation of C1-C2, which routinely occurs due to incompetence of the TAL. Rheumatoid involvement and trauma to the TAL are the most common reasons for anterior subluxation of the atlantoaxial joint. In a different type of atlantoaxial rotatory subluxation, the pivot point is one C1-C2 joint, whereas the contralateral C1 lateral mass is shifted anterior to C2. The TAL is usually attenuated or frankly disrupted in this variety of rotatory subluxation. Atlantoaxial rotatory subluxation usually occurs in children and is a common cause of torticollis (**Fig. 9.1**). This is routinely caused by trauma or infection of the upper respiratory tract, which weakens the ligamentous and facet capsular structures of C1-C2. The flat C1-C2 facet joints do not provide intrinsic stability and are specialized to allow rotation. Minimal trauma and minor pharyngeal inflammation can therefore lead to C1–C2 rotatory subluxation.

Most C1-C2 rotatory subluxations in children reduce spontaneously. The torticollis deformity may be treated with a short course of a cervical collar or low-weight traction with a head halter. If these maneuvers do not reduce the deformity, then open reduction and internal fixation is contemplated. The articulation is best visualized, reduced, instrumented, and fused from a posterior approach. The most powerful method of reduction and instrumentation is through anchoring a screw into each lateral mass of C1 and pedicles of C2 to directly manipulate the vertebrae with these "joysticks."

## Expectations

Anatomic reduction of the atlantoaxial articulation with resolution of the torticollis deformity is expected (**Fig. 9.2**). With direct access to the joints and focused manipulation through the segmental fixation into C1 and C2, perfect reduction is anticipated.

## Indications

The indications for this technique of direct reduction and internal fixation with polyaxial lateral mass screws in C1 and pedicles screws in C2 connected through rods are irreducible rotatory subluxations of C1-C2 that are unresponsive to nonoperative treatment (**Fig. 9.3**).

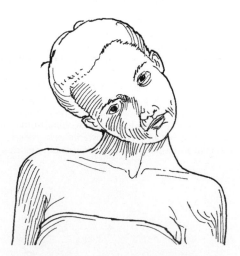

**Fig. 9.1** *A 10-year-old girl 5 months after a car crash with a fixed torticollis. This severe deformity continued despite multiple attempts of closed reduction and immobilization even with a halo.*

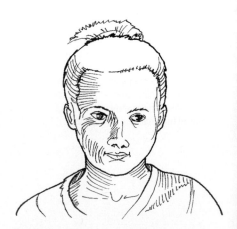

**Fig. 9.2** *The same girl as in* **Fig. 9.1** *one day after open reduction and internal fixation of the C1-C2 joints.*

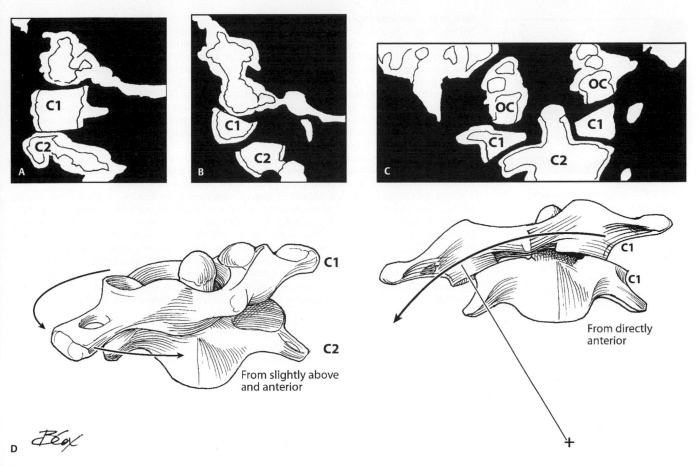

**Fig. 9.3** *Representations of preoperative computed tomography (CT) scans with reformatted reconstructions. (A) Left C1-C2 joint with the lateral mass of C1 posterior to the C2 superior articular surface. (B) Contralateral right C1-C2 joint with the lateral mass of C1 anterior to the C2 superior articular surface. (C) Coronal view with asymmetry of C1-C2 articulation (OC = occiput). (D) Mechanisms of dislocation.*

### Contraindications

The contraindications are those subluxations/dislocations that reduce and are stable with nonoperative methods.

### Special Considerations

Visualization and complete mobilization of the C1-C2 articulation requires full access to the posterior aspect of the C1-C2 joint, which is covered by the C2 nerve root. Thus, the C2 nerve root needs to be circumferentially mobilized. Also, it is extremely important to understand the course of the vertebral artery (VA), which runs from C3 to the occiput (**Fig. 9.4**).

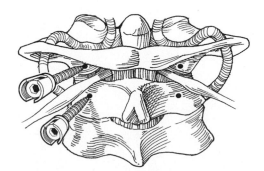

**Fig. 9.4** *The course of the vertebral artery (VA) in relation to the C2-C3 facet joint, the starting point for the C2 pedicle screw and the C1 lateral mass screw.*

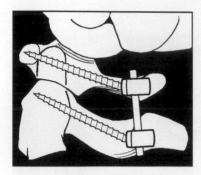

**Fig. 9.5** *Final construct with bilateral C1 lateral mass and C2 pedicles screws connected to rods in a reduced position.*

**PITFALLS**

• If the rotatory subluxation is not acute, significant fibrous and bony callus within the joint may cause difficulty with reduction. Also, the joints may be "stuck" by the complete dislocation of the articular surfaces. Breaking up the callus within the joint and distraction of the articular surfaces through the screws overcomes this challenge.

### Tips, Pearls, and Lessons Learned

An important tip for mobilizing the C2 nerve is the control of the venous plexus, which surrounds the nerve as it courses posterior to the C1-C2 facet joint. It is necessary to gain complete control of this plexus so that the nerve can be retracted both cephalad and caudal to completely visualize the joint. If the C2 nerve is retracted without coagulating the venous plexus, significant blood loss and poor visualization may complicate this procedure.

The vertebral artery is placed at risk with traditional transarticular (TA) C1-C2 screws. Up to 18% of C1-C2 joints anatomically cannot be fixed with TA screws due to the path of the VA crossing the trajectory of the screw. The VA is most at risk during the start of the screw path anterior to the inferior articular process of C2. Because the start of this TA screw (which is the same as a C2 pars screw) is very low (just cephalad to the C2-C3 facet joint), the VA is crossing from medial to lateral just anterior to this starting point. Because the pedicle screw starts cephalad to the TA screw, in many instances the VA has crossed from medial to lateral caudal to this point, and because the pedicle screw path is approximately 30 degrees medial, it is running away from the course of the VA. Thus, this C2 pedicle screw places the VA at less risk.

Although it may be tempting to begin the C1 lateral mass screw in the posterior arch of C1, this must be resisted. Again, this is due to the course of the VA (which runs in a groove along the cephalad aspect of the C1 posterior arch). The VA may dip caudally, significantly thinning the bony connection of the posterior arch to the C1 lateral mass. A deceptively wide posterior arch of C1 may hide the VA anterior to a thin wafer of bone, making screw insertion extremely dangerous. If the screw is started on the lateral mass of C1, it is a very safe screw. The spinal cord is not at risk because the screw starting point is in the anterior aspect of the spinal canal. The vertebral artery is not at risk because it is very lateral and cephalad to this entry point. The major difficulty with accessing this insertion point, however, is the venous plexus surrounding the C2 nerve root. The key to easily introducing the C1 lateral mass screw is fully mobilizing the C2 nerve root.

### Key Procedural Steps

• Posterior exposure of C1-C2 with mobilization of the C2 nerve roots
• Disimpaction of the C1–C2 joints and removal of the articular surfaces
• Insertion of the polyaxial screws into the lateral masses of C1 and the pedicles of C2
• Anatomical reduction of the atlantoaxial joints by using the screws as "joysticks" as well as levering instruments into the articular surfaces
• Seating of rods into the polyaxial screws to fix C1–C2 in an anatomic position (**Fig. 9.5**)
• Application of bone graft into the denuded atlantoaxial joints bilaterally

### Bailout, Rescue, Salvage Procedures

If this screw technique cannot be implemented for whatever reason, then posterior fusion with a cable or wire construct can be performed. A Brooks or modified posterior spinous process wiring technique may be utilized if the posterior elements of C1 and C2 are intact. Postoperatively, however, the patient requires halo immobilization because this form of fixation is profoundly weaker than the described polyaxial screw/rod construct.

# 10

## Posterior Cervical Wiring

*Howard B. Levene and Jack I. Jallo*

### Description

Posterior cervical wiring is a relatively simple and inexpensive technique for achieving cervical stability by providing a posterior tension band that resists flexion. At one time the preferred procedure for posterior cervical stabilization, the technique has since fallen out of favor in light of the popularity of lateral mass screw fixation. However, the technique remains a valuable supplemental or salvage procedure. There are three general types of wiring: (1) spinous process wiring, (2) facet wiring, and (3) sublaminar wiring. Although sublaminar wiring continues to be useful for atlantoaxial fixation, it generally has been abandoned for subaxial cervical spine fixation due to the comparatively high risk of neurologic injury when compared with modern fixation systems.

Spinous process wiring and facet wiring share the fundamental ability to fuse adjacent levels through the creation of a posterior tension band. Wires are passed through a bony element (spinous process or facet) and either looped over another bony element or passed through another bony element. Autograft/allograft/artificial biomaterials can be used to supplement the fusion technique.

There are multiple techniques for simple interspinous wiring: Rogers wiring, Whitehill modification of the Rogers Wiring, Benzel-Kesterson modification of Rogers wiring, Bohlman triple-wire technique, and the Murphy-Southwick modification of the Rogers technique.

Facet wiring techniques include Cahill oblique facet wiring and Callahan non-oblique facet wiring.

### Expectations

The Rogers method and its various modifications are expected to provide cervical stability to a single subaxial cervical motion segment. To stabilize additional levels, the procedure can be repeated. The Murphy-Southwick modification of the Rogers technique is designed to stabilize additional segments.

### Indications

Cervical wiring is indicated for subaxial instability resulting from trauma, neoplasm, degeneration, or infection (posttreatment). Cervical wiring is indicated when stability is restored with re-creation of a posterior tension band to prevent progression of deformity, to alleviate pain, or to promote bony fusion.

### Contraindications

These wiring techniques are contraindicated when there is an incomplete posterior bony ring, poor bone quality, or stability requirements (extension, rotation, lateral motion) beyond what can be delivered by posterior wiring.

### Special Considerations

When choosing posterior wiring, it is important to remember that wiring provides almost no stability in extension, lateral bending, or axial rotation.

### Special Instructions, Position, and Anesthesia

Careful preoperative consultation with anesthesia colleagues is required. For intubation, the surgeon should arrange for fiberoptic laryngoscopic intubation. Prior to positioning, neuromonitoring (somatosensory evoked potential [SSEP], motor evoked potential [MEP]) should be checked for baseline values. Changes in baseline signals during positioning are addressed with repositioning, steroid administration, or abandonment of the procedure. When positioning, the patient is prone with neutral cervical spine or slight extension to the cervical spine. Mayfield pins or cervical traction are options.

### Tips, Pearls, and Lessons Learned

Posterior wiring requires that the posterior elements are intact. Avoid this technique in cases of severe instability. Use it as a stand-alone device only when the anterior and middle load-bearing columns are intact and a posterior tension band needs to be restored. A rigid cervical collar or halo may be required for stability during fusion. Facet wiring can be used when the lamina or spinous process of the adjacent rostral segments are missing. When using autograft, ribs make good posterior strut grafts versus iliac crest due to their natural curvature. Stainless steel, titanium, and polyethylene cables are available; 16- to 20-gauge metallic wires are the preferred sizes. Stainless steel wires have the best tensile strength. Titanium is more susceptible to fatigue notching than stainless steel, but it has a better magnetic resonance imaging (MRI) profile. Polyethylene cables exhibit more creep than metal alloys, but have the best MRI

cables are then passed through these holes and are used to affix two strut grafts along the posterior elements on each side (**Fig. 10.4**). The Murphy-Southwick modification of the Rogers technique allows for fusion of two adjacent motion segments. Holes are drilled into each respective spinous process as above and wires are placed and tightened to bind all three spinous processes.

In facet wiring, the wires attach the facets to either adjacent facets or to an adjacent spinous process. By creating a tension band from the facet to the spinous process, rotational stability is augmented as in a

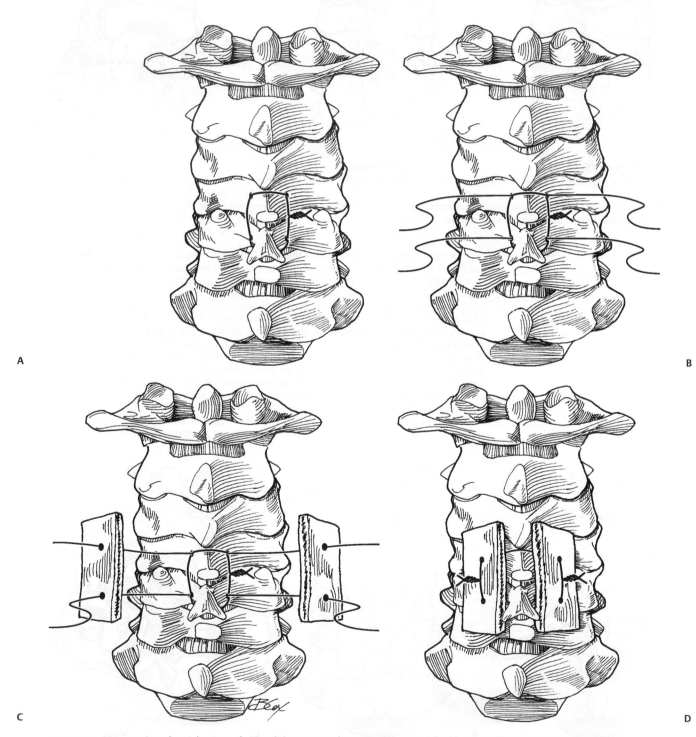

A

B

C

D

**Fig. 10.4** *Bohlman and McAfee triple-wire technique. **(A)** Begin as in the Rogers technique. **(B)** Additional cables are passed through the superior and inferior holes. **(C)** Additional cables are threaded through the graft. **(D)** Construct is tightened.*

reduced facet dislocation. Expose as above, except that the lateral masses/facets must be fully exposed. Remove the facet joint capsules and enter the facet with a small elevator and curette or drill away the articular cartilage. Drill a small hole perpendicular to the plane of the facet. Protect the nerve root and vertebral artery with small dissector. For the Cahill oblique wiring, place the wire and loop through spinous process below. Repeat contralaterally (**Fig. 10.5**). For the Callahan wiring technique, the wires loop through a bony graft (rib or iliac crest) and do not connect with the spinous processes (**Fig. 10.6**).

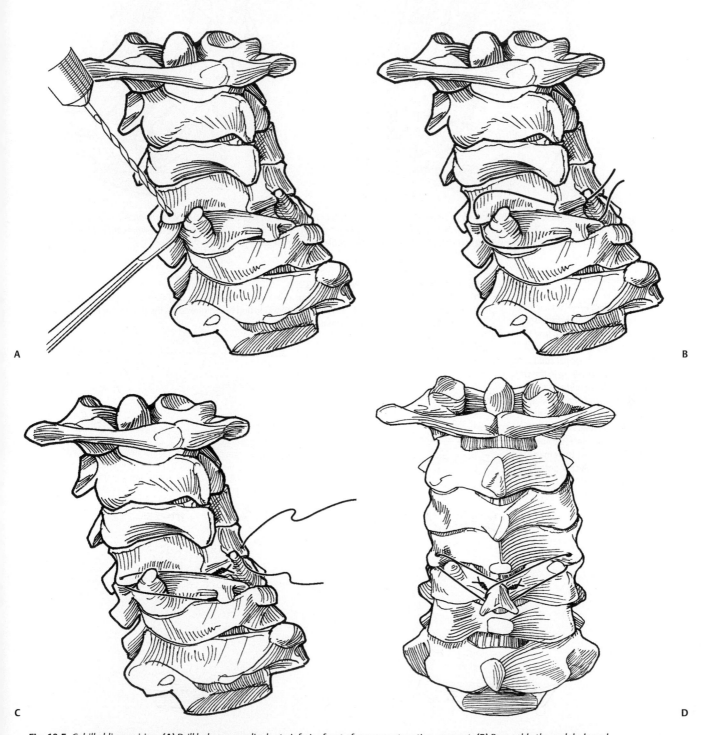

**Fig. 10.5** *Cahill oblique wiring. **(A)** Drill holes perpendicular to inferior facet of uppermost motion segment. **(B)** Pass cable through hole and loop over spinous process at inferior level. **(C)** Repeat contralaterally. **(D)** Construct is tightened.*

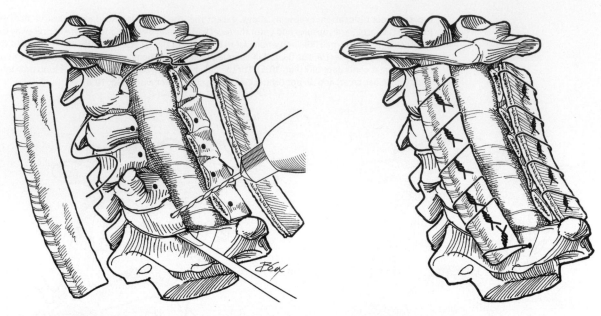

A                                                                                        B

**Fig. 10.6** *Callahan facet wiring. **(A)** Drill holes perpendicular to inferior facet of each motion segment. Pass a cable through each hole in a cranial-caudal direction. One cable is used per hole. **(B)** Cables are tightened around a strut graft. Take care to spare the most caudal facet joint by using a cable through the spinous process rather than passing a cable through the facet joint.*

PITFALLS

- Avoid overtensioning wires, which may result in a hyperextension deformity. Overtensioning wires may also lead to wire breakage or pullout. (Use 8 to 12 inch-pound torque for normal adult bone.) Unilateral facet wiring in the setting of a bilateral facet subluxation may result in rotary instability and will not confer adequate stability. When fusing, do not disrupt facet joints at cranial or caudal nonfused segments. Do not allow metals of different alloys to be in contact, as they will create an electric potential and promote corrosion.

**Bailout, Rescue, Salvage Procedures**

If a posterior element fracture is present, one can incorporate an additional level above or below in the fusion construct. Alternatively, other fixation and fusion techniques may be utilized such as pedicle screws, lateral mass screws, or rarely laminar clamps.

# 11

## Cervical Lateral Mass Screw Placement (C3–C7)

*Yu-Po Lee, Choll W. Kim, and Steven R. Garfin*

### Description
To safely place screws within the cervical lateral mass while avoiding injury to the surrounding neurovascular structures.

### Key Principles
Unicortical and bicortical screws may be placed safely within the lateral masses of the cervical spine (C3–C7).

### Expectations
Lateral mass screws and rods provide rigid segmental fixation in cases of trauma or to enhance fusions.

### Indications
Cervical instability, following a multilevel anterior corpectomy and strut grafting, and following posterior cervical laminectomy.

### Contraindications
- Aberrant vertebral artery anatomy
- Fracture of the lateral mass
- Absent or small lateral mass (C7)

### Special Considerations
Detailed preoperative imaging using plain radiographs and magnetic resonance imaging (MRI) is necessary prior to surgery to adequately assess local anatomy, including the location of neural structures and the vertebral arteries. Computed tomography (CT) is helpful in certain cases for better assessment of the bony anatomy.

### Special Instructions, Position, and Anesthesia
If the procedure is to be performed in an unstable spine, awake intubation and positioning is recommended. Electrophysiologic monitoring is also helpful. Place the patient prone in the reverse Trendelenburg position with a Mayfield pin headrest or foam pillow. The neck may need to be slightly flexed in patients with a large occiput that is preventing access to the cervical vertebrae. Avoid forceful or excessive flexion. Also, placing the head at the foot of an AMSCO table (Steris Corp., Mentor, OH) is often helpful if using fluoroscopy. Tuck in the patient's arms at the sides. Use 3-inch tape to provide longitudinal traction to the shoulders. This aids in radiographic visualization of the cervical spine.

### Tips, Pearls, and Lessons Learned
Taking an x-ray once the patient has been positioned is helpful for checking the alignment of the cervical spine and for planning the incision. This avoids having to reposition the patient after he/she has been prepped and draped or having to enlarge the incision or violating facet joints that were not intended to be fused. The most prominent spinous processes to palpation are C2, C7, and T1. Also, C6 is the last bifid spinous process, and the vertebral arteries do not usually run in the transverse foramen of C7. Care should be taken in the exposure to stay midline in the ligamentum nuchae. Straying laterally into muscle causes bleeding that will impede visualization of the lateral masses. Care should also be taken not to dissect the muscles off of the spinous process of C2, as this could lead to potential C2-C3 instability. The drill for the lateral mass screw is aimed 15 degrees cephalad and 30 degrees laterally relative to the vertebrae. Adjustments in the position of the neck and in the table may make it difficult to judge the orientation of the vertebra. Placing a Penfield No. 4 elevator (Miltex, Tuttlingen, Germany) in the facet joint can be helpful in clarifying the orientation of the facet joint and thus the proper trajectory of the drill. Also, it is important to remember that the lateral mass of C7 is smaller and a steeper trajectory is often needed.

### Difficulties Encountered
Should lack of stable fixation become a problem with a unicortical screw, bicortical fixation may improve screw purchase. Also, a salvage screw may improve screw fixation. The most inferior screw must not violate the facet joint, as this may lead to pain at the adjacent level.

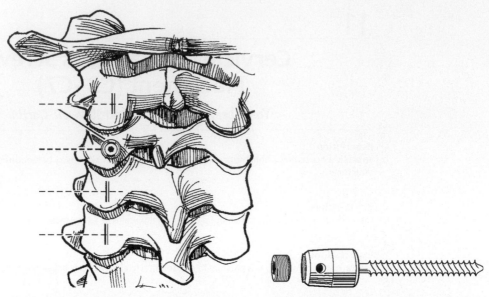

A                                                                                                                                                                      B

**Fig. 11.1** *(A) The portal of entry for the lateral mass screws should be in the middle of the lateral mass in the cephalad-caudad plane and 1 mm medial to midline in the medial lateral plane. (B) A lateral mass screw.*

### Key Procedural Steps

Make a midline incision at the desired level. Proceed through the ligamentum nuchae to the spinous processes. Use a subperiosteal dissection to expose the posterior elements and the lateral masses. Care should be taken not to violate the facet joints that are not to be fused. The starting point for the lateral mass screws should be in the middle of the lateral mass in the cephalad-caudad plane and 1 mm medial to midline in the medial lateral plane (**Fig. 11.1**). Use a 2-mm pneumatic burr to penetrate the cortex. Use a 2.5-mm drill with a 14-mm stop to drill the hole. A 14-mm screw is usually sufficient for bicortical fixation. The drill should be aimed 15 degrees cephalad and 30 degrees laterally (**Fig. 11.2** and **Fig. 11.3**). This should avoid injury to the vertebral artery, which generally lies in the midline of the lateral mass, and the nerve roots, which run inferiorly as they exit the neuroforamen. The hole depth is measured and tapped; 3.5-mm polyaxial screws with favored angles are helpful for placement of the connector rods. If bicortical fixation is desired, start with a 10-mm drill and increase 2-mm in sequential fashion until the other cortex is breached.

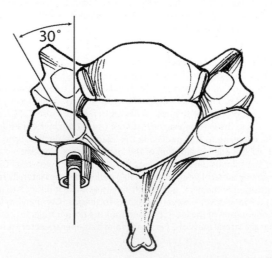

**Fig. 11.2** *The angle of insertion in the coronal plane should be 30 degrees from the sagittal plane. This limits the incidence of vertebral artery injury.*

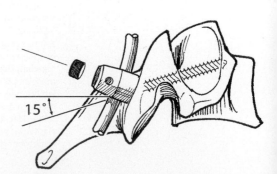

**Fig. 11.3** *The screw should be aimed 15 degrees cephalad relative to the vertebral body to avoid violation of the facet joint.*

PITFALLS

• Inadequate lateral mass size (C7), poor fixation, vertebral artery violation, nerve root injury, and injury to the adjacent facet joints.

**Bailout, Rescue, Salvage Procedures**

Should the vertebral artery be violated during the procedure, hemostasis is achieved by packing the site with thrombin-soaked Gelfoam and bone wax. Instrumentation on the contralateral side should be avoided to ensure that at least one vertebral artery remains intact. In situ fusion with halo fixation can be used as an alternative fusion technique. Interspinous process wiring and anterior fixation should also be considered.

If poor screw purchase is encountered within the lateral mass, the use of a larger-diameter salvage screw may offer greater purchase. Conversion to a Roy-Camille technique or cervical pedicle screws (C7) should also be considered.

# 12

# Cervical Subaxial Transfacet Screw Placement

*Jeffrey M. Spivak*

## Description

This fixation technique is not commonly used, as there are no clinical series of posterior cervical fusions reported using this method alone. However, this technique can be quite useful for isolated facet joint fusions, and has been described as a salvage technique in cases of failed lateral mass fixation.

## Key Principles

A full understanding of the anatomic orientation of the cervical subaxial facet joints is imperative for the proper use and execution of this fixation technique. The cervical facet joints are flat and angled cephalad at approximately 60 degrees in the coronal plane.

Standard techniques for lateral mass screw insertion involve directing the screw path laterally and cephalad, avoiding any penetration of the facet joint. Subaxial facet screw fixation requires a caudal direction of the screw, perpendicular to and therefore across the facet joint surface.

## Expectations

Transfacet screw fixation can be used as an isolated fixation technique or, more commonly, as a supplementary method of fixation in combination with anterior plate fixation following anterior diskectomy or corpectomy. The technique is technically demanding, with little room for error, but it can be used to salvage inadequate lateral mass fixation. Biomechanical data have shown that transfacet screw placement provides stronger resistance to pullout than bicortical lateral mass screws, with the most pronounced difference noted at the C7-T1 level. Comparison testing of fixated motion segments to resistance to physiologic motion (flexion-extension, lateral bending, axial rotation) has not been done for the two fixation techniques, and the strength of direct transfacet fixation alone to resist these forces is unknown.

## Indications

Use of subaxial facet screw fixation is indicated as an adjunct to cervical spine fusion. The technique can be used to support an anterior decompression and fusion procedure or as an isolated posterior fusion. It can be used in conjunction with other posterior fixation techniques including spinous process wiring and sublaminar wiring when these posterior elements are available. The technique can also be used as part of a multilevel posterolateral fixation construct in combination with lateral mass or pedicle fixation using rod or plate longitudinal members. It is very useful as a salvage technique for failed lateral mass fixation (**Fig. 12.1**).

## Contraindications

Use of subaxial facet screw fixation is contraindicated in cases where one or both of the lateral masses is comminuted, incompetent, or disconnected from the remainder of the vertebra secondary to either a traumatic or neoplastic process. In cases requiring decompression of the neural foramen posteriorly via partial facetectomy and foraminotomy, this technique is not likely to be suitable due to the smaller amount of remaining facet joint surface following the decompression.

## Special Considerations

For cases requiring fusion due to trauma or neoplasm, preoperative evaluation with computed tomography (CT) scanning including sagittal reconstructions is necessary to assess the bony integrity of the lateral masses and facet joint to be sure that posterolateral fixation of any type is a viable option for providing stability.

## Special Instructions, Position, and Anesthesia

Prone positioning with rigid hold of the head using skull pin fixation is recommended. Adequate cervical alignment should be achieved before the skin incision if possible. If not, intraoperative reduction and realignment must be achieved before screw placement. Subaxial cervical facet screws are used only for fixation, not for segmental realignment.

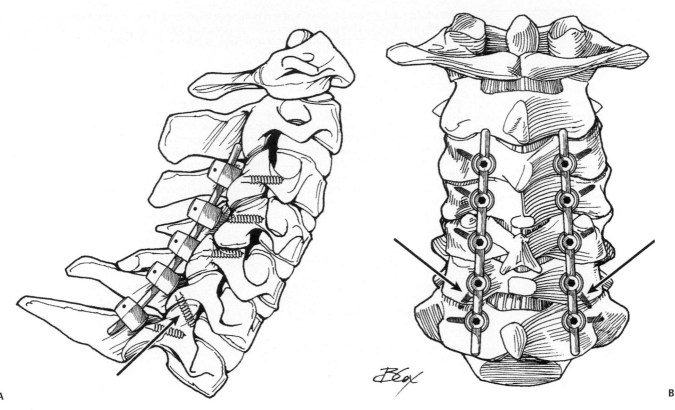

**Fig. 12.1** *Lateral view (A) and PA view (B) of transfacet fixation at C6-C7 as a salvage for failed right C6 lateral mass fixation. The caudal screw fixation (arrows) can be seen well in both views.*

A

B

### Tips, Pearls, and Lessons Learned
Fluoroscopic guidance for screw placement is extremely useful to be sure that the joint is crossed near its midportion and to ensure adequate surrounding bone stock to avoid iatrogenic facet fracture. Fluoroscopy is also helpful to ensure that the next caudal facet joint is not disrupted at its anterior aspect due to too caudal screw angulation.

Fluoroscopic visualization by level without parallax is important to ensure proper screw insertion. The left and right facet joints at each level should be visualized as one structure without incongruent overlap. Deformities of the motion segment can be compensated for by adjusting the position of the operative table or the fluoroscopy unit to visualize the facet joints properly. The alignment of the facets should be visualized and evaluated preoperatively once the patient is positioned and before prepping and draping and beginning the procedure.

Use of a transfacet screw as part of a multilevel lateral mass fixation construct will place the screw-head offset from the regular lateral mass screw head positioning within the plate. This may require some compromise of optimal screw insertion point and angulation to keep it within the plate construct. Multiaxial screw and rod systems, with increased flexibility for screw head position and screw angulation, are preferred for this type of mixed fixation construct.

### Difficulties Encountered
The main difficulty with this type of screw placement is achieving adequate fixation across the facet joint. Use of intraoperative lateral fluoroscopy is extremely helpful to ensure proper trajectory and screw length.

### Key Procedural Steps
As with cervical lateral mass screws, exposure of the posterior neck should allow for full definition of the lateral border of the lateral mass and the posterior aspect of the facet joint to be bridged. This joint capsule should be removed and the posterior facet decorticated, but the capsules of the joints above and below must be meticulously maintained if they are not to be fused.

The proper screw insertion point for a cervical transfacet screw is described as 1 mm medial and 1 to 2 mm caudal to the midportion of the lateral mass. The screw path is directed as perpendicular as possible to the facet joint, approximately 40 degrees caudally from the posterior lateral mass surface, and 20 degrees

PITFALLS

• The caudal trajectory of the subaxial facet screw may get in the way of surrounding lateral mass screws. The head of a cephalad lateral mass screw may interfere with transfacet screw preparation and insertion and may be so close together when inserted that rod insertion is problematic. The caudal transfacet screw may interfere with optimal trajectory of a suprajacent lateral mass screw. To prevent this, the most caudal transfacet screw should be placed first, as the caudal end of the fixation is most prone to failure.

laterally to avoid the exiting nerve root and transverse foramen; 3.5-mm-diameter cortical bone screws are utilized, which is a standard size in most manufacturers' cervical screw-rod and screw-plate sets. Screw length should allow for fixation across the anterior cortex of the caudal lateral mass.

### Bailout, Rescue, Salvage Procedures

This technique is most commonly used itself as a bailout for failed segmental lateral mass fixation. When it is used as such and fails, as by fracture of the inferior articular process, the only potential monosegmental bailout would be with the use of pedicle screw fixation. Connection of pedicle screws to lateral mass or transfacet screws requires the use of offset connectors and rod-based systems, and cannot be done as part of segmental plate fixation. Additional lateral mass fixation used above or below a transfacet screw often provides adequate additional fixation along with onlay bone grafting.

Failure of this technique when using a primary procedure for monosegmental fixation may be salvageable with the use of lateral mass fixation if adequate bone stock is available, or by pedicle screw fixation if the surgeon has adequate experience with this technique in the midcervical spine. Fixation and fusion of additional levels above or below is also a potential salvage technique. Fixation of the contralateral side, with or without midline (spinous process) fixation, may also be sufficient and obviate the need for inclusion of any additional levels.

# Cervical Pedicle Screw Placement

*Kuniyoshi Abumi*

### Description
To place a screw safely into the cervical pedicle with avoidance of injury to the surrounding neurovascular structures.

### Key Principles
Cervical pedicle screws have nearly twice the pullout strength of lateral mass screws. In addition, cervical pedicle screw instrumentation provides a greater stabilization effect than other cervical internal fixation procedures.

### Expectations
Cervical pedicle screws may be used in several settings in which the cervical lamina or lateral masses are inadequate because of fracture, tumor destruction, postsurgical disturbances, or marked osteoporosis. Cervical pedicle screw fixation, due to its rigid anchorage within the cervical pedicle, provides an opportunity for greater correctability of kyphotic deformity than lateral mass screw fixation.

### Indications
- Cervical or occipitocervical instability, and kyphosis

### Contraindications
- Absent, extremely small, or destroyed pedicle
- Aberrant vertebral artery anatomy

### Special Considerations
Preoperative imaging studies include computed tomography (CT) to help delineate bony anatomy. Reconstructive CT in the oblique plane provides useful information on the size of the neural foramen. Magnetic resonance imaging (MRI) and magnetic resonance angiography facilitate determining the precise location of the vertebral arteries. In about 5% of the population, the foramen transversarium of C7 contains the vertebral artery. This should be appreciated prior to pedicle screw insertion.

### Special Instructions, Position, and Anesthesia
The patient is placed in the prone position with a Mayfield headrest and shoulder taping to pull the shoulder girdles caudally for proper lateral fluoroscopy image.

### Tips, Pearls, and Lessons Learned
Intraoperative lateral fluoroscopy is helpful to determine the level of screw entry point in the sagittal plane, screw depth, and trajectory. Laminoforaminotomy of the subaxial vertebrae allows tactile identification of the cephalad, medial, and caudad pedicle borders, especially for the C7 pedicle when adequate lateral fluoroscopic image may not be available.

### Difficulties Encountered
An alternative fixation method or possibly unilateral pedicle screw fixation should be considered if a pedicle breach is encountered.

### Key Procedural Steps

#### Placement of C2
The starting point of C2 pedicle screw placement is the cranial medial portion of the C2 lateral mass (**Fig. 13.1**). A nerve retractor should be placed within the canal to confirm the medial border of the C2 isthmus and pedicle. A 2- to 3-mm high-speed diamond burr may be used to create an entrance hole on the lateral mass of C2. A pedicle probe insertion is recommended prior to tapping and screwing. The direction is approximately 15 to 20 degrees medially in the horizontal plane (**Fig. 13.2**) and perpendicular to the anterior surface of the axis (**Fig. 13.3**). The ventral cortex of C2 may be penetrated by the screw.

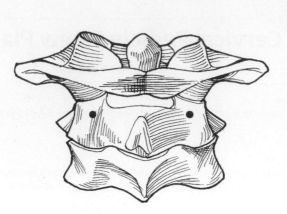

**Fig. 13.1** *Starting point of C2 pedicle screw.*

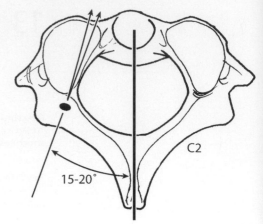

**Fig. 13.2** *C2 screw direction in the horizontal plane.*

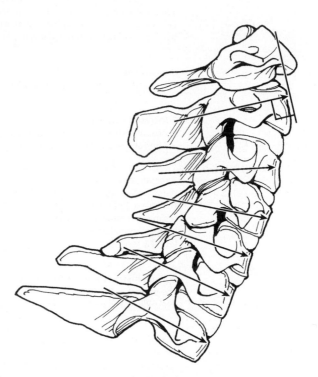

**Fig. 13.3** *Screw direction in the sagittal plane.*

### Placement of C3–C7

The lateral margin of the lateral mass has a notch approximately at the level of the pedicle. Entry points for C3–C7 pedicle screws are 3 to 4 mm medial to the notch and lateral to the center of the lateral mass and just below the inferior margin of the inferior articular process of the cephalad vertebra (**Fig. 13.4**). The anatomic direction of the pedicle from C3 to C6 in the horizontal plane is 40 to 50 degrees medially oriented in most patients and 30 to 40 degrees medially oriented at C7. However, screws may be inserted with less medial angulation than the anatomic angle (**Fig. 13.5**). The convergence of screw in the sagittal plane should be slightly cephalad for the C3 and C4 pedicle, and neutral for the C5, C6, and C7 pedicles (**Fig. 13.3**). The channel for screw placement can be checked with a ball-tipped pedicle sounder prior to screw insertion.

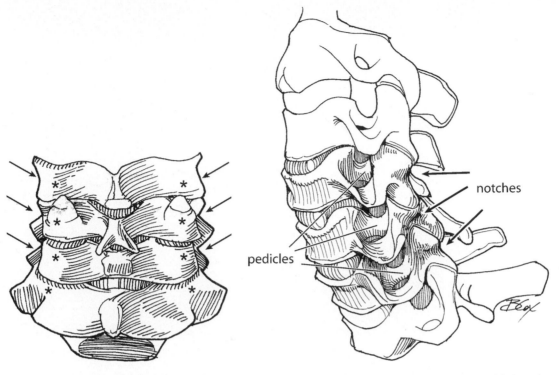

A                                                                                                                    B

**Fig. 13.4** *(A) Starting points of C3–C7 pedicle screw placement. Each arrow indicates a notch on the lateral margin of the lateral mass. Asterisks show the screw starting points. (B) Lateral view of notches and pedicles.*

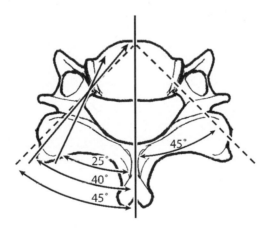

**Fig. 13.5** *C3–C7 screw direction in the horizontal plane.*

PITFALLS

• Inadequate pedicle size, intraoperative pedicle breach, vertebral artery violation, nerve injury, and root lesion by iatrogenic foraminal stenosis.

**Bailout, Rescue, Salvage Procedures**

If violation of the vertebral artery occurs, quickly place bone wax to stop bleeding. Instrumenting the other noninjured side must be aborted due to the potential for bilateral vertebral artery injury. Realizing the purchase within the lateral masses may be less than optimum, one may consider a lateral mass screw on the contralateral side followed by the application of a rigid orthosis. If significant instability is still a problem, the fusion may be extended either further cranially and caudally than the originally anticipated fusion levels. If a nerve root lesion occurs due to iatrogenic foraminal stenosis by reduction of anterior vertebral displacement or by correction of kyphosis, a foraminotomy without screw removal may be conducted.

# 14

# Anterior Cervical Diskectomy and Foraminotomy

*Kern Singh, Alexander R. Vaccaro, Todd J. Albert, and Peter M. Fleischut*

## Description

Pathologic processes, including trauma and age-related degeneration, may affect the cervical spine, resulting in the clinical presentation of radiculopathy or myelopathy. Anterior cervical diskectomy and foraminotomy is an effective technique for neural decompression secondary to herniated disks and spondylotic spurs.

## Key Principles

Adequate neural decompression via a diskectomy requires a precise annulotomy, thorough diskectomy, and meticulous foraminotomy.

## Expectations

A thorough diskectomy and meticulous end-plate preparation facilitate neural decompression, disk space distraction, and successful interbody graft incorporation.

## Indications

Failure of nonoperative treatment to relieve persistent or recurrent radicular arm pain, progressive neurologic deficit, and myelopathy.

## Contraindications

Bleeding disorders and posterior neural compression secondary to hyperlordosis, ligamentous infolding, and osteophytic formation.

## Special Considerations

Preoperative imaging is essential to determine the etiologic and anatomic sites of neural compression. Plain radiographs, in addition to magnetic resonance imaging (MRI), myelography, or postmyelogram computed tomography (CT) imaging, are essential for identifying sites of neural compression.

## Special Instructions, Positioning, and Anesthesia

The operating room table should be placed into a slightly reverse Trendelenburg position allowing for venous drainage. The patient's neck may be extended by placing a small roll vertically between the scapulae. Caudal traction to the shoulders is gently applied using adhesive tape. Good lighting and the use of loupes or a microscope facilitates the diskectomy and decompression. Total intravenous narcotic anesthesia is utilized, allowing for the measurement of somatosensory evoked potentials, motor evoked potentials, and dermatomal evoked potentials in a specific nerve root distribution.

## Tips, Pearls, and Lessons Learned

Anatomic landmarks may aid in the placement of the surgical incision. Typically, the hyoid bone overlies the C3 vertebral body, the thyroid cartilage overlies the C4–5 intervertebral disk space, and the cricoid ring overlies the C6 level. Disk space localization is performed with a radiopaque marker and a lateral radiograph (**Fig. 14.1**). An annulotomy is then made outlining the disk–end-plate junction using a sharp scalpel. Curettes must always stay in the disk space while "peeling" the disk and end-plate cartilage to avoid damaging the esophagus or other soft tissue structures (**Fig. 14.2**). Perforation of the end plate should be avoided to minimize bleeding. A 3-0 angled curette is helpful for getting behind the uncinate process and for creating a path for the 1- and 2-mm Kerrison punch to resect the uncinate process. Adequacy of the foraminotomy can be determined by passing a nerve hook anterior to the exiting nerve root without significant resistance. Routine removal of the posterior longitudinal ligament (PLL) is unnecessary, and there have been reports that postoperative epidural hematoma and other complications may occur with this technique.

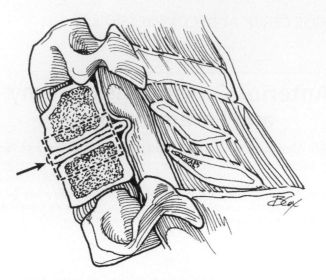

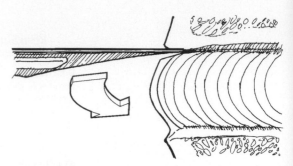

**Fig. 14.1** *Representation of a lateral radiograph of the cervical spine used for localization.*

**Fig. 14.2** *Sharp annulotomy and radical diskectomy with a scalpel.*

### Difficulties Encountered

In cases of severe spondylosis, disk space visualization may be difficult. Osteophytes and the anterior inferior corner of the superior vertebra can be removed using an osteotome or a high-speed burr (**Fig. 14.3**). This maneuver increases "the window" or space for adequate and safe removal of the disk. The use of sequentially larger curettes may help in disk extraction. A small Cobb may be twisted while positioned intradiskally, allowing for distraction of the disk space and cracking of the posterior anulus.

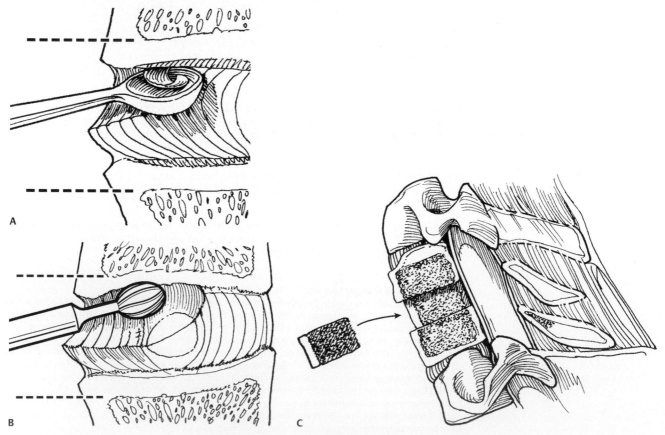

**Fig. 14.3** *(A,B) Decortication of the end plates and (C) contouring of the harvested bone graft.*

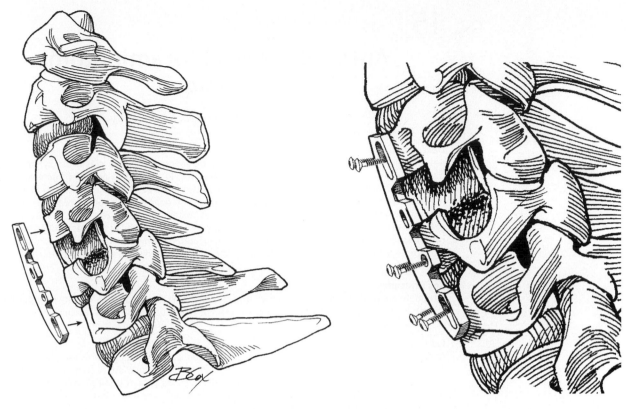

**Fig. 14.4** *(A,B) Placement of the plate across the prepared disk space that is to be fused.*

A

B

PITFALLS

- The incidence of vocal cord paralysis from recurrent laryngeal nerve injury ranges from 1 to 11%. Possible etiologies include traumatic division, neuropraxia, compression from postoperative edema, and injury from thermal necrosis. Midline soft tissue injury to the trachea, esophagus, and pharynx are uncommon. Dysphagia following anterior cervical surgery is common but temporary and is estimated to occur transiently in 8% of patients. Vascular injuries may be prevented by avoiding overzealous retraction and by using blunt-edged retractors. The likelihood of pseudarthrosis may be minimized by performing a meticulous diskectomy and thorough decortication of the end plates.

**Key Procedural Steps**

- Soft tissue dissection
- Localizing lateral radiograph (**Fig. 14.1**)
- Harvest bone graft (if allograft is not being used) while x-ray is taken (usually 7- to 9-mm tricortical graft)
- Sharp annulotomy and radical diskectomy with a scalpel and then an O-curette (**Fig. 14.2**)
- 3-0 angled curette to palpate behind the vertebral body
- 1-mm followed by a 2-mm Kerrison punch to perform the uncinate resection
- Decortication of the end plates and contouring of the harvested bone graft (or allograft) (**Fig. 14.3**)
- Repeat steps for any other disk space levels.
- Place the plate across the prepared disk space to be fused (**Fig. 14.4**).

**Bailout, Rescue, Salvage Procedures**

Treatment of an inadequate decompressive foraminotomy may be achieved via a posterior foraminotomy versus a revision anterior foraminotomy. Pseudarthrosis may be treated by either a repeat anterior diskectomy and interbody fusion or via a posterior arthrodesis.

# Anterior Cervical Foraminotomy Technique

*Neil R. Malhotra and M. Sean Grady*

### Description

Anterior cervical foraminotomy is performed when there are isolated one-level radicular symptoms without findings to support the need for complete diskectomy. In contrast to posterior foraminotomy, the anterior approach provides access to anterior osteophytes and free disk fragments with minimal nerve manipulation. Cervical foraminotomy performed from an anterior approach permits removal of offending spondylotic bone spur or compressive extranuclear disk material in combination with direct visualization of the nerve root. Cervical foraminotomy can significantly improve disability that has resulted from neural compression due to osteophyte formation and disk herniation. When radiculopathy is the primary presenting symptom, foraminotomy can result in significant reduction in radiculopathic symptoms.

### Key Principles

Although cervical diskectomy effectively addresses myelopathy, it is foraminotomy, with clear decompression of the nerve root, that most effectively addresses unilateral upper extremity radiculopathy.

### Expectations

Failure to address foraminal free disk fragments and osteophytes will plague the patient and surgeon alike. The key pathology can be accessed and removed via foraminal exploration. Decompression of the nerve root leads to excellent outcomes in the appropriately selected patient population. Always counsel the patient about the risk of postoperative sympathetic plexus injury and Horner-type syndrome, as well as hoarseness, cerebrospinal fluid leak, and swallowing difficulties.

### Indications

Isolated unilateral radiculopathy, in conjunction with imaging that supports the finding of a free disk fragment, indicates the need for, and potential benefit of, anterior cervical foraminotomy.

### Contraindications

Anterior cervical foraminotomy is contraindicated in patients with neck pain and myelopathy. In myelopathic patients anterior cervical diskectomy and fusion is appropriate with appropriate pathology. Additionally, in the setting of posterior compression, or significant spondylolisthesis at adjoining levels, anterior foraminotomy is contraindicated.

### Special Considerations

Preoperative imaging, including magnetic resonance imaging (MRI), and possibly plain x-ray, in conjunction with attention to the physical exam and a description of the location of pain permits tailoring of surgery to most benefit the patient. Perform flexion extension x-ray if a question of instability exists. Consider computed tomography (CT) scan through surgical levels if other imaging does not adequately resolve questions concerning bony pathology.

### Special Instructions, Position, and Anesthesia

The patient is placed supine on the operative table with a gel roll under the scapulae to aid extension and exposure of the operative field. A foam doughnut or horseshoe headrest placed under the head enables maximal safe extension and minimizes jaw intrusion into the operative field. Perioperative antibiotics should be administered 30 minutes prior to the skin incision. Fiberoptic intubation is generally not needed. Anesthesia colleagues should minimize the use of airway monitors such as temperature probe when alternative options exist. Shoulders should be taped down to maximize cervical exposure and permit adequate cross-table lateral x-ray to be taken for localization. Arms should be tucked at the patient's side. Intraoperative physiologic monitoring is not needed.

### Tips, Pearls, and Lessons Learned Dealing with Difficulties Encountered

- The skin incision should be on the side of the radiculopathy to permit greatest exposure of the pathologic foramen.
- Horizontal skin incisions, incorporating an existing skin wrinkle, result in the most aesthetically pleasing scar for the patient.

- A vertical incision through the platysma allows the greatest freedom in the surgical approach to multiple levels and minimizes stress on the healing wound.
- Lateral retraction of the longus colli permits excellent exposure.
- Upturned curette or Penfield No. 4 elevator (Miltex, Tuttlingen, Germany) permits palpation of the transverse process (TP). It is the TP that will act as a crucial outer landmark for the approach.
- The imaginary line formed by connecting the medial aspect of the transverse process above and below the disk level of the operation acts as an excellent lateral border of the exposure and minimizes risk of injury to the vertebral artery (**Fig. 15.1**). It is imperative to determine the location of the vertebral artery based on the preoperative imaging (**Fig. 15.2**).
- Do not remove the longus colli lateral to the vertebral body as risk to the overlying sympathetic trunk is increased (**Fig. 15.3**).
- A bent spinal needle, with stylet, can be used to localize the disk level on fluoroscopy or cross-table x-ray prior to annulotomy.
- A Kerrison punch is excellent for removing the longus colli from the medial aspect of the operative field.

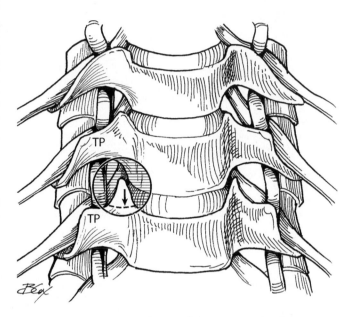

**Fig. 15.1** *Anterior exposure and approach for a patient with right C4-C5 foraminal stenosis. Arrow indicates the site of uncinate process takedown with 2-mm cutting burr. TP, transverse process.*

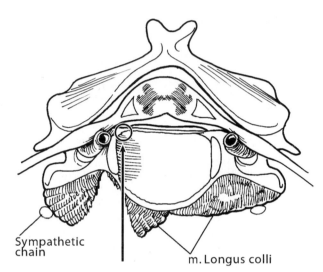

**Fig. 15.2** *Axial view of a vertebral body demonstrating the approach for an anterior foraminotomy. Operative approach includes drilling down through the uncinate process to the starting point of the foraminotomy. Special attention must always be paid to the nearby vertebral artery.*

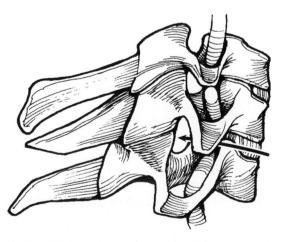

**Fig. 15.3** *This lateral view demonstrates the slight angle (arrow) one should take when drilling down the uncinate process.*

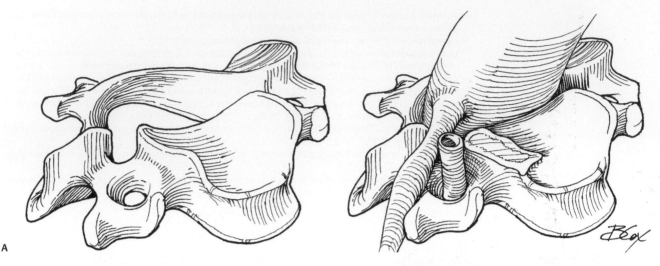

**Fig. 15.4** *(A) Oblique view of motion segment demonstrating bony anatomy. (B) Superimposed vertebral artery and nerve root.*

PITFALLS

- One must understand the trajectory of the nerve root and the location of surrounding structures (e.g., pedicle, vertebral artery) to provide adequate but safe decompression of the exiting nerve root (**Figs. 15.3 and 15.4B**). Focal decompression of the nerve root leads to a significant reduction of symptoms. Wide decompression is both unnecessary and risks injury to the surrounding structures.

- In the cervical spine, the nerve root exits above the pedicle of its like-numbered vertebra and closely hugs the inferior portion of the above pedicle (**Fig. 15.4**).
- The microscope should be employed from this point forward.
- A 2-mm cutting burr is excellent for creating a cylinder down to the posterior longitudinal ligament (PLL). The PLL can be pierced with an upturned curette and then resected with a 1-0 or 2-0 Kerrison rongeur.
- The 2-mm cutting burr can be used to drill off the uncinate process.
- The right-angled blunt nerve probe is excellent for exploration of the foramen.
- If a path into the foramen cannot be safely created, a temporary increase in Caspar retraction can be employed to further open the space.
- The footplate of the 2-mm Kerrison punch can be placed into the foramen for completion of the decompression.
- Always reexplore the foraminotomy cavity with the nerve hook to confirm adequate decompression.

### Key Procedural Steps

Always check and double check to confirm that you are decompressing the most symptomatic nerve root. Placement of the Caspar pins in the body above and below the foramen to be decompressed aids retraction and permits an ideal view of the nerve root being explored. An operative microscope, if not in the field already, should be brought in to aid in the evaluation of the nerve root and foramen. Start the foraminotomy by first exploring the space with the upturned curette. Placing the footplate of the Kerrison along the nerve root allows decompression to be performed. Frequently assess the degree of decompression with a blunt nerve hook to ensure that you resect only compressive bone.

### Bailout, Rescue, Salvage Procedures

Should the patient remain symptomatic, and imaging supports further exploration, one should consider a posterior keyhole foraminotomy or a complete anterior cervical diskectomy. Performing posterior foraminotomy ensures that the nerve is essentially circumferentially decompressed. With adequate anterior decompression the posterior approach should only very rarely need to be employed.

# 16

## Posterior Longitudinal Ligament Takedown

*Iain H. Kalfas*

### Description
Resection of the posterior longitudinal ligament (PLL) following anterior cervical discectomy or corpectomy.

### Key Principles
Resection of the PLL provides optimal access to the epidural space.

### Expectations
Following anterior cervical diskectomy or corpectomy, resection of the PLL allows for the removal of subligamentous or free disk fragments as well as providing for a more optimal removal of ventral epidural osteophytes. Access to the lateral neural foramina is also improved. Failure to remove the PLL may result in an incomplete decompression of the epidural space.

### Indications
Anterior cervical surgery for significant epidural compression (**Fig. 16.1**).

### Contraindications
Anterior cervical surgery without significant epidural compression. Ossification of the PLL may be a relative contraindication to removal of the PLL depending on its severity.

### Special Considerations
Magnetic resonance imaging (MRI) or computed tomography (CT)/myelography is required preoperatively to demonstrate the spatial relationship of the disk herniation or osteophyte(s) to the epidural space as well as the degree of epidural compression.

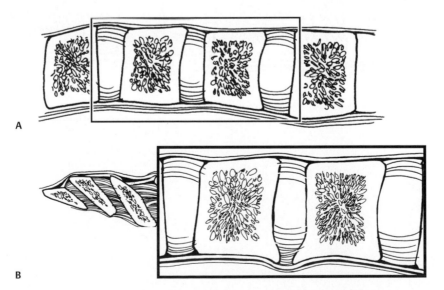

**A**

**B**

**Fig. 16.1** *(A) Lateral view demonstrating the relationship of the PLL to the vertebrae and the underlying dura. (B) Lateral view demonstrating a ventral epidural osteophyte. The PLL is projected into the dura.*

### Special Instructions, Position, and Anesthesia

The patient is positioned supine with only a mild degree of cervical extension. Fiberoptic intubation is used if the patient's symptoms are worsened during preoperative cervical extension. Intravenous steroids may be administered preoperatively for prophylaxis. Electrophysiologic monitoring is a consideration in procedures requiring removal of the PLL.

### Tips, Pearls, and Lessons Learned

The technique is more easily performed using the optimal illumination and visualization provided by a head light or a surgical microscope. The initial opening of the PLL can be made with a nerve hook inserted between the fibers of the PLL. The hook is then pulled upward, producing a small opening in the PLL. The opening can then be enlarged with a 1-mm Kerrison rongeur.

### Difficulties Encountered

Removal of the PLL rarely results in a durotomy. If this occurs, it is managed by placing a layer of Gelfoam over the defect. If the durotomy is large, a short period of lumbar subarachnoid drainage may be required.

Removal of the PLL can also result in epidural bleeding. Except in the isolated cases of ossification of the posterior longitudinal ligament (OPLL), it is rarely significant. Epidural bleeding can usually be controlled with bipolar electrocautery and gentle epidural pressure with Gelfoam and cottonoid pledgets.

### Key Procedural Steps

Following the diskectomy or corpectomy, the PLL is opened with a nerve hook or No. 11 blade. The PLL is pulled upward to produce a small tear that will allow for insertion of a 1-mm Kerrison rongeur. As the opening is enlarged, the dura is visualized. It is differentiated from remaining thin leaflets of PLL by a glistening appearance and the lack of any longitudinal striations. Failure to easily pass the rongeur under the adjacent vertebrae is also an indication that the PLL has not been incised completely.

As the decompression progresses, a 2- or 3-mm Kerrison rongeur can be used to undercut the adjacent vertebral end plates (**Fig. 16.2**). This allows for a more complete removal of intervertebral osteophytes as well as access to free disk material (**Fig. 16.3**). Removal of the PLL also provides access to the neural foramina. The proximal 2 to 3 mm of the root can be directly decompressed following PLL resection.

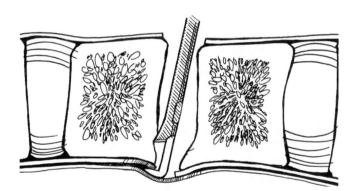

**Fig. 16.2** *Removal of the PLL allows for insertion of a Kerrison rongeur into the epidural space for a more optimal removal of the osteophyte.*

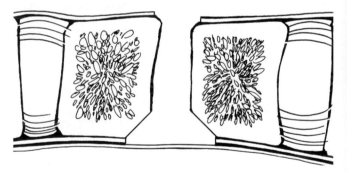

**Fig. 16.3** *Lateral view demonstrating the extent of decompression following removal of the PLL. (Courtesy of J. Kanasz.)*

# 17

# Exposure of the Vertebral Artery

*Daniel K. Resnick*

### Description
The vertebral artery runs through the foramen transversarium of the first six vertebral bodies, loops around the superolateral margin of the lamina of C1, and then enters the skull through the foramen magnum. The vertebral artery is vulnerable to injury following facet subluxation injuries, as well as during anterior cervical diskectomy (and anterior microforaminotomy), lateral mass and C3–C6 pedicle screw placement, and exposure and fixation of the craniocervical junction. Occasionally, exposure of the vertebral artery may be required for direct repair or occlusion following iatrogenic injury.

### Key Principles
Appreciation of the anatomy of the vertebral artery and the surrounding bony structures is essential for complication avoidance. Anatomic variation is most commonly seen at the level of C2, where 15 to 20% of patients may have aberrant vessels that preclude pars interarticularis or pedicle screw placement. Preoperative study and knowledge of alternative fixation techniques decrease the incidence of vertebral artery injury. The most important principle in managing a vertebral artery injury is to avoid a bilateral injury at all costs.

### Expectations
Management of vertebral artery injuries requires immediate control of hemorrhage, the use of alternative fixation techniques, prompt assessment of cerebrovascular competence, and if necessary repair or occlusion of the vertebral artery.

### Indications
Iatrogenic injury of the vertebral artery.

### Contraindications
Once hemostasis is ensured, further efforts to explore the vertebral artery are reserved for cases with demonstrated or suspected neurologic compromise.

### Special Considerations
The loss of a single vertebral artery is usually well tolerated. The loss of both vertebral arteries is usually fatal. Embolism and pseudoaneurysm formation are late complications of injury that may require arterial reconstruction, bypass, or occlusion.

### Special Instructions, Positioning, and Anesthesia
In the case of iatrogenic injury, the patient is positioned for the index procedure. If elective exploration is performed, the patient may be positioned supine with the head turned away from the operative site. Close monitoring of blood pressure to preserve cerebral perfusion pressure is mandatory.

### Tips, Pearls, and Lessons Learned
Complication avoidance is much preferred to complication management. Careful preoperative assessment of the location of the vertebral artery in relationship to anticipated sites of operative manipulation is essential. If a vertebral artery injury is identified or suspected, the contralateral vertebral artery must be preserved. This may result in unilateral fixation (side of the injury) or the need for external immobilization.

Immediate postoperative assessment of cerebrovascular anatomy and reserve should be coordinated with an experienced cerebrovascular neurosurgeon.

### Difficulties Encountered
Blood loss may be rapid and significant. Depending on the site of injury, bleeding may be controlled with tamponade, packing with hemostatic agents, or simply by screw placement. Local exploration and attempts at repair may be possible in rare instances. Such attempts should not be undertaken without prior cerebrovascular experience and an adequately prepared operating room staff. Endovascular techniques for occlusion or stenting of the artery should be considered as valuable treatment options.

### Key Procedural Steps
If exploration of the artery is undertaken, the surgeon must be prepared to deal with the risk of significant bleeding, hemodynamic lability, and the risk of embolization.

### Bailout, Rescue, Salvage Procedures

Injuries to the vertebral artery at or above C2 usually are encountered during the initial exposure (injuring the vessel along the rostral border of the C1 lamina) or by inadvertent laceration of the artery by a drill, tap, or screw. If the vessel is injured during the initial exposure, the site of injury is obvious and direct tamponade followed by local dissection will expose the area of injury. If the bleeding is through a hole in the bone, screw placement will generally achieve hemostasis. If the injury occurs during a posterior fixation procedure below C2, injury is likely related to screw placement. Hemostasis should be obtained with screw placement; the ipsilateral construct is rapidly completed, and the contralateral vertebral artery is preserved. Postoperative imaging is obtained. Conventional angiographic study is preferred, as the visualization of the artery is unaffected by metallic artifact, and therapeutic maneuvers such as stenting or occlusion may be performed contemporaneously. If the artery is occluded, anticoagulation or bypass should be considered in cooperation with a cerebrovascular specialist. In the asymptomatic patient, no therapy may be required. Revascularization options may also include endovascular techniques and bypass procedures such as the occipital artery–posterior inferior cerebellar artery bypass.

If an injury occurs during an anterior procedure, such as during an anterior cervical diskectomy or an anterior microforaminotomy, then exploration may be feasible. Exploration may be considered when hemostasis cannot be adequately obtained locally, or when immediate preservation of the artery is deemed to be essential (dominant vertebral artery, known contralateral occlusion) and the surgeon has some experience with vascular repair.

The vertebral artery may be exposed over several segments from an anterolateral approach. It may be accomplished through an extension of the standard anterior cervical approach. The incision is made along the border of the sternocleidomastoid, and may be extended to just posterior to the mastoid process. The precervical fascia is divided and the plane medial to the sternocleidomastoid is exploited to expose the prevertebral fascia overlying the spine. The longus colli is mobilized to expose the transverse processes (**Fig. 17.1**) and the transverse foramina are opened using a drill or Kerrison rongeurs. For more rostral exposure of the vertebral artery, a more lateral approach is preferred (**Fig. 17.2**). The sternocleidomastoid muscle is detached from the mastoid process and reflected caudally (leave a cuff of muscle attached

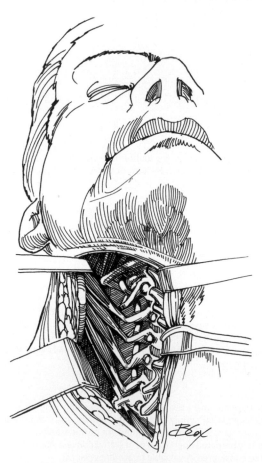

**Fig. 17.1** *Anterior approach to the vertebral artery through an extended anterior cervical exposure and elevation of the longus colli.*

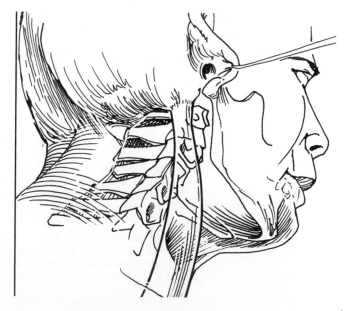

**Fig. 17.2** *Orientation for the lateral approach to the vertebral artery.*

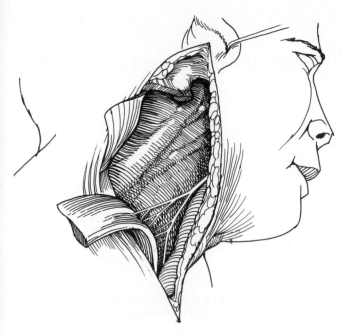

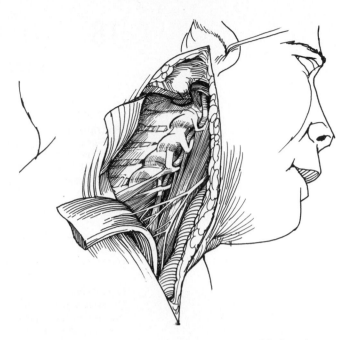

**Fig. 17.3** *Reflection of the sternocleidomastoid muscle with preservation of the spinal accessory nerve.*

**Fig. 17.4** *The vertebral artery is exposed as it runs around the lateral mass of C1 and may be exposed further caudally by opening the foramen transversarium of the caudal vertebral bodies.*

to the mastoid for later closure). Identification and preservation of the spinal accessory nerve will avoid a postoperative shoulder drop (**Fig. 17.3**). As the sternocleidomastoid muscle is retracted, the transverse processes of the upper three or four vertebral bodies will be palpable, as will the pulsatile vertebral artery. Serial section of the splenius capitis and levator scapula muscles will expose the lateral aspect of the vertebral artery as it runs in the transverse foramen and then loops across C1 (**Fig. 17.4**).

# 18

# Anterior Cervical Corpectomy

*James C. Farmer*

## Description

Anterior cervical corpectomy is a method of decompressing the cervical spinal cord and nerve roots. It is performed by removing the disk above and below the vertebral body that is to be resected, followed by the vertebral body itself (complete corpectomy) (**Fig. 18.1**). Under some circumstances only one disk is removed along with a portion of the adjacent vertebral body/bodies (partial corpectomy).

## Key Principles

Anterior osteophytes, ossification of the posterior longitudinal ligament, as well as disk herniations positioned behind the vertebral body can be resected utilizing careful surgical technique. Excellent decompression of the spinal cord and nerve roots can be achieved. Sagittal deformities such as kyphosis can be corrected through this technique.

## Expectations

Following a corpectomy, all anterior compression of the spinal cord and nerve roots should be relieved. If kyphosis exists preoperatively, it can be corrected allowing restoration of normal cervical lordosis. On occasion, supplemental posterior stabilization may be required.

## Indications

- Cervical spondylotic myelopathy
- Preexisting cervical kyphosis with spinal cord or nerve root compression
- Vertebral burst or compression fractures
- Vertebral body neoplasms
- Cervical diskitis or osteomyelitis
- Cervical disk herniations with fragments migrated behind the vertebral body

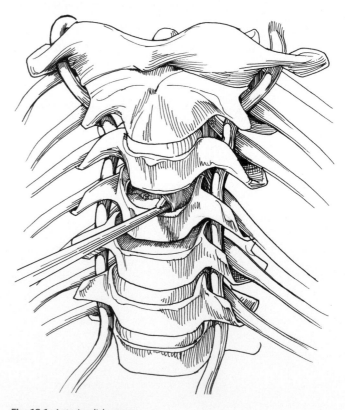

**Fig. 18.1** *Anterior diskectomy.*

## Contraindications
- Previous radiation to the anterior neck
- Aberrant vertebral artery anatomy
- Severe chin on chest deformity making the anterior approach impossible
- Medical contraindications to a general anesthetic

## Special Considerations
Magnetic resonance imaging (MRI) remains the modality of choice when treating patients with cervical disorders. MRI with flexion and extension sagittal images can be helpful in evaluating positional effects on cervical stenosis as well as evaluating the reduction of instability. Computed tomography (CT), which can be combined with myelography, provides the best imaging of bony structures. A CT scan is paramount when evaluating ossification of the posterior longitudinal ligament (OPLL) to adequately assess the degree of ossification as well as the number of levels involved.

Myelography can evaluate the effects of flexion and extension dynamically on spinal cord and nerve root compression.

## Special Instructions, Position, and Anesthesia
The patient is positioned supine with the arms at the side and carefully padded and protected. A roll is placed between the shoulders to allow the head to be positioned in a neutral to a slightly extended position. It is important to avoid overextension of the neck as this can cause spinal cord impingement and possible injury. Gardner-Wells tong traction can be used. Spinal cord monitoring is recommended. In patients with significant spinal cord compression or instability, fiberoptic intubation may be necessary.

## Tips, Pearls, and Lessons Learned
Obtaining proper imaging studies as well as a careful preoperative evaluation of these studies is paramount for optimal surgical treatment. Determination of the number of levels involved as well as the extent of compression at each individual level is essential. Additionally, careful evaluation of the location and course of the vertebral artery is necessary to avoid iatrogenic injury. At the time of surgery, complete diskectomies prior to resection of the vertebral bodies facilitate assessment of the depth of the vertebral body as well as the location of the spinal canal. In cases of ossification of the posterior longitudinal ligament where the ossification is extremely adherent to the dura, direct resection can be dangerous. Successful decompression can be performed by removing the posterior longitudinal ligament on either side of the ossified area, and allowing it to float away anteriorly from the cord (anterior floating technique) without necessitating direct resection, and high risk of dural tear and subsequent spinal fluid leak. When performing the corpectomy, a high-speed burr can be used to resect most of the vertebral body, leaving only a thin rim of posterior cortical bone. The posterior cortical bone can be removed using either a small curette or a Kerrison rongeur.

## Difficulties Encountered
It is imperative to identify the uncovertebral joints bilaterally when performing the decompression. This enables the surgeon to maintain orientation to the midline, facilitating an adequate decompression of the spinal canal, and avoiding dissecting too laterally with the risk of injury to the vertebral artery. Careful resection of the posterior cortex and posterior longitudinal ligament is necessary to avoid injury to the dural sac and spinal cord. Significant bleeding can occur during resection of the vertebral body and can make visualization difficult at times. This can be controlled with the judicious use of bone wax and hemostatic agents such as Gelfoam, Surgicel, and Avitene.

## Key Procedural Steps
During the performance of multilevel corpectomies, adequate surgical exposure is paramount. During surgical exposure, the raising of subplatysmal flaps as well as the takedown of fascial structures along the surgical interval provide optimal exposure and enable mobilization of the soft tissue structures along the anterior spine. The operating room microscope provides optimal illumination and excellent visualization of the surgical field for both the surgeon and the assistant. Loupe magnification and a headlight also enable safe neural decompression. Standard diskectomies should be performed above and below the vertebral body to be resected. Visualization of the posterior longitudinal ligament and uncovertebral joints on each side is necessary for an adequate decompression. The initial portions of the corpectomy can then be performed either with a rongeur or with various high-speed burrs (**Fig. 18.2**). The width of the decompression should be on average 15 to 16 mm. Again, identification of the uncovertebral joints during the decompression facilitates assessment of the widest extent of decompression that can be performed should it be needed. The posterior longitudinal ligament does not routinely need to be excised unless it is felt that a compressive lesion posterior to the posterior longitudinal ligament exists or in the case of an OPLL. With OPLL the surgeon may elect to remove the entire ossified ligament, or in cases where it is felt to be exceedingly adherent to the dura, the anterior floating method can be utilized (**Fig. 18.3**).

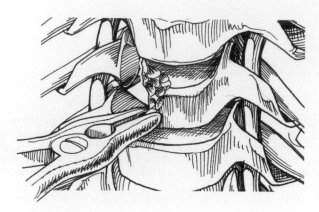

**Fig. 18.2** *The corpectomy can be initiated with 3-mm Leksell rongeurs to two-thirds depth of the vertebral body.*

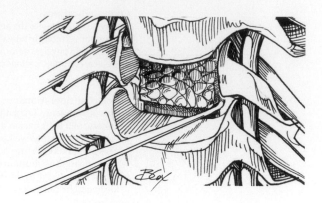

**Fig. 18.3** *Thinned posterior cortex can be removed with a forward-angled curette.*

PITFALLS

- Iatrogenic injury to the vertebral artery can occur due to either an aberrant vertebral artery or to excessive lateral decompression.
- Dural tear, spinal fluid leak, or neurologic injury can occur during resection of the posterior vertebral body and posterior longitudinal ligament.
- Graft extrusion and hardware failure can occur in cases of prior posterior decompressive procedures or multilevel corpectomy; a posterior stabilizing procedure with instrumentation may be necessary to adequately protect the anterior construct.

Once the decompression is completed, the end plate should be prepared and burred down to some underlying bleeding cancellous bone. Maintaining a small posterior lip along vertebral bodies helps prevent graft extrusion in the canal. The graft should be carefully placed and then traction removed to assess the fit and stability of the graft. Grafting options include a tricortical iliac crest bone graft, autograft fibula, allograft fibula, and interbody cages with cancellous bone graft. If an anterior plate is to be used, it is important to remove the distractive forces across the head and neck prior to placement of the plate. Screws should not be placed into the graft, as this may cause the graft to break. Prior to placement of the graft, the neural foramina should be assessed, and, should it be necessary, foraminotomies performed with a Kerrison.

**Bailout, Rescue, Salvage Procedures**

In the case of graft extrusion or hardware failure, an urgent revision anterior procedure should be performed with revision of the plate or graft, and likely a subsequent posterior stabilization procedure. In the case of a dural tear with spinal fluid leak, options include a primary repair versus use of fibrin glue. Primary repair can be difficult due to the small size of the working space. In cases where it is felt that there will be a high likelihood of a persistent spinal fluid leak, a lumbar drain may be necessary. In the case of a vertebral artery injury, options include local control with the use of hemostatic agents versus a direct repair or ligation of the injured vessel.

# 19

# Transoral Odontoid Resection and Anterior Odontoid Osteotomy

*Amgad Hanna, Eli M. Baron, and James S. Harrop*

### Description

The transoral procedure uses an anterior midline approach, through the oropharynx, to gain access to the osseous anterior craniocervical junction.

### Expectations

This procedure, combined with posterior stabilization, provides decompression and stabilization of craniocervical pathology and affords immediate mobilization in a cervical collar with a low surgical morbidity. Careful selection of candidates is important. As with all surgical patients, for those with poor health, optimization of preoperative nutritional status is essential. Nasopharyngeal incompetence is a frequent postoperative finding, but typically recovers in a delayed manner.

### Indications

- Rheumatoid patients with spinal compression symptoms and irreducible anterior neuraxial compression at the craniocervical junction (**Fig. 19.1**). The compression could be due to a soft tissue mass (pannus) or vertical migration of the dens (**Fig. 19.2**).
- Irreducible chronic nonunion of a fractured odontoid process
- Extradural tumors, e.g., chordoma
- Intradural lesions: meningiomas, schwannomas, neurenteric cysts when a far lateral approach is not accessible
- Rarely for vascular pathology, aneurysm clipping (anterior-inferior cerebellar artery [AICA]), when these lesions cannot be approached endovascularly or posterolaterally

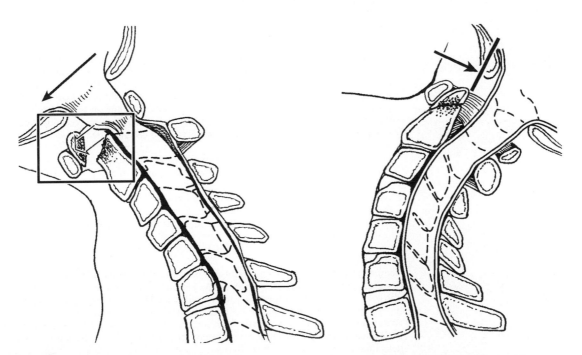

A

B

**Fig. 19.1** *Representations of preoperative plain radiographs in flexion* **(A)** *and extension* **(B)** *in a patient with rheumatoid arthritis, revealing C1–C2 instability, which reduces in extension.*

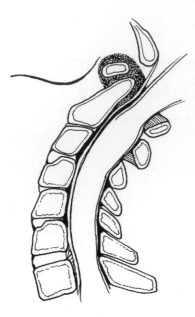

**Fig. 19.2** *Representation of a preoperative sagittal T2-weighted MRI showing compression of the cervicomedullary junction by the rheumatoid pannus.*

## Contraindications
- Dental or periodontal abscess
- Reducible lesions; need only posterior stabilization, without decompression
- Inability to open the mouth >25 mm, which could be due to associated temporomandibular joint disease. This is a relative contraindication; these lesions can be approached through a transmandibular approach.

## Special Considerations
- There is a potential for instability after this procedure due to resection of the anterior osseous and ligamentous structures. Although some people do not routinely perform a posterior internal fixation, we recommend posterior arthrodesis as an adjunct to this procedure.
- The vertebral arteries are 24 mm from the midline at the arch of C1, 11 mm from the midline at the foramen magnum and at the C2-C3 junction. However, this anatomy could be distorted by pathology or congenital abnormalities.
- Patients with irregular dentition may require a gum guard to be fashioned prior to surgery to fit the retractor and the dentition. Edentulous patients may require special adjustments in the retractor to avoid slippage during the procedure.

## Special Instructions, Position, and Anesthesia
- Preoperative magnetic resonance imaging (MRI)/magnetic resonance angiography helps plan the procedure by identifying the degree of compression, the anatomy and dominance of the vertebral arteries, and the relationship of the internal carotid arteries to the anterior arch of C1.
- Topical hydrocortisone ointment (1%) to the oral cavity before and after surgery reduces significantly the amount of perioral swelling.
- Somatosensory and motor evoked potentials should be considered to monitor neural function.
- Intraoperative guidance could be achieved by fluoroscopy, intermittent intraoperative x-ray imaging, or image-guidance by intraoperative navigation.
- A nasogastric tube helps to prevent postoperative wound contamination.
- The endotracheal tube should be left in place for 24 to 48 hours after surgery, or until the surgeon is sure that the airway is not compromised.
- Postoperative palatal dehiscence should be immediately closed, whereas late (>1 week) postoperative pharyngeal dehiscence is better left to granulate because of friable edges with diversion of particulate food via the nasogastric tube or gastrostomy. However, direct repair may be attempted in early postoperative pharyngeal dehiscence.

## Tips, Pearls, and Lessons Learned
- If the interdental distance is ≥25 mm with mouth opening, the transoral approach is feasible.
- Perioperative antibiotics, usually cephalosporins, are used to decrease the rate of infection. Infection rate is also diminished by protecting the mucosal edges during the surgery to allow the apposition of cleanly incised healthy edges at the end of the procedure, obliterating the dead space by two-layer closure of the posterior pharyngeal wall, and avoidance of particulate food until the wound has healed.
- Release of the tongue retractor blade from time to time during the procedure helps to prevent postoperative swelling. The surgeon always needs to avoid catching the tongue between the teeth and the retractor.
- Magnification is achieved by surgical loupes, operative microscope, or endoscopy.
- The anterior tubercle of atlas with the attached longus colli and anterior longitudinal ligament is an important landmark to the midline.
- The lateral exposure should not exceed 2 cm from the midline to avoid injury to the vertebral arteries, hypoglossal nerves, or eustachian tubes.
- A freely pulsating dura or soft tissue is a good sign of adequate decompression.

## Key Procedural Steps
Fiberoptic laryngoscopy with nasotracheal or orotracheal intubation is less hazardous than tracheostomy. However, elective tracheostomy is sometimes indicated, especially with preoperative brainstem dysfunction or persistent postoperative swelling. Lateral position has been used by some surgeons to access both the mouth for decompression and the back for fusion. However, it presents the surgeon with unfamiliar anatomic relationships, both from the front and from the back. The transoral approach is therefore typically performed with the patient in a supine position with the head slightly extended. Head extension moves the dens caudally in the operative field. The head is held either fixed in a Mayfield headrest or without fixation. The mouth and oropharynx are prepared with 1% Betadine or cetrimide. The upper esophagus is packed with a collagen sponge or gauze to minimize the ingestion of blood.

A right-handed surgeon stands at the patient's left side of the head, and anesthesia is placed at the foot of the table. The nurse stands in front of the surgeon to the left of the patient, and the assistant on the right side of the patient (**Fig. 19.3**). An image intensifier can be brought in and positioned for a lateral view. The operating microscope is placed at the head of the patient. Special retractors are used for better

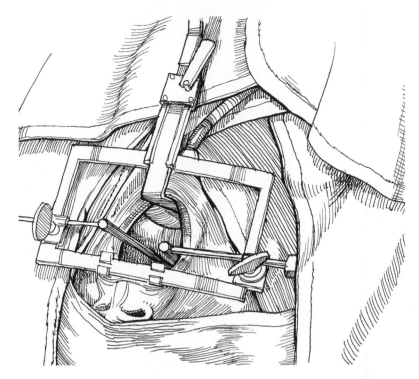

**Fig. 19.3** *Operative setup, showing the positions of different members of the operative team. The operative microscope is brought in from behind the surgeon (at the head of the patient).*

visualization: Dingman, McIvor, Spetzler-Sonntag, or Crockard self-retaining retractor. The soft palate is retracted and sometimes needs to be divided for better exposure (**Fig. 19.4A**). If visualization below C2 is necessary, it may be necessary to split the mandible.

The posterior pharyngeal wall is infiltrated with 1% lidocaine with epinephrine. The posterior pharyngeal mucosa is incised in the midline using the anterior tubercle of atlas as a landmark. The muscles are then elevated from the anterior surface of the clivus, the anterior arch of C1, and the anterior surface of C2. Some surgeons recommend exposing laterally until the medial aspect of the C1-C2 joint is seen. About 14 mm of the anterior arch is removed to expose the dens and pannus (**Fig. 19.4B**). This is achieved by a high-speed drill

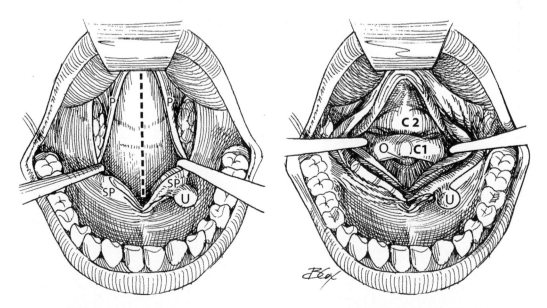

A                                                                                              B

**Fig. 19.4** *(A,B) Intraoperative views after splitting the uvula (U) and soft palate (SP), and after incision of the posterior pharyngeal wall (P), and resection of the anterior arch of C1, revealing the odontoid process (O) of C2.*

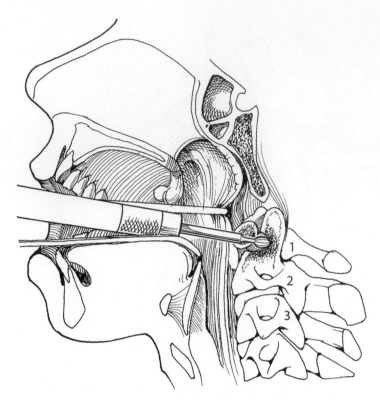

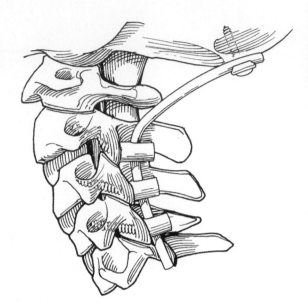

**Fig. 19.5** *Representation of an intraoperative fluoroscopic view of the final part of drilling of the dens. 1 = C1; 2 = C2; 3 = C3.*

**Fig. 19.6** *Postoperative lateral view after anterior decompression and posterior craniocervical instrumentation.*

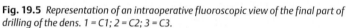

PITFALLS
• Failure to recognize or treat cerebrospinal fluid (CSF) leak could be complicated by meningitis.
• The internal carotid artery may have a variable relationship with the anterior arch of C1.

or Kerrison rongeurs. The odontoid is then resected craniocaudally to avoid spinal cord compression during resection of an amputated odontoid. The major part of the dens is removed using a 3-mm cutting burr, and then the posterior cortical bone is removed using a diamond drill **(Fig. 19.5)**. It is usually hard to differentiate the ligaments from the inflammatory pannus. The osseous pannus and ligaments are dissected from the dural surface to achieve decompression. Bipolar coagulation, nerve hook, 2-mm angled curettes, 1- or 2-mm Kerrison rongeurs, and dissectors are used to aid in the decompression. Resection is continued laterally until the lateral curvature of the dural sac is identified, or the dura is pulsating without osseous compression. Posterior stabilization should then be performed **(Fig. 19.6)** or the patient is kept in a halo-vest.

**Bailout, Rescue, Salvage Procedures**
• Inadequate exposure cranially: split the soft palate
• Inadequate exposure caudally: split the mandible
• Vertebral artery bleeding can be controlled by packing. Bone wax can be used. Venous bleeding can be controlled by Gelfoam, Surgicel, Avitene, or fibrin glue.
• Dural tears: we recommend using both fascial autograft (fascia lata), and artificial dural substitutes, with fibrin glue. The dural grafts tend to slide caudally, and they should be stabilized with small clips in the corners. Postoperatively, the patient should be sitting in bed. Lumbar drainage may not be necessary unless postoperative CSF leak is noted.

# 20

# Anterior Open Reduction Technique for Unilateral and Bilateral Facet Dislocations

*G. Alexander Jones and Edward C. Benzel*

### Description
Unilateral or bilateral cervical facet dislocations may be reduced during a ventral fusion and fixation procedure. This technique is arguably safer than closed reduction with traction or manipulation under anesthesia, and, if successful, may eliminate the need for a staged ventral and dorsal procedure.

### Expectations
Several techniques are described here. They may be safely used to restore anatomic alignment prior to fixation and fusion.

### Indications
Open reduction is an option as a primary means of reducing cervical facet dislocations. It may also be used in the event that cervical traction is unsuccessful in restoring alignment.

### Contraindications
Care should be taken to perform a complete diskectomy and to take down the posterior longitudinal ligament prior to reduction. If this is not done, the reduction maneuver could cause a fragment of disk or bone to impact the spinal cord during the reduction process, with potentially devastating consequences.

It is emphasized that in the case of a severely comminuted facet fracture, an open ventral reduction is less likely to be successful.

### Special Instructions, Position, and Anesthesia
Uncommonly, the dislocation may prove difficult, if not impossible, to reduce, thus requiring an additional dorsal approach. Radiographic confirmation of the reduction should be obtained prior to placement of a bone graft and plate. This may be accomplished with intraoperative plain radiographs or fluoroscopy.

Patients who are not already intubated upon arrival in the operating room should be submitted to an awake fiberoptic intubation to minimize the risk of further neurologic injury. Distraction of the interspace can be accomplished in a controlled manner during the operative procedure. This obviates the need for traction.

### Tips, Pearls, and Lessons Learned
Several techniques may be used for reduction. Caspar distraction pins may be inserted into the vertebral bodies, with the shafts positioned at a divergent angle of 10 to 20 degrees (**Fig. 20.1**). Bringing the pins into a parallel orientation and placing them in the distracter, followed by controlled distraction, often results in disengagement of the facets (**Fig. 20.2**). The rostral level is then translated dorsally, occasionally with the application of moderate pressure, to restore alignment.

In place of the distracter, the wrenches/pin drivers used for pin application may be left on the pins. This facilitates additional freedom of movement in the coronal plane. Placing a solid object, such as a small bone

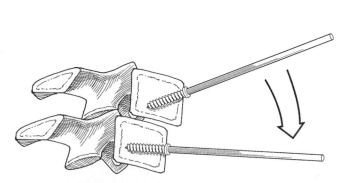

**Fig. 20.1** *Placing distraction pins at a 10- to 20-degree angle with respect to each other in the sagittal plane permits the creation of a kyphosis to disengage the facets.*

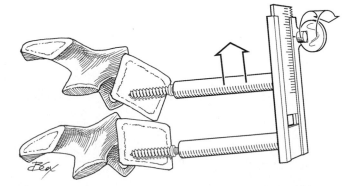

**Fig. 20.2** *Slight distraction can also be used to cause the facets to disengage. Dorsal force application to the rostral vertebra assists in reduction of the dislocation.*

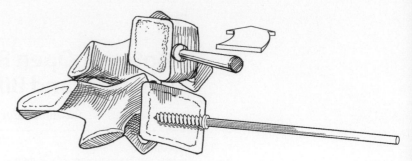

**Fig. 20.3** *Placing the pins at a 15-degree angle with respect to each other in the coronal plane allows reduction of a rotational deformity when distraction is applied.*

tamp, between the vertebral bodies ventrally provides a solid fulcrum on which the bending moment may be applied. If osteopenia is a concern, longer pins may be placed with bicortical purchase.

In the case of a unilateral dislocation, the distraction pins should be applied with a divergent angle in the coronal plane to allow the rotational deformity to be reduced after distraction (**Fig. 20.3**).

Alternatively, a small curette may be inserted in the interspace and braced against the rostral end plate of the caudal vertebral body. The handle is rotated rostrally while the tip remains stationary. As the motion is begun, the predominance of the resultant force is that of distraction, but as the curette gains a greater angle relative to the end plate, it forces the rostral vertebral body dorsally (**Fig. 20.4**).

Another option involves the use of a vertebral body spreader. Distraction across the disk space is applied first, and then the spreader is rotated in a rostral direction to restore alignment (**Fig. 20.5**).

**Key Procedural Steps**
A standard anterior cervical diskectomy and fusion (ACDF) approach is used. The importance of a complete, aggressive diskectomy prior to reduction cannot be overemphasized. The posterior longitudinal ligament

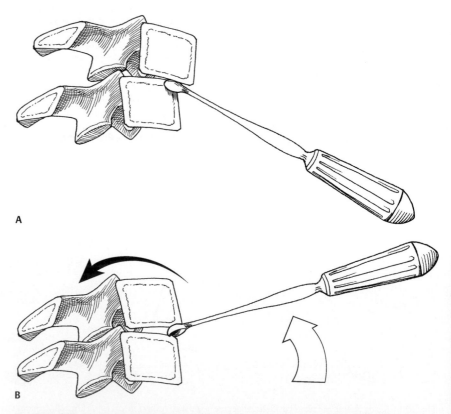

**Fig. 20.4** *(A)* A curette (or similar device) can be used to create distraction, followed by *(B)* dorsal translation of the rostral vertebra, to reduce the deformity.

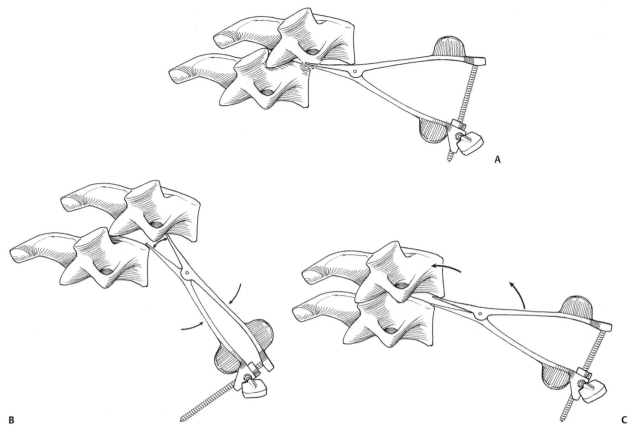

**Fig. 20.5** *(A) A disk interspace spreader can be used to reduce deformities by placing the spreader in the disk interspace at an angle. (B) Distraction is then applied to disengage the facet joints, followed by rotation (C) to reduce the deformity.*

PITFALLS
• The dislocation may prove to be difficult to reduce. Therefore, it is best to be armed with several techniques that may be utilized at the time of surgery.
• Overdistraction during the reduction process may result in further neurologic injury. Because a flexion-distraction injury with facet dislocation is a three-column injury (and therefore inherently unstable), a ventral plate should always be used.

should be resected across its entire width to facilitate manipulation of the vertebral bodies. Once these steps are complete, the dislocation may be reduced, foraminotomies performed if needed, a bone graft placed, and a plate applied.

**Bailout, Rescue, Salvage Procedures**
If there is a sagittal plane deformity (kyphosis) at the injured level, the caudal portion of the rostral body may be resected with a high-speed drill to allow access to the disk space (**Fig. 20.6**).

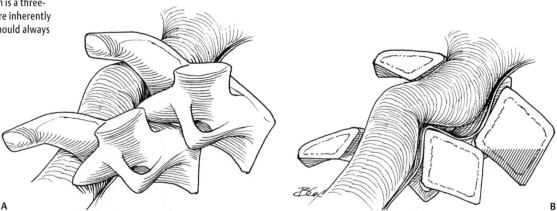

**Fig. 20.6** *(A,B) A dislocation may necessitate the removal of a portion of the ventrocaudal aspect of the rostral vertebral body (shaded area) to visualize the disk interspace, and allow the translation required for reduction of the dislocation.*

# 21

# Odontoid Screw Placement

*Darrel S. Brodke*

### Description
Reduction and fixation of a type II or high type III odontoid fracture with a precisely placed lag/compression screw.

### Key Principles
Anatomic alignment at the fracture site by initial positioning or intraoperative reduction is vital to the success of this procedure. The lag screw must be able to glide through the vertebral body and firmly purchase the odontoid fragment to gain firm compression at the fracture edges.

### Expectations
Screw fixation of the odontoid fracture should significantly improve fracture-healing rates over those treated in halo-vest immobilization, and avoid the limitations of a primary C1-C2 fusion, with associated loss of motion.

### Indications
Patients with acute or subacute (less than 6 months old) type II or high type III odontoid fractures, particularly those at higher risk of pseudarthrosis, are ideal for this technique.

### Contraindications
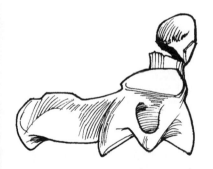
- Fractures older than 6 months
- Reverse (anterior) oblique fracture line, angling from posterior rostral to anterior caudal (**Fig. 21.1**)
- Significant osteoporosis or fracture comminution
- Inability to gain anatomic reduction
- Inability to gain appropriate screw placement, due to body habitus (barrel chest) or associated disease process (ankylosing spondylitis)

**Fig. 21.1** *A reverse (anterior) oblique fracture, not amenable to odontoid screw fixation.*

### Special Considerations
Patients older than 50 years of age, with fractures displaced greater than 4 to 5 mm, have the highest rate of nonunion with halo fixation. They should be considered for immediate odontoid screw fixation. Likewise, younger patients with high-risk lifestyles and elderly patients who may poorly tolerate 3 months in a halo vest may be considered for immediate fixation. Those patients who do undergo 3 months in a halo and have persistent motion at the fracture site may still heal with screw fixation. Although there is often some loss of motion following odontoid fracture treatment by any means, the motion remains better than with C1-C2 fusion, which is associated with a 50% loss of rotation of the neck.

### Special Instructions, Position, and Anesthesia
The patient should be positioned supine on the operating table with the head in traction. This can be accomplished with the Mayfield three-pin head-holder, Gardner-Wells tongs, and a pad under the head and between the shoulder blades, or with halter traction. The arms may be gently taped down to the sides with mild traction, though the shoulders rarely block visualization. If the endotracheal tube can be positioned off to the side in the mouth, this will allow improved visualization of the odontoid in the anteroposterior (AP) plane.

### Tips, Pearls, and Lessons Learned
- Get as close to anatomic reduction as possible prior to the prep and drape. This can be accomplished by adjusting the height of the head on towels or foam, or by placing towels under the shoulder blades. Both rotation of the neck and forward translation of the head, as compared with the chest, may be required to reduce the fracture and allow access for screw placement.
- Use biplane fluoroscopy to obtain quick AP and lateral views of the odontoid throughout the procedure (**Fig. 21.2**). A bight block, wad of gauze, or a wine cork with cutouts for the teeth may be used to hold open the mouth, improving AP visualization.

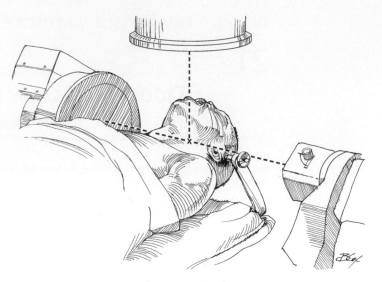

**Fig. 21.2**  *Intraoperative positioning with biplane fluoroscopy.*

- Ensure access to the screw trajectory above the chest, and confirm on the lateral fluoroscopy view prior to prep and drape (**Fig. 21.3**).
- Approach through a C5-C6 level skin incision (on the right for a right-handed surgeon).
- Enter the C2 body at the C2-C3 disk, under the anterior edge of the body. This may require removing a small amount of the C3 body anteriorly, as well as some of the C2-C3 disk annulus, to get the correct trajectory.
- Further reduction may be achieved by using a radiolucent retractor that also enables the assistant to place anterior to posterior pressure on either the C2 vertebral body or the odontoid fragment.

### Difficulties Encountered

Patient body habitus or position may inhibit access to the proper trajectory for screw placement. If the chest is barrel shaped, the drill will not be able to get low enough. If the neck has a fixed flexed position, the proper screw placement is also blocked. Fracture pattern may inhibit screw fixation. If the fracture has a reverse oblique orientation, angling from posterior rostral to anterior caudal (**Fig. 21.1**), attempts at fracture compression will cause loss of reduction. Inability to obtain fracture site compression will lead to a higher rate of failure. Additional difficulties may be encountered if there is poor fluoroscopic visualization. Taking the time to ensure good AP and lateral fluoroscopic views before beginning the procedure is a key element to success.

### Key Procedural Steps

Following intubation and placement of cranial traction, the C-arms are positioned for perfect AP and lateral views of the odontoid. The head and neck are then positioned for anatomic alignment of the fracture. This may require both rotation and translation of the head. The screw trajectory is then checked on the lateral view with a Kirschner wire (K-wire) laid alongside the neck, to ensure that the sternum is cleared and the screw can be placed appropriately. The neck is prepped for a right-sided anterior approach at the C5-C6 level.

A standard anterior approach to the cervical spine is performed, between the midline structures and the carotid sheath. Once down between the longus colli muscles, blunt dissection is continued up to the C2 vertebral body, and a radiolucent retractor is used to allow an AP fluoroscopic view. The C3 vertebral body is notched and the anterior annulus of the C2-C3 disk is removed in midline. A guidewire or drill is advanced through the undersurface of the anterior-inferior corner of the C2 body.

Under AP fluoroscopic control, the drill is advanced up through the C2 body, aiming for the midpoint of the odontoid tip. The lateral view is used to confirm a trajectory aimed up through the midportion of the odontoid to the tip. The drill is advanced to the fracture site. If the fracture is well reduced, the drill is advanced across, into the proximal fragment, then slowly and carefully through the tip of the odontoid, feeling the change in bone density as the cortex is met and then penetrated. If reduction is required, this is performed before advancing the drill.

A decision is now made to place either a partially threaded or a fully threaded screw. The partially threaded screw is a natural lag screw, allowing compression at the fracture site. A fully threaded screw requires over-drilling of the body fragment to become a lag screw and allow compression. If a partially threaded screw is to be used, the length is measured off of a depth gauge or the drill. The odontoid fragment is tapped and

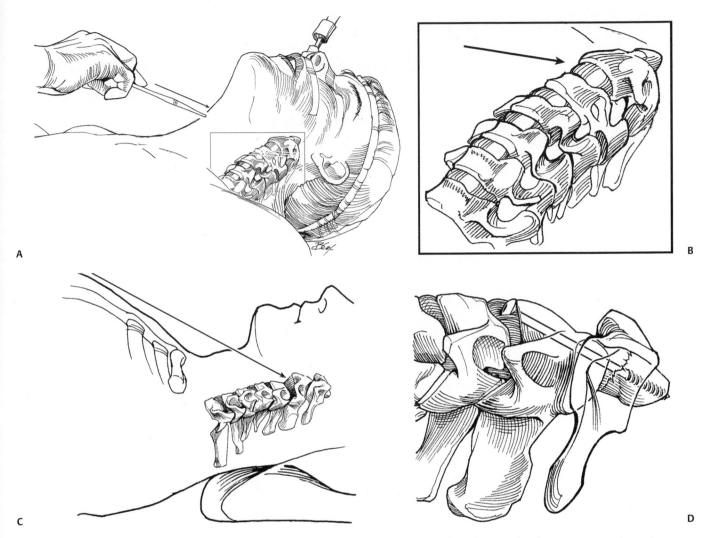

**Fig. 21.3** *(A–D)* Odontoid screw placement requires neck extension and occasionally some forward translation, so that the screw trajectory is anterior to the chest wall.

**PITFALLS**

- Malreduction of the odontoid fracture prevents fracture site compression and adequate stability. Re-displacement or pseudarthrosis are likely to occur.
- Significant osteoporosis, comminution at the fracture site, or failure to gain purchase on the cortical bone at the tip of the odontoid fragment also prevents compression and diminishes stability.
- Incorrect starting position can lead to poor screw position and fixation or re-displacement of the fracture.
- A guidewire may be used to gain and hold initial position and over-drill. If there is a slight bend in the guidewire, as the drill is advanced it will bind the wire and advance it out through the tip of the odontoid.

the screw is placed, gaining purchase on the cortical tip. If a fully threaded screw is to be used, the C2 body is overdrilled with a drill the same size as the outer diameter of the screw and advanced up to the fracture sight. The odontoid fragment is then tapped and the screw advanced up through the tip of the odontoid, obtaining purchase on the cortex. As the screw is then advanced, the head of the screw contacts the base of C2, the tip achieves purchase on the proximal fragment, pulling it distally, and the fracture edges are compressed.

### Bailout, Rescue, Salvage Procedures

During initial setup and fracture reduction, increasing or decreasing the amount of traction may help. Just before drilling the odontoid fragment, further reduction can be obtained with help from the anesthesiologist with anterior to posterior pressure through the mouth on the anterior ring of C1, or posterior to anterior pressure from underneath. If the fracture is high in the odontoid, the threads of a partially threaded screw may cross the fracture preventing compression. Either cutting the tip of the screw to shorten, or use of a fully threaded screw with overdrilling to the fracture site prevents this problem. If problems occur before or during the procedure, it may be necessary to abandon attempts at fixation of the fracture and switch to a primary C1-C2 posterior fusion.

# Anterior C1, C2 Arthrodesis: Lateral Approach of Barbour and Whitesides

*Eli M. Baron, Alexander R. Vaccaro, and Peter M. Fleischut*

## Description

The lateral retropharyngeal approach to the upper cervical spine was developed by Kelly and Whitesides as an alternative approach to the anterior cervical spine, avoiding the complexities of anterior extrapharyngeal approaches, which require an approach medial to the carotid sheath or dislocation of the mandible. This approach is actually done posterior to the carotid sheath, avoiding branches of the carotid artery and the facial nerve. Additionally, the approach allows access from C1 to T1 and avoids the potentially higher morbidity of a transoral/transpalatal approach.

## Expectations

To perform a stand-alone C1-C2 anterior arthrodesis via a bilateral lateral approach.

## Indications

Instability at C1-C2 requiring anterior fixation or when an anterior approach is required for a diagnosis. The approach is advantageous over a transoral approach where fixation is necessary for instability and a posterior approach is contraindicated (presence of posterior infection or incompetent posterior elements). It also may be useful as a salvage technique following failed posterior arthrodesis.

## Contraindications

- Vertebral artery injury
- Local infection
- Inexperience with regional anatomy

## Special Instructions, Position, and Anesthesia

The patient is placed in the supine position. Fiberoptic nasotracheal intubation is preferred in cases of significant instability. Intraoperative neurophysiologic monitoring, including somatosensory evoked potentials and transcranial motor evoked potentials, if available, is used during positioning and throughout the procedure. Dental occlusion should be maintained to keep the angle of the mandible from limiting the area of dissection.

Biplanar fluoroscopy or frameless stereotaxy may be useful during guidewire insertion, drilling, and screw placement to ensure proper instrumentation placement while limiting the risk of neurovascular injury.

For positioning, if not contraindicated, the neck should be rotated to the opposite side and extended as much as possible. The ear lobe can be sewn anteriorly to the cheek to facilitate exposure of the field. Postoperative prophylactic tracheostomy should be considered in cases where there is significant retropharyngeal dissection. Performance of the tracheostomy after the procedure is usually more convenient.

## Tips, Pearls, and Lessons Learned

Preoperative imaging and planning are essential prior to performing the procedure. This includes computed tomography (CT) imaging for studying bony anatomy and estimating screw length. CT angiography and magnetic resonance angiography (MRA) are useful noninvasive modalities for assessing the position and patency of the vertebral arteries.

## Difficulties Encountered

- Avoid the parotid gland, which may be seen superficially at the cranial end of the incision. Dissection into the gland may result in facial nerve injury or parotid fistula. Also, deep at the cephalad end of the incision lies the posterior belly of the digastric muscle. Care should be taken to avoid retraction against this muscle to minimize risk of injury to the facial nerve, which lies between the digastric muscle and the base of the skull.
- Excessive medial retraction on the nasopharynx may result in mucosal laceration and subsequent contamination of the field.
- Excessive retraction may contribute to postoperative dysphagia and possible cranial nerve injury, including the hypoglossal and superior laryngeal nerve.
- Excessive retraction on the spinal accessory nerve should be avoided to minimize risk of sternocleidomastoid or trapezius weakness.

## Key Procedural Steps

A hockey-stick incision is made from the tip of the mastoid process and taken distally along the sternocleidomastoid muscle (**Fig. 22.1**). The greater auricular nerve is identified as it crosses the

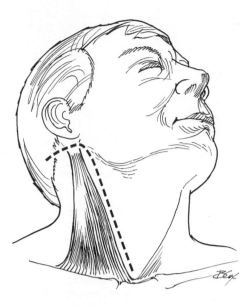

**Fig. 22.1** *Hockey-stick incision (dotted line) used for the lateral approach to the upper cervical spine.*

sternocleidomastoid muscle and dissected proximally and distally to increase its laxity, facilitating retraction. If needed, it may be divided with a resultant small sensory deficit around the ear. The external jugular vein is also ligated and divided.

The platysma is then divided in line with the prior incision, followed by division of the deep cervical fascia investing the sternocleidomastoid muscle. The sternocleidomastoid muscle is detached from the mastoid process. This is done by dividing it transversely as it inserts onto the mastoid process, and then everting it. The spinal accessory nerve is then identified, approximately 3 cm from the tip of the mastoid process. The nerve should then be protected.

The internal jugular vein is then identified in the carotid sheath and dissected from the spinal accessory nerve for greater mobilization. The sternomastoid branch of the occipital artery is located next, distal to the spinal accessory nerve and is ligated. Both the spinal accessory nerves and the internal jugular veins are dissected proximally to the digastric muscle. The dissection then continues posterior and lateral to the carotid sheath and medial to the spinal accessory nerve and sternocleidomastoid muscles (**Fig. 22.2**).

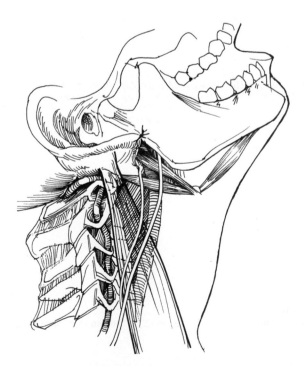

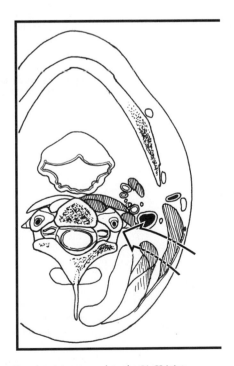

A                                                                                                                                    B

**Fig. 22.2** *(A) Lateral approach to the upper cervical spine. (B) Transverse section showing approach to the C1-C2 joint. Muscles to be retracted or transected are shaded.*

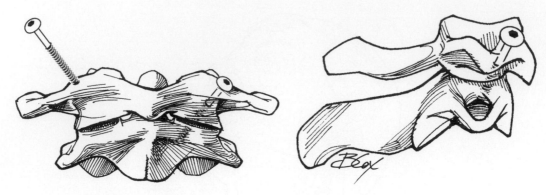

**Fig. 22.3** *Anterior (A) and lateral (B) views of screw trajectory through the C1-C2 facet joints.*

A

B

The dissection then continues transversely along the anterior border of the transverse processes. The retropharyngeal space is then accessed with blunt dissection, which is further used to clear the prevertebral fascia. The C1 arch is easily located by palpation based on the prominence of its transversely oriented anterior arch. C2 has a prominent vertical ridge at its base. A subperiosteal dissection of C1 and C2 is then performed where the longus colli and longus capitis muscles are stripped laterally. The longus colli muscle may be detached from its origin on the anterior surface of C1-C2 to maximize exposure. The intertransverse membrane at C1-C2 should be preserved. The approach and dissection is then repeated on the contralateral side. Subsequently the facets are exposed through blunt dissection. A small cutting burr and cervical curettes are used to denude the C1-C2 articulation, and the joint space is packed with autogenous iliac crest bone graft.

Afterward, screw fixation is performed. A 2-mm guidewire is placed at the anterior base of the C1 transverse process, aiming 25 degrees from superolateral to inferomedially in the coronal plane and 10 degrees posteriorly in the sagittal plane. At the starting point, the guidewire should be in line with the ipsilateral mastoid process. Biplanar fluoroscopy should confirm wire placement. Drilling is then performed with a cannulated drill, first using a 2.7-mm cannulated drill bit over the guidewire followed by a 3.5-mm cannulated drill bit that is taken through only the C1 lateral mass for a lag technique. The procedure is then repeated on the contralateral side. A 3.5-mm tap is used, followed by a 3.5 × 26 mm cannulated screw, in the average adult. Preoperative CT measurements, however, are essential in estimating appropriate screw length (**Fig. 22.3**).

Meticulous hemostasis is obtained, followed by reapproximation of the sternocleidomastoid muscle to the periosteum overlying the mastoid process. A drain should then be placed followed by closure of the platysma and skin. At this point prophylactic tracheostomy should strongly be considered. Postoperatively the patient should be maintained in a Philadelphia collar.

**Bailout, Rescue, Salvage Procedures**
The definitive salvage procedure for a failed C1-C2 anterior arthrodesis is a posterior occipitocervical arthrodesis. Should a vertebral artery injury occur, packing with Gelfoam or Surgicel should be done for tamponade, and intraoperative neurovascular consultation should be obtained. The contralateral procedure should be aborted.

# Anterior Cervical Plating: Static and Dynamic

*Wade K. Jensen and Paul A. Anderson*

## Description

Anterior cervical plating provides stabilization of the cervical spine after arthrodesis. Theoretical advantages of plate fixation include improved initial stability, decreased complications from bone graft dislocation, end-plate fracture, and late kyphotic collapse. Whether anterior cervical plates result in higher fusion success is controversial, although recent reports confirm the efficacy of one- and two-level fusions. Modern plates have the capacity of screw capture, thereby preventing loosening, and require only unilateral screw purchase. Plate systems can be static or dynamic. Static plates have a rigid connection between screw and plate and do not allow motion during healing. Dynamic plates allow change in plate position to accommodate changes in the interbody graft that occurs following implantation.

## Key Principles

During healing of interbody cervical fusions graft, resorption of 1 to 2 mm per interspace occurs. Theoretically, plates may unload the graft or shield it from stress, and may lead to nonunion or plate failure. This is seen more commonly in longer fusion.

Cervical spine plates are classified as follows: (1) unrestricted backout, and (2) constrained (static) and semiconstrained plates that include two subclasses of (a) rotational and (b) translational. Unrestricted backout plates are of historical note. These were nonlocked, required bicortical screw purchase, and were associated with screw backout. They are therefore not currently recommended. The constrained or static plates are locked screw interface that allow unicortical fixation without screw backout (**Fig. 23.1**). Dynamic or semiconstrained plates have been developed that allow axial settling to accommodate a potential biologic or mechanical shortening of the anterior strut graft (**Fig. 23.2**). Rotational plates allow rotation or toggle at the plate–screw interface. The translational plates offer locked bone–screw interfaces with the ability to translate along the long axis to accommodate shortening (**Fig. 23.3**). Several mechanisms are available including plates that have oval holes allowing translation through the holes, whereas others have screws fixed to the plate and translation occurs by plate shortening.

Anterior cervical plates are load-sharing devices that require a graft or other interbody device. Cadaveric biomechanical load transmissions through the graft were found to be higher with a dynamic (68–80%) versus static plate (53–57%). This was accentuated when the graft was undersized (dynamic 50–57% versus static 17%). Therefore, one may hypothesize that a dynamic plate will lead to high union rates when the graft is appropriately loaded. The lack of load sharing over time in static plates may lead to hardware fatigue or loosening. Still unknown, however, is the critical amount of load sharing to allow bony union. What is

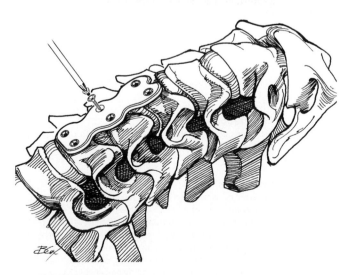

**Fig. 23.1** *Placement of a statically locked plate.*

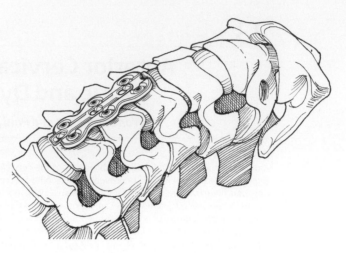

**Fig. 23.2** *Placement of a dynamic plate, allowing translation.*

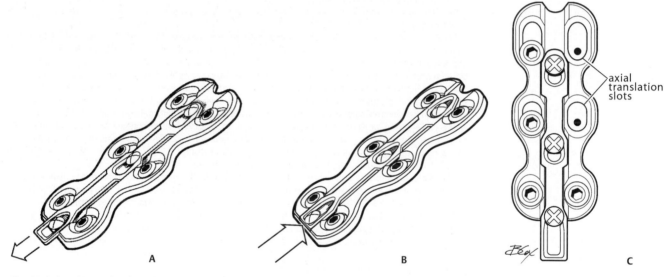

**Fig. 23.3** *(A–C) Examples of translation along the long axis to accommodate shortening.*

known is that strain rates of less than 5 to 6% lead to union, and strain rates of >10% lead to nonunion. Thus, plate fixation must limit strain and optimize load sharing to allow healing.

### Expectations

Anterior cervical plates result in high fusion rates, prevent graft collapse, and maintain spinal alignment. A low rate of hardware-related complications should occur.

### Indications

Anterior cervical plate fixation has a wide range of indications. It is used to stabilize unstable conditions from trauma or other destructive lesions such as tumors. Its most common use is following decompression for degenerative conditions. It is thought to result in higher fusion success for two- and three-level cases. Its use following single-level fusion is controversial. Although evidence of efficacy in fusion success is conflicting, several investigations have demonstrated that plating for single-level cases results in a lower incidence of graft complication and maintains lordosis to a greater degree than do nonplated cases. Anterior plates can be used after both diskectomy and corpectomy.

Adequate evidence is not available to determine the role of dynamic versus static plates. Longer constructs such as three- or four-level fusions appear to have a high failure rate with static plates, with the usual failure mechanism being screw loosening at the caudal end and graft dislodgment or intussusception. In these cases, if an anterior plate is used, the authors recommend a translation plate.

### Contraindications

Static plates have a relative contraindication for use in long multilevel reconstructions secondary to early failure. Dynamic plating has been shown biomechanically to be weaker in trauma patients with significant posterior involvement. A recent study suggests that dynamic plates were stable until the posterior longitudinal ligament (PLL) was sacrificed, which then resulted in significantly more range of motion (ROM) in flexion and extension, and more axial ROM. Clinically it is unknown if this is an important effect. In a randomized study of patients with combined anterior and posterior injury, anterior static plates resulted in similar outcomes compared with posterior cervical plates. The efficacy of translational plates in these patients is unknown.

Anterior plates should be used with caution in patients with osteoporosis, renal osteodystrophy, or severe kyphotic deformities, or in patients in a highly unstable condition with total ligamentous destruction, severe comminution, or missing posterior elements.

### Special Considerations

If patients have osteoporosis or rheumatoid arthritis that compromises fixation, one may consider either supplemental posterior fixations or more rigid immobilization postoperatively with close radiographic follow-up.

### Special Instructions, Position, and Anesthesia

Anterior diskectomy and fusion is performed with the patient in the supine position on a standard table. The head is held with a horseshoe head holder, with the neck slightly extended. A shoulder roll can be placed either transversely or longitudinally, based on surgeon preference, to aid in neck extension. Three-inch cloth tape is used to lower the patient's shoulders bilaterally. The endotracheal tube should be taped on the right side of the mouth. Verify that once positioned, the patient is symmetric before sterile preparation and draping. In trauma patients, reduction should be performed prior to plating.

### Tips, Pearls, and Lessons Learned

Plates should be placed in the midline and have screws as close to the fused disk space as possible. Lateral placement can result in vertebral artery injury or intraforaminal screw placement. The plate should lie as flush as possible on the spine. This often requires machining of the osteophytes or bony prominences.

Plate length should be chosen to keep the plate 5 mm or more away from the adjacent level to avoid adjacent level ossification. Screws orientation should be parallel to the end plates to avoid crossing an unfused disk. To keep the plate oriented to the midline, the plate should be firmly held in place. If the surgeon is not sure of the position, an anteroposterior radiograph should be obtained. Most systems have temporary fixation pins that can maintain orientation while drilling and screw placement. If the patient is small, particularly small Asian women, sometimes even the smallest screws in the set are too long, so shorter screws need to be available.

To avoid iatrogenic spinal cord injury, make sure that when drilling any pilot hole to check the length of the drill bit protruding from the drill guide.

### Difficulties Encountered

Dysphagia is a common complication after anterior cervical diskectomy and fusion (ACDF) with plate fixation. A recent study has shown that to minimize dysphagia, osteophytes should be removed that would prevent the plate from sitting flat against bone. Low-profile plates have been shown to minimize dysphagia postoperatively.

### Key Procedural Steps

Once decompression is completed and the graft is properly placed, then plate placement is performed. Good carpentry of the graft–host interface is paramount for stability. The anterior osteophytes are burred down to allow a flat surface for the plate to sit. The plate size should be carefully chosen so the screws are placed adjacent to the end plates nearest the diskectomy/corpectomy. Lower profile plates have a lower incidence of dysphagia and should be used if possible. Screw length can be gauged from the vertebral body depth determined when the graft was fashioned, commonly 14 mm. Verify that the drill protruding from the drill guide is 14 mm prior to drilling to avoid catastrophic complications. If placing bicortical screws, use fluoroscopy to verify drilling and screw placement. Hold the plate in the midline while drilling so the plate does not shift. Eccentric plate placement can result in vertebral artery injury or screw placement that is intraforaminal. Lastly, obtain intraoperative radiographs to verify position of the plate prior to closure. Immobilization is controversial and depends on the injury, procedure performed, and fixation obtained intraoperatively.

### Bailout, Rescue, Salvage Procedures

If screws have poor purchase, larger diameter or longer screws can be placed. Another option is bicortical screw placement. Alternatively, posterior fixation can augment the anterior plate.

If hardware is loose or screws are seen to be backing out, early revision is recommended.

# 24

# Costotransversectomy

*John E. Tis and Timothy R. Kuklo*

## Description

Several diseases of the spine require resection of all or part of the vertebral body and concurrent exposure of the posterior elements. These include some benign and malignant tumors that require biopsy or resection, congenital kyphosis and kyphoscoliosis, hemivertebra resection, and rigid scoliosis. The traditional approach has been to perform a combined anterior and posterior approach in a staged fashion. The anterior approach is necessary to remove all or part of the vertebral body, and the posterior approach is then performed to complete the resection of the posterior elements or provide stabilization with rigid posterior instrumentation. Costotransversectomy was first described by Menard to treat a paraspinal abscess associated with tuberculosis. Since then, it has also been described as a method to treat thoracic disk herniations, spinal nerve root tumors, ventrally based space-occupying intraspinal lesions, and all of the conditions listed above that have traditionally required anterior and posterior access to the spine. This approach provides adequate exposure of the anterior column to allow resection of the vertebral body and limited anterior fusion with visualization of the thecal sac to allow resection of anterior spinal tumors or prevent cord impingement during deformity correction.

## Key Principles

Although costotransversectomy has been shown to have similar complication rates to anterior and combined anterior/posterior approaches in experienced hands, it is a technically challenging procedure associated with potentially significant blood loss. Surgeons should be experienced in both anterior and posterior approaches before attempting a costotransversectomy.

## Indications

Vertebral column resection is indicated for any disease that requires exposure or removal of part or all of the anterior or middle columns of the thoracic spine, such as the following:

- Congenital kyphosis and kyphoscoliosis
- Rigid, large curve scoliosis requiring vertebral osteotomy
- Thoracic disk herniations
- Metastatic or primary tumors of the spine that require debulking or excision
- Anterior intraspinal tumors
- Paraspinal abscess drainage

It is especially indicated for anterior exposure in patients who cannot tolerate a thoracotomy such as the elderly, or other patients with limited pulmonary reserve and in those patients in whom the surgeon wishes to avoid contamination of the thoracic cavity.

## Contraindications

Conditions that require extensive anterior exposure and fusion may be better approached through an anterior (transthoracic) approach.

## Special Considerations

A thorough understanding of the three-dimensional anatomy of the thoracic spine and costovertebral articulation is essential. Each rib has bilateral superior and inferior costovertebral articulations that contribute to the thoracic spine's inherent stability.

Preoperative planning includes obtaining adequate radiographs to localize the pathologic process to be approached and obtain a rib count so that the correct rib(s) will be removed at the time of surgery. In the case of certain tumor resections (renal cell carcinoma, hemangioma, hemangiosarcoma), consideration may be given to preoperative arterial embolization to reduce blood loss.

## Special Instructions, Position, and Anesthesia

This approach has been described with the patient in either the prone or lateral decubitus position. We prefer the prone position, especially if concurrent posterior instrumentation is to be performed. The patient is placed on a well-padded open Jackson frame or radiolucent table in the prone position with the abdomen allowed to hang freely. The radiolucent table has the advantage of allowing rotation around the central longitudinal axis ("airplaning" the table). The arms are placed with the shoulders abducted 90 degrees and

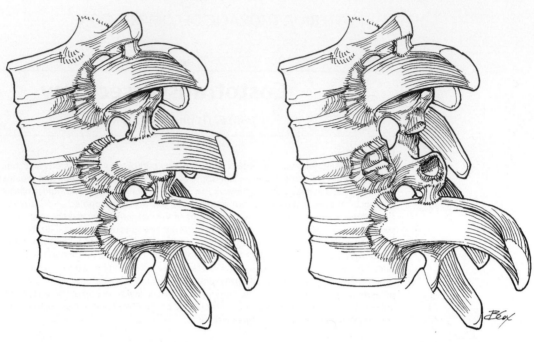

**Fig. 24.1  (A)** *Coronal view of the relationship among the rib, same-level vertebra, and cephalad adjacent vertebra.* **(B)** *Resection of one rib provides exposure to the same level vertebral body, the caudal portion of the superior adjacent vertebral body, and the interposed disk.*

the elbows flexed 90 degrees. General endotracheal anesthesia is used, and the neck is placed in a neutral to slightly flexed position. Alternatively, a Wilson frame may be used on a radiolucent table. The frame is elevated to its maximum height during the exposure and resection, and lowered during instrumentation and deformity correction. Spinal cord monitoring is placed (somatosensory and motor evoked potentials), and central intravenous access is established along with an arterial line. Mean arterial pressure is kept at 70 mm Hg during the dissection and at the resting level during any deformity correction. The back is sterilely prepared and draped widely out to the posterior axillary line.

### Tips, Pearls, and Lessons Learned
Removal of a rib head exposes the vertebra of the same number as well as the inferior portion of the adjacent, cephalad vertebral body (**Fig. 24.1**). Removal of the sixth rib head exposes the T5-T6 disk. Generally, only 2 to 4 cm of one or two ribs needs to be resected to allow access to the lateral aspect of two vertebrae. The rib heads to be resected should be at the level of the hemivertebra, disk, or tumor to be removed or the apex of the deformity. More extensive vertebral resections or more anterior dissection, such as that required for en bloc tumor resection, may require three or more ribs to be removed. The goal is to obtain adequate subperiosteal exposure of the vertebra(e) to be resected without violating the thoracic cavity. If more than three ribs are removed or bilateral resections are performed, this will cause instability requiring posterior instrumentation. If only a thoracic diskectomy is planned, the costovertebral joint and lateral end plates are drilled instead of performing rib resection. This allows limited exposure of the annulus that is sufficient to remove a single thoracic disk.

### Difficulties Encountered
Pleural violation is not uncommon and should be recognized, closed (if possible), and a chest tube placed at the end of the procedure. This complication is more common in the case of tumors, infection, or previous surgery that creates pleural scarring. It is occasionally necessary to intentionally violate the pleura to gain anterior access.

Neurologic compromise can occur if the spinal cord is impinged during correction of a deformity. The thecal sac should be visualized, decompressed, and protected before deformity correction is initiated.

Significant bleeding may also be encountered, particularly after the rib head is resected, if the intercostal artery is not ligated or retracted. Frequently, the intercostal artery and nerve are identified and ligated prior to resection of bone to improve exposure and decrease blood loss. Substantial bleeding may also be encountered during vertebral resection after cancellous bone is resected and can be controlled with products such as bone wax and Gelfoam (Pharmacia and Upjohn Company, Kalamazoo, MI) or Surgicel (Johnson and Johnson, New Brunswick, NJ). An autogenous blood recovery system such as Cell Saver (Haemonetics, Braintree, MA) should be used, and sufficient blood products available to replace blood lost during the procedure.

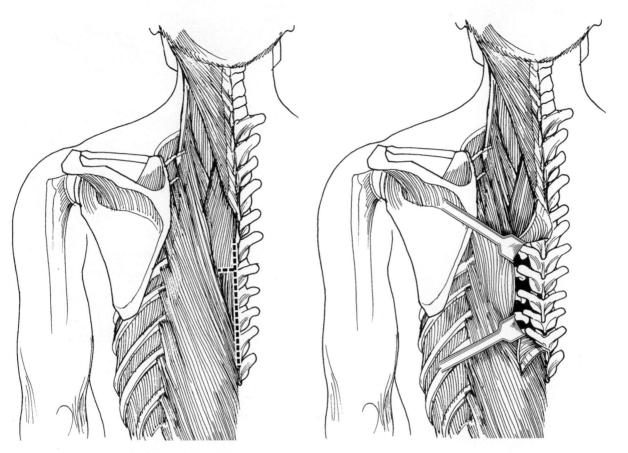

A                                                                                                          B

**Fig. 24.2** *The posterior thoracic musculature, scapula, and posterolateral approaches to the spine. (A) The posterior midline approach utilizing subperiosteal dissection out to the transverse processes and transection of the paraspinous musculature. (B) The lateral approach made just lateral to the paraspinous musculature.*

Exposure to the upper four thoracic vertebrae is made difficult by the presence of the scapula, which must be retracted laterally after the rhomboid and trapezius muscles are divided medially. Unless bilateral costotransversectomy is performed, anterior exposure is limited at all levels. Care should be taken to develop a plane between the anterior longitudinal ligament (ALL) and the pleura, or damage to the great vessels may occur. If a bilateral approach is planned or more than three ribs need to be resected to provide exposure, the adjacent vertebrae should be instrumented prior to vertebral resection to provide stabilization. This can also help with deformity correction.

### Key Procedural Steps
A straight longitudinal approach starting just lateral to the paraspinal muscle mass has been described, but this makes posterior instrumentation difficult, and the authors prefer using a midline approach and performing subperiosteal dissection out to the transverse process and then transversely splitting the paraspinous muscles with electrocautery to expose the ribs (**Fig. 24.2**). It may be possible in a thin patient where only limited exposure is needed to retract the paraspinal muscles laterally without dividing them. A needle or other radiopaque object is placed at the intended level of resection and portable radiographs or fluoroscopy is used to confirm the level. Pedicle screws or hooks and a contralateral temporary rod may be placed at the adjacent segments if instability is anticipated.

Generally, the medial 4 to 5 cm of the ribs to be resected are subperiosteally exposed, and the intercostal neurovascular bundle on the inferior aspect of the rib is retracted caudally. As previously noted, the bundle may be ligated and divided if necessary. The rib and transverse process at the desired level(s) are also resected. The costotransverse ligaments are divided sharply, and the transverse process is removed at its junction with the lamina. The rib, which has already been subperiosteally exposed, is resected with a rib cutter approximately 2 to 4 cm (or more if needed for exposure) from the vertebra at its prominent posterior angle (**Fig. 24.3**). It is important to note that the pedicle lies immediately anterior to the cut transverse process. Subperiosteal dissection along the path of the pedicle will bring the surgeon to the vertebral body, avoiding the inferior and superior neural foramina and the more caudally located segmental vessels that run along the center of the vertebral body (**Fig. 24.4**). Once the dissection has been carried as far anteriorly as the particular situation requires, subperiosteal dissection is extended inferiorly to the waist of the

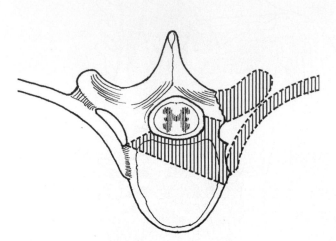

**Fig. 24.3** *Cross-section of the costotransversectomy approach. The shaded area depicts bone that may be removed using this approach to expose the spinal canal.*

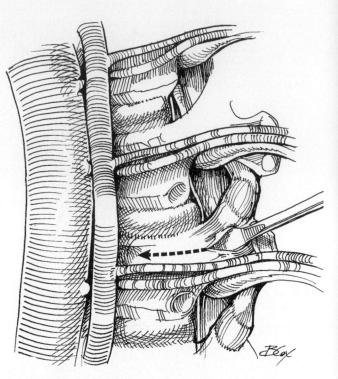

**Fig. 24.4** *Coronal view of the "safe" path for periosteal dissection along the pedicle, avoiding the inferior segmental vessel and the neural foramina inferiorly and superiorly.*

body and superiorly to the disk. Most of the vertebral body, the cephalad disk, and a portion of the adjacent cephalad vertebral body will now be exposed. This should be sufficient for vertebral or pedicle biopsy or limited resection.

### Vertebral Osteotomy, Resection, or Spinal Cord Decompression

One or two additional ribs and transverse processes may need to be removed. It is important to identify the neural foramina and exiting nerve root, which, as noted, may have been resected lateral to the neural foramina. The nerve root is followed back to the cord and both are protected while the bone of the superior pedicle, overlying lamina, and the dorsal cortex of the vertebral body are removed with rongeurs and the thecal sac is directly visualized. The posterior longitudinal ligament (PLL) may be removed or left in place to protect the dura. Decompression for kyphosis correction requires resection of all or most of the dorsal cortex of the vertebral body. A wedge of the vertebral body is then decancellated to correct the deformity or resect the tumor, depending on the situation. At the completion of the procedure, the field is filled with saline and checked for air leaks. If one is discovered, the defect is closed and a chest tube is placed.

### Hemivertebra Excision

After removal of one or two ribs, a small periosteal elevator such as a Penfield No. 1 (Miltex, Tuttlingen, Germany) is used to carry the dissection anteriorly to the anterior longitudinal ligament (ALL). A blunt retractor is placed with the tip at the anterior apex of the vertebral body, and the lamina and pedicle of the hemivertebra are removed with a rongeur while the nerve root is protected. The superior and inferior disks and end plates are exposed and removed before the vertebral body to aid in hemostasis. The vertebral body is then removed as completely as possible and the PLL resected while the ALL is preserved. The adjacent bodies are then allowed to close the gap. This may be performed manually or with the aid of instrumentation (**Fig. 24.5**).

### Bailout, Rescue, Salvage Procedures

- Failure to adequately expose the vertebral body may result in incomplete vertebral excision, necessitating incision of the pleura and possibly a formal transthoracic approach. Either of these procedures requires closure of the defect and placement of a chest tube.
- Uncontrollable cancellous bleeding may be controlled with bone wax, packing, and closure of the defect.
- Instability may need to be addressed with placement of posterior instrumentation; either hooks or pedicle screws may be utilized. This is ideally performed before resection of the ribs and transverse processes.

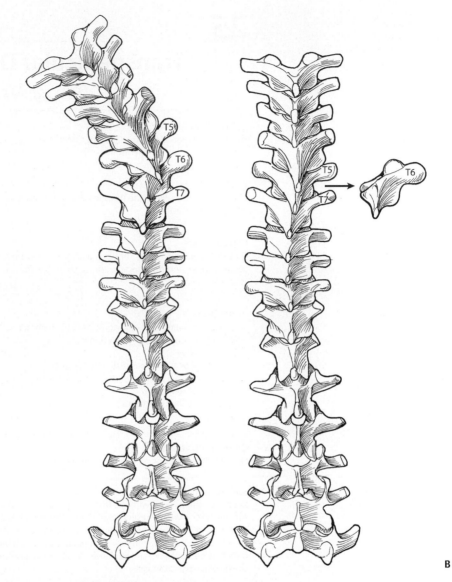

**Fig. 24.5** *(A) Right T6 hemivertebra. (B) Removal of right T6 hemivertebra.*

A

B

**PITFALLS**

- Transection or damage to the exiting nerve root or adjacent cord
- Anterior longitudinal ligament violation resulting in vascular or visceral injury
- Uncontrollable bleeding
- Instability after resection of greater than three ribs or bilateral ribs

- Intraoperative somatosensory and motor evoked potentials should be utilized throughout the procedure to detect potential spinal cord injury. In the case of significant evoked potential changes, or spinal cord injury, consideration should be given to more complete decompression and better visualization of the thecal sac. Any impingement should be corrected and mean arterial pressure returned to resting levels. If the potential is still abnormal or no impingement is visualized, the deformity correction should be reversed and stabilized with instrumentation, a wake-up test performed, and consideration given to initiation of the North American Spinal Cord Injury Study (NASCIS) III steroid protocol.

### Acknowledgments

The opinions or assertions contained herein are the private views of the authors and are not to be construed as official or as reflecting the views of the United States Army or the Department of Defense. Author Tis is an employee of the United States government. This work was prepared as part of his official duties and as such, there is no copyright to be transferred.

# 25

# Transpedicular Decompression

*Kingsley R. Chin*

### Description
A technique that allows surgeons to "safely" access the intervertebral disk and lesions in the pedicle and vertebral body, and to decompress the neural elements through a posterior approach.

### Key Principles
The protective walls of the pedicles provide a safe pathway to access the pedicles, vertebral bodies, and intervertebral disks.

### Expectations
This technique decreases the risks and potential morbidity that would be associated with costotransversectomy or an anterior thoracic approach for the same pathology. In cases of intrapedicular lesions, it is the technique of choice.

### Indications
- Resection or biopsy of intrapedicular or vertebral body lesions
- Fracture stabilization or reduction
- Tuberculosis
- Transdural or anterolateral disk herniation
- Decompression of anterolateral spinal cord compression in the setting of spinal instability requiring posterior stabilization
- Resection of hemivertebra
- Diskectomy for posterior release of idiopathic scoliosis

### Contraindications
Focal midline anterior spinal cord compression.

### Special Considerations
Access to the pedicle without fluoroscopic assistance will necessitate either a laminotomy to probe the medial pedicle wall or resection of the proximal rib head or transverse process to access the lateral pedicle wall. Patients with a fusion mass and a laminectomy membrane may necessitate the use of fluoroscopy to access the pedicle. Patients with rotatory kyphoscoliosis may need a combination of fluoroscopy and direct palpation as described above to follow the pedicle trajectory for risk of breakthrough and injury to the displaced great vessels.

### Special Instructions, Position, and Anesthesia
Placing the patient in the prone position on a Jackson table to facilitate maneuverability of the fluoroscope is preferred, but the choice of position may be based on stabilization techniques and other factors. Motor and sensory evoked potential monitoring is preferred. A double-lumen tube is used to allow single lung ventilation if needed. General anesthesia is preferred, with or without supplementation with local long-acting anesthetic.

### Tips, Pearls, and Lessons Learned
Review the preoperative axial images to understand the pedicle anatomy and map the location of the pathology. Three-dimensional reconstruction is advised. To access the pedicle under direct vision, remove the rib head and transverse process, or perform a laminotomy. Removal of the lateral pedicle walls, transverse process, and rib head enables greater access to the midline. If uncomfortable localizing the pedicle visually, use a gearshift to localize and penetrate the pedicle under biplanar fluoroscopic guidance followed by a 4.2 tap to core out a path as you would for pedicle screw placement. The gearshift should not advance beyond 80% of the distance to the anterior cortex to avoid anterior cortical penetration. Frequent fluoroscopy is suggested to monitor the leading depth of penetration during decompression. Anterior column support may be improved with a concomitant transpedicular placement of autogenous bone graft or other osteobiologics.

### Difficulties Encountered
Excessive cancellous bleeding may occur. Use hemostatic aids liberally and work expeditiously. Medial wall breech may cause dural tear, neural injury, and excessive epidural bleeding, necessitating a laminotomy or

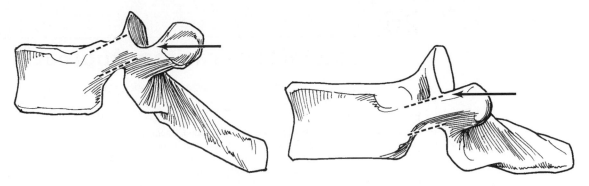

**Fig. 25.1** *Variations in the location of the pedicle relative to the base of the transverse process in* **(A)** *upper and* **(B)** *lower vertebrae.*

laminectomy. Use of intraoperative ultrasound diminishes the risk of inadequate decompression of midline structures, although this is rarely necessary in practice.

### Key Procedural Steps

Fluoroscopy is used to localize the incision. A midline incision is used but only the ipsilateral erector spinae muscles are dissected free off the posterior elements unless bilateral transpedicular approaches are planned. The exposure should include the entire lamina, transverse process, and rib-head/costovertebral junction of the selected vertebra. Biplanar fluoroscopy can be used to localize the pedicle, which is situated directly inferior to the superior articular process and at the level of the top of the transverse process in the upper thoracic spine, but at the level of the middle to lower half of the transverse process in the lower thoracic spine (**Fig. 25.1**). The posterior cortex of the pedicle is opened with a high-speed burr. Sequentially larger curettes are used to develop the medullary canal of the pedicle down to the vertebral body. Sequential fluoroscopic views are used to assess the depth of decompression at intervals. Alternatively, a faster decompression can be achieved with a high-speed burr along a channel that was previously developed with a gear shift and tapped. Once the appropriate depth is reached and localized fluoroscopically, the transpedicular channel should allow passage of angled curettes at 45 degree angles to each other to remove bone through the opposite pedicle, or to impact loose fragments of bone anteriorly (**Fig. 25.2**)

### Bailout, Rescue, Salvage Procedures

If adequate decompression is not achieved transpedicularly, remove more of the lateral pedicle or perform an extrapedicular approach. A costotransversectomy provides even greater access. If decompression is still inadequate, consider access from the contralateral pedicle if the lesion is accessible or convert to an anterior decompression. An unrepairable dural leak can be treated locally with Duragen and a sealant agent followed by a lumbar subarachnoid drain.

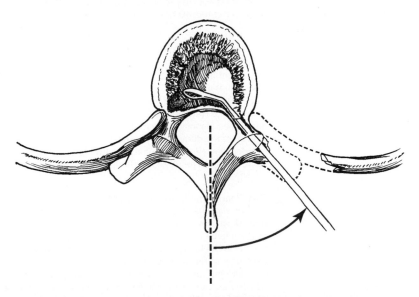

**Fig. 25.2** *To allow access to the interior of the vertebral body, it may be necessary to resect the rib, rib head, and transverse process.*

# 26

# Lateral Extracavitary Approach

*Howard B. Levene and Jack I. Jallo*

## Description

The lateral extracavitary approach has been developed to approach the posterior lateral and anterior lateral aspects of the spine and dura without the need of an anterior thoracic or abdomen exposure. The approach allows the surgeon to manipulate instruments in a direction away from the dura. The lateral extracavitary approach was originally developed for Pott's disease but has proven effective for diskectomy, vertebrectomy, biopsy, and fusion.

## Expectations

This approach affords the spine surgeon visualization of the posterior lateral and anterior lateral vertebral body. If a corpectomy is performed, the surgeon can visualize the posterior lateral and anterior lateral dural surfaces. The surgeon can perform a diskectomy, vertebrectomy, biopsy, or fusion with instrumentation through one incision. If posterior instrumentation (i.e., thoracic pedicle screws) is desired, the incision allows the additional placement of instrumentation. The surgical approach is technically challenging. The procedure requires expertise, experience, and a comfortable knowledge of thoracic and retroperitoneal anatomy.

## Indications

A lateral extracavitary approach is indicated for anterolateral dural compression. Compression may arise from trauma, neoplasm, infection, or degenerative changes. The approach is ideal when an anterolateral decompression is necessary to perform a vertebrectomy, diskectomy, biopsy, and or fusion.

## Contraindications

Patients who have had thoracic or pulmonary trauma or cardiopulmonary limitations may not be good candidates for any type of surgical intervention. Patients with severe abnormalities of the ribcage or spine (e.g., severe scoliosis) are less than ideal candidates for an extracavitary approach.

## Special Considerations

Exposure at the limits of the approach (T1–T5 and L5-S1) is difficult. For lower lumbar dissections, dissection of the lumbar nerves off the iliopsoas muscle is required. The artery of Adamkiewicz has an unpredictable origin. Preoperative spinal angiography may be considered. Approaching the spine from the contralateral side to the artery of Adamkiewicz may be desirable. The fascia of the middle to lower thoracolumbar spine forms an aponeurosis, which when incised to expose the erector spinae muscle, often creates a large potential space. The space must be closed meticulously to prevent seroma formation. For exposure of a single vertebrae, the ribs above and below must be excised.

## Special Instructions, Position, and Anesthesia

The operating table may be angled to provide better visualization. It is important, therefore, to make sure the patient is well secured to allow rotation. When nerve roots are encountered, gentle retraction using vessel loops are useful. Tracing intercostal nerves/arteries back to the dura will identify the pedicles above and below the entrance to the foramen. Neuroelectrophysiology (somatosensory evoked potential [SSEP], motor evoked potential [MEP]) monitoring is highly advisable as an early-warning method for neural irritation. When planning for anterior grafting, it is advisable to leave the posterior cortex intact, if possible, to protect the dura. Close consultation with the anesthesiologist is required. Some authors have recommended single-lumen intubation with high-frequency ventilation. Prior to closure, fill the wound with saline to inspect for a pneumothorax or air leaks.

## Tips, Pearls, and Lessons Learned

The approach has limits depending on the level of the spine. The confines of the upper thoracic spine include the narrowing of the thoracic inlet, and the presence of great vessels, mediastinum, and lung apices. At the middle to low thoracic spine, the diaphragm is an impeding anatomic structure. Anatomic constraints in the lumbar spine include the abdominal viscera, kidneys, and great vessels. Unique anatomic challenges of the lumbosacral junction include the narrow pelvic inlet and the iliac vessels. During dissection, dividing the intercostal nerves distally allows better access to the foramen. Dividing the intercostal nerves creates a tolerable band of hypesthesia and avoids a dysesthetic pain syndrome from stretch injuries. Some difficulties inherent in the procedure include persistent bleeding, which may require fresh frozen plasma (FFP) if there is greater than 2 L of blood loss.

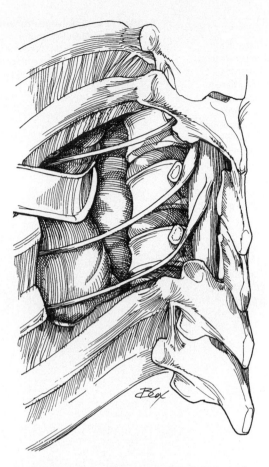

**Fig. 26.1** *Lateral view of the retracted paraspinal muscle bundle medially and the myocutaneous flap laterally, the lateral dural sac and exiting nerve roots, and the lateral vertebrae.*

### Key Procedural Steps

The anesthesiologist must be alerted to the possibility of lung intubation. Central IV access or large-bore IV access and an arterial line are recommended. For nononcologic cases, Cell-Saver is recommended. The patient may be positioned on chest rolls and secured tightly. The ipsilateral chest roll can be placed medially to allow the scapula to fall away for high thoracic approaches. Depending on the levels to be approached, consider a Mayfield pin frame versus face pad support. Create a midline curvilinear hockey-stick skin incision three segments above and below the target level for a corpectomy and fusion. For a diskectomy, only 1.5 segments above and below the target level are required for adequate exposure. Alternatively a paramedian linear incision can be used for exposure. For autograft, the incision is extended to the lateral crest for bone harvesting. The exposure allows visualization of the spinous processes, laminae, and transverse processes. There will be aponeurotic attachments at the transverse process. Dissect laterally to find the lateral margin of erector spinae muscles and retract the superficial soft tissues medially. For exposure up to C7, identify and separate the fascial planes of the trapezius and rhomboids and reflect them laterally as a myocutaneous flap. For exposure of the lateral thoracic or thoracolumbar junction, rib removal is required frequently at and below the vertebral level of interest. The rib may be dissected in its entirety (subperiosteal circumferentially) or dissected as a vascularized bone graft with preservation of the neurovascular bundle. During dissection, identify nerves and tag them with vessel loops. Intercostal nerves may be sacrificed proximal to the dorsal root ganglion for exposure (**Fig. 26.1**).

Dissect the lateral pedicle and vertebral body taking care to preserve the pleura. A high-speed drill or a rongeur are used to remove the pedicle. For a diskectomy, a combination of pituitary rongeurs and curettes are used. A Woodson tool can be used to palpate the anterior surface of the annulus to confirm adequate disk removal.

For a corpectomy, proceed with a high-speed drill to remove the anterior portion of the vertebral body. Take care to leave a thin rind of bone anteriorly, laterally, and posteriorly. Continue bone resection to the contralateral pedicle. At the conclusion of the dissection, break the posterior vertebral margins to decompress the neural elements. It is important to note that with the dura mater exposed, manipulation of compressive lesions by instrument maneuvers away from the dura is advocated. Wound drains are regularly placed.

## PITFALLS

- This approach requires extensive knowledge of thoracolumbar anatomy. The great vessels are close to the operative field and there is a danger of excessive bleeding. Any dural tears encountered should be primarily repaired. Consider cerebrospinal fluid (CSF) drainage if needed. Beware of the potential of iatrogenic neurologic injury to the cord and nerve roots. Incomplete decompression is a risk. Violating the pleura may result in a pneumothorax or hemothorax. Be aware of the possibility of postoperative ileus.

- This operation is not recommended in patients with severe cardiac or pulmonary disease, or a life expectancy of less than 3 months. For patients who refuse blood or blood products, one should reconsider this approach.

### Bailout, Rescue, Salvage Procedures

For soft tissue bleeding, cauterize and pack as necessary. For damage to the great vessels, an emergent vascular surgery consult is recommended. When compressing/packing bleeding tissue, take care to avoid compressing the dura. If the bleeding is uncontrollable, the wound can be packed and closed, and a separate approach can be performed at a later time. If a pneumothorax or hemothorax is suspected, a chest tube should be placed.

# 27

# Supralaminar, Infralaminar Transverse Process Hook Placement

*Steven C. Ludwig*

### Description
The safe placement of hooks within the thoracic spine allows for surgical correction and stabilization of a variety of spinal disorders. Anchor site selections include a down-going supralaminar hook, up-going infralaminar hook, and either an up- or more commonly down-going transverse process hook.

### Key Principles
Spinal instrumentation systems are characterized by a rod (longitudinal component) that is segmentally fixed to the spine via a hook or screw (anchor).

### Expectations
Three-dimensional corrective forces may be delivered to the spine for deformity correction, graft compression, or spinal stabilization. Despite the merits of segmental fixation, careful attention must be directed toward the preparation of a fusion bed because all rigid implant systems will fail if a solid fusion is not achieved.

### Indications
Scoliotic and paralytic deformity as well as all types of spinal instability including trauma, degenerative, neoplastic, and congenital. Laminar hooks may help shield pedicle screws and prevent late screw failure.

### Contraindications
Severe osteoporosis, active posterior infection, and significant loss of anterior column stability without reconstruction. These pathologies put posteriorly placed instrumentation under excessive stress and lead to fixation failure.

### Special Considerations
Careful preoperative planning is essential to determine the site of hook placement. Paired hooks in an apposing claw configuration provide a secure fixation point, especially at the ends of a construct.

### Special Instructions, Position, and Anesthesia
Prone position on a variety of frame choices including Relton-Hall frame, Wilson frame, or Jackson table. Consider controlled intraoperative hypotension in the absence of significant cord compression and electrophysiology monitoring.

### Tips, Pearls, and Lessons Learned
Preoperative and intraoperative communication with the surgical staff concerning the levels and types of hook facilitates the placement of the instrumentation.

### Difficulties Encountered
An alternative method of segmental fixation or a change in the instrumented level should be performed if violation of the lamina or transverse process makes hook placement unsafe.

### Key Procedural Steps
Thoracic laminar hooks can be placed against the superior or inferior edge of the lamina. Laminotomy windows are performed, using a skinny nose Leksell rongeur. Depending on the level, the interspinous/supraspinous ligaments are taken down to expose the ligamentum flavum. At the extremes of instrumentation placement the supraspinous and interspinous ligaments should be preserved. Also, one may place hooks on each side of the spine without removing the interspinous ligaments. Following removal of the

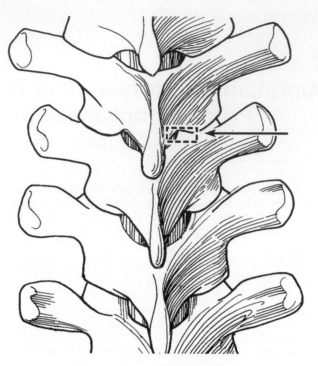

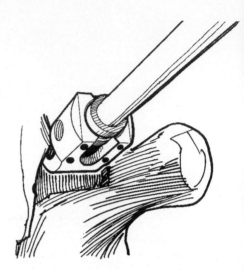

**Fig. 27.1** *Supralaminar hook requires a small intralaminar laminotomy. A small medial facetectomy may also be required to allow for hook seating.*

**Fig. 27.2** *Placement of an infralaminar hook with gentle upward positioning.*

interspinous ligaments, the ligamentum flavum is removed until epidural fat is visualized. Using a 2-mm Kerrison, the laminotomy site is widened laterally. One or two millimeters of the superior facet may be removed to allow for proper hook seating (**Fig. 27.1**). Care is taken to bite away only the ligamentum flavum and preserve the epidural fat to avoid epidural bleeding. A trial laminar hook is grasped with a hook holder and placed into the space created. Infralaminar hooks can be directly placed under the lamina in an up-going fashion (**Fig. 27.2**). The blade of a supralaminar hook should be inserted by rotation about the arc of the hook to facilitate the placement and minimize spinal canal hook intrusion (**Fig. 27.3**). Hook purchase is checked manually with a gentle posterior-anterior maneuver.

Downward- or upward-facing transverse process hooks are inserted over the superior or inferior edge of the transverse process, respectively. The edge of the transverse process is cleared in a subperiosteal fashion using electrocautery. A curved transverse process hook starter is used to enter the region along the anterior aspect of the transverse process, into a small triangular space bounded anteriorly by the rib head and laterally by the costotransverse process articulation (**Fig. 27.4**). A trial transverse process hook is placed into space and hook purchase is checked manually with a gentle posterior-anterior maneuver.

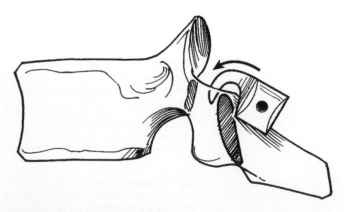

**Fig. 27.3** *Supralaminar hook placement.*

PITFALLS

• Avoid placing two laminar hooks at the same levels to prevent iatrogenic spinal canal stenosis from hook placement. Beware of fracturing the transverse process and losing a segmental point of fixation by creating an intraosseous defect with the transverse process hook starter. Transverse process hook placement may not be possible in the lower thoracic spine because the transverse processes become smaller in size and more vertically oriented. Rotation of a supralaminar hook into the spinal canal prevents the risk of forcing the hook into the spinal canal. When creating the laminotomy sites, epidural bleeders can be controlled with the use of a thrombin-soaked Gelfoam patty and thrombin-Gelfoam powder.

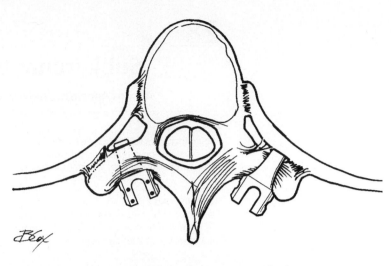

**Fig. 27.4** *Appropriate position of thoracic transverse process hook.*

### Bailout, Rescue, Salvage Procedures

Alternative methods of fixation include the use of pedicular fixation when the anatomic morphometry of the pedicles make this technique a viable option. The upward-facing hook option may allow for the placement of a pedicle hook instead of an infralaminar hook. The addition of a pedicular-screw hook is available as an additional means of fixation. Be aware that placement of pedicle hooks is frequently not possible at the lower thoracic levels because of a more sagittal facet orientation. Transverse process screws directed bicortically through the transverse process and into the rib head may be a good alternative method of fixation if the type of instrumentation allows for this option.

# 28

# Sublaminar Wire Placement

*Alexios Apazidis, Sanjeev Sabharwal, and Michael J. Vives*

## Description

Sublaminar wires are often used in conjunction with longitudinal members (rods) to provide rigid segment stability to the posterior spine. Sublaminar wires are an efficient means of manipulating the spinal column in the coronal, transverse, and sagittal planes.

## Key Principles

The risk of bone/implant failure is lessened due to the multitude of points of fixation contact available with this form of instrumentation. Wire placement at the extremes of the instrumentation construct resists implant pullout in the sagittal plane.

## Expectations

Sublaminar wire placement is extremely safe in well-trained hands. Substantial translational correction in the coronal plane is possible in flexible scoliotic curves (**Fig. 28.1**). A recent study demonstrated similar operating times for scoliosis cases using apical sublaminar wires versus pedicle screws.

## Indications

Any multilevel posterior fusion construct with intact posterior elements.

## Contraindications

Sublaminar wires should not be placed in regions of spinal stenosis, swelling of the neural elements, or levels of posterior element fracture or deficiency.

## Special Considerations

Once the wire is passed, it should be twisted over the respective posterior lamina to prevent inadvertent canal migration.

## Special Instructions, Position, and Anesthesia

The radius of curvature of the bent sublaminar wire should be at least equal to the width of the lamina. The primary bend can be made over the handle of a Cobb elevator, with a compensatory bend to facilitate wire passage. The wires should be passed just beneath the lamina in a caudal to cranial direction. Central passage of the wires under the lamina avoids the potential for nerve root injury from lateral wire deviation and minimizes the risk of encountering epidural bleeders. The spinous processes of the instrumented vertebrae are removed with a double-action bone cutter to adequately visualize the ligamentum flavum. A thin Leksell rongeur is used to create a midline defect in the ligamentum flavum, which is further enlarged with Kerrison rongeurs to allow safe passage of the sublaminar wire.

## Tips, Pearls, and Lessons Learned

Develop a routine for wire passage where the inferior tail of the sublaminar wire is placed either medial or lateral to the superior tail at the time of wire bending, prior to twist locking the wire ends. Some favor placing the inferior tail laterally, because the free ends of the wire can puncture the surgeon's gloves. Remember always to separate the wire ends at the time of rod placement prior to wire tightening to avoid the technical difficulty of trying to slip a wire end between the rod and bone after the wire is well seated. When twist locking the wire ends, rotate the wire ends away from the midline. If wires are placed at levels above or below the instrumentation, they should be twist tightened in a direction away from the fusion mass. For long constructs utilizing sublaminar wires as the primary fixation, wiring alternate levels instead of every level does not compromise the stability of the construct, provided that the most proximal two levels are consecutively wired. This practice would theoretically decrease the risk of cord injury and reduce surgical time.

## Difficulties Encountered

The potential for neurologic compromise is extremely low in sublaminar wire placement. At any point during passage of the wires, if there is any resistance at all, the wire should be removed, repositioned, and then gently reinserted. Forceful insertion of sublaminar wires may result in significant inadvertent thecal sac compression. If there is excessive epidural bleeding, gentle tamponade with Gelfoam or use of bipolar electrocautery can be utilized.

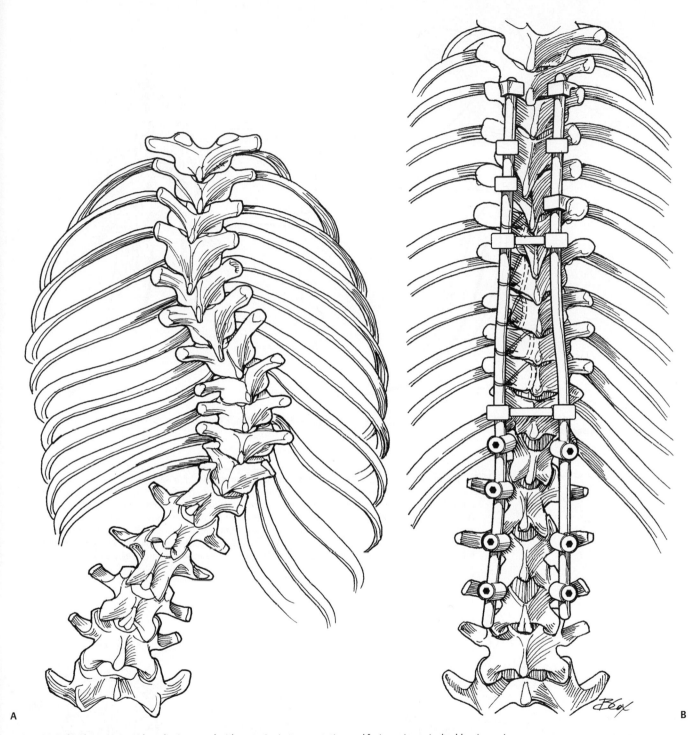

**Fig. 28.1** *(A,B) A patient with scoliosis treated with posterior instrumentation and fusion using apical sublaminar wires.*

**Key Procedural Steps**

Expose the ligamentum flavum at the levels of anticipated wire placement. Luque double-bent wires or doubled 16- or 18-gauge wires are pre-bent at one end into a semicircular arc. To avoid inadvertent jolting and canal penetration, the sublaminar wires are usually the last bony anchors that are inserted just before performing corrective maneuvers for spinal deformities. The wires are passed in four steps: introduction, advancement, roll-through, and pull-through. The wire should be introduced at the midline of the inferior edge of the lamina. The tip of the wire should remain in contact with the undersurface of the lamina as it is advanced cranially (**Fig. 28.2**). The wire should be rolled so the tip emerges at the upper end of the lamina

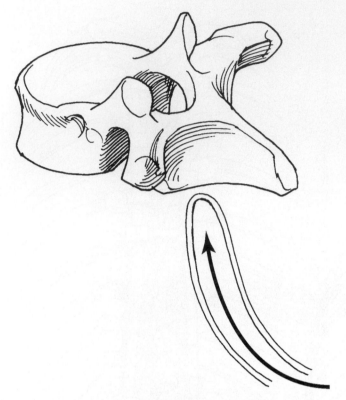

**Fig. 28.2** *The tip of the wire should remain in contact with the undersurface of the lamina as it is advanced cranially.*

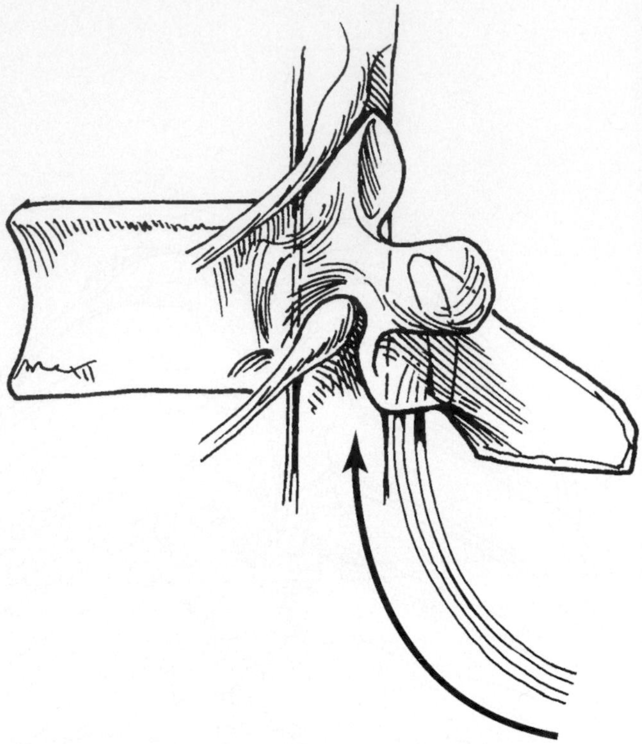

**Fig. 28.3** *Lateral view of the wire in the spinal canal.*

in the midline. The looped leading edge can then be grasped with a nerve hook or narrow needle holder. The wire is then pulled through by keeping a firm posterior force on the leading and trailing edge of the wire (**Fig. 28.3**). The wire ends are then bent to conform to the posterior lamina as described above (**Fig. 28.4**). At the time of rod placement, the wire ends are separated to allow the rod to rest between them. The wires are then tightened by twisting in a clockwise direction using a jet wire twister (**Fig. 28.5**). Retightening of the wires is often necessary before they are shortened with a wire cutter. The twisted wire ends are then twist-folded in the direction of wire twisting toward the midline posterior elements (**Fig. 28.6**).

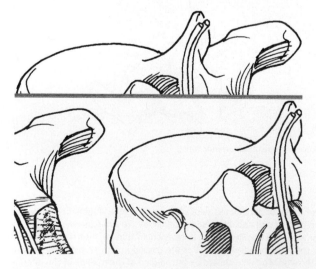

**Fig. 28.4** *The wire ends are bent to conform to the posterior laminae.*

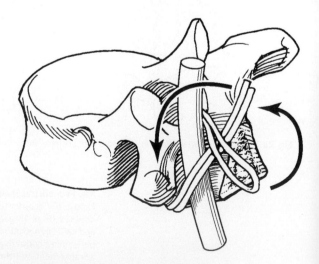

**Fig. 28.5** *Wires are tightened around the rod.*

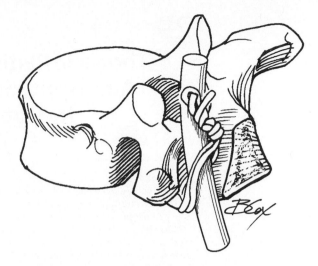

**Fig. 28.6** *The twisted portion of the wire is then twist-folded in the direction of the wire toward the midline posterior elements.*

**PITFALLS**

- Neurologic injury (spinal cord, nerve root) is the most common reported complication caused by the passing of the sublaminar wires. The most common reported symptom is temporary hyperesthesia caused by nerve root trauma. An infrequent complication is bony failure via wire pull-through, especially in the osteopenic patient. An adequate laminotomy is required to facilitate wire passage; however, the size should be limited to prevent compromise of the mechanical strength of the lamina. Overzealous tightening of the wire can also lead to wire breakage.

**Bailout, Rescue, Salvage Procedures**

If a wire cannot be placed without undue effort, the wire should be removed and passage should be reattempted after evaluating the passage route for evidence of obstruction. All wires should be removed if there is any evidence of permanent electrophysiologic or neurologic decline or weakness during a Stagnara wake-up test. If bony failure results at the time of wire tightening, an alternate level of spinal fixation should be chosen or transpedicular fixation, if applicable, can be performed.

# 29

# Thoracic Pedicle Screw Placement: Anatomic, Straightforward, and In-Out-In Techniques

*Timothy R. Kuklo*

## Description

Thoracic pedicle screws have become increasingly common for the treatment of spinal deformity, trauma, and tumors due to their superior fixation and improved correction. Theoretic concerns of increased neurologic complications from thoracic pedicle screw placement have not been proven.

Maximizing pedicle screw and construct advantages requires an understanding of pedicle screw biomechanics, including screw characteristics and insertion techniques. In addition, an understanding of bone quality, pedicle morphometry, and screw salvage options is necessary. This is best illustrated by the fact that the pedicle, rather than the vertebral body, contributes approximately 80% of the stiffness and approximately 60% of the pullout strength at the screw–bone interface.

## Key Principles

The major screw design variables include thread pitch, shaft design, inner (minor) and outer (major) diameter, head size and design, and material composition. In general, the most important variable to improve thoracic pedicle screw fixation is the outer diameter, whereas the inner to outer diameter ratio (ID/OD) has a smaller effect. Increasing pitch (more threads per inch) has only a minor effect. Approximately 75% of the pullout strength is achieved by crossing the neurocentral junction, or physeal scar, whereas anterior cortical purchase has a small additional effect on pullout, but is generally not recommended due to potential complications. Engagement of 50 to 80% of the vertebral body on a lateral radiograph appears optimal.

Intrapedicular thoracic pedicle screw placement is superior to an extrapedicular (in-out-in) placement, which achieves only 64% of the pullout strength compared with intrapedicular placement. Further, a straightforward trajectory (directing the pedicle screw parallel to the superior vertebral end plate) is biomechanically superior to an anatomic trajectory (directing the pedicle screw along the sagittal anatomic pedicle axis approximately 20 to 25 degrees caudad) (**Fig. 29.1**). However, if a straightforward trajectory is not achieved due to pedicle wall violation or some other condition, then a salvage strategy using the anatomic trajectory will again achieve 60 to 70% of the pullout strength compared with the ideal straightforward trajectory.

When performing construct testing, pedicle screw constructs again provide improved construct stiffness; however, lateral pullout is the weakest testing mode for thoracic pedicle screws. Cross-links improve construct torsional stability when using thoracic pedicle screws.

## Indications

Spinal deformity, trauma or tumors, especially with destabilizing procedures such as vertebral osteotomies, resection, or correction.

## Contraindications

Inadequate-sized or compromised pedicles.

## Special Considerations

A thorough understanding of surgical anatomy is paramount to successful thoracic pedicle screw placement. As recently as several years ago, the thoracic pedicle was thought to be a rather homogeneous, ovoid structure throughout the thoracic spine. However, we now know that the anatomy of the pedicle is quite complex and varies from region to region in the thoracic spine. Pedicle height, or sagittal pedicle isthmus width, varies from 12.0 to 20.0 mm (mean 15.8 mm) at T12 to 7.0 to 14.5 mm (mean 9.9 mm) at T1, and is never the limiting factor. Pedicle width is the critical anatomic variable. In the adult lower thoracic spine (T10–T12), the average pedicle width averages from 6.3 to 7.8 mm, often larger than the average pedicle width at L1 and L2. Pedicle width then decreases with a more cephalad vertebral level, and is usually the smallest at T4–T6. The interpedicular distance, or canal width, is also widest in the lower thoracic spine and subsequently decreases more cephalad until approximately T4, where it is often the narrowest. Thus T4 may be one of the most difficult thoracic pedicle screws to place, especially with a coronal deformity.

The coronal or transverse pedicle axis varies from cephalad to caudad, with the greatest transverse angle being at T1. Clinically, pedicle screw insertion depends on this axis, as well as the preferred start

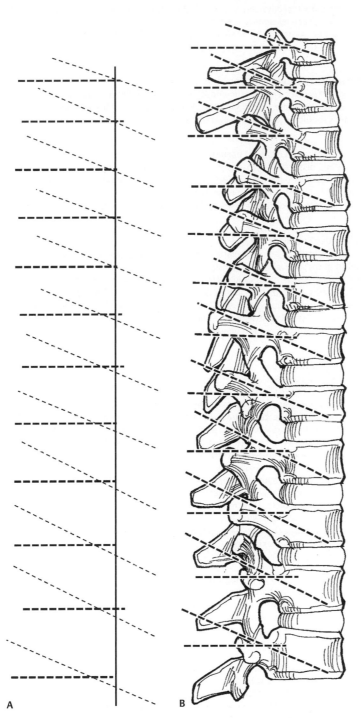

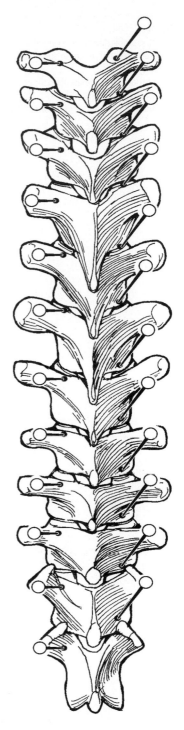

**Fig. 29.1** *(A) Lateral schematic of straightforward and anatomic trajectories.*
*(B) Lateral image of thoracic pedicle screw placement utilizing the straightforward and anatomic trajectory techniques.*

**Fig. 29.2** *Dorsal starting points for straightforward and anatomic trajectories.*

point (**Fig. 29.2**). The sagittal pedicle axis has received less attention, with the pedicle inclination routinely averaging between 20 and 25 degrees throughout the thoracic spine, with only small differences between males and females. The medial wall is also between two and three times thicker than the lateral wall throughout all thoracic levels.

Studies using cadaver computed tomography (CT) measurements, both before and after pedicle screw insertion, show that the pedicle undergoes plastic deformation if the outer diameter of the screw is larger

## PITFALLS

- Pedicle violation medially or inferiorly resulting in nerve root or spinal cord injury
- Anterior cortex violation resulting in vascular or visceral injury
- Pedicle screw pullout or failure of fixation

than the endosteal diameter, or if it is within 80% of the outer cortical diameter. Further, plastic deformation always precedes pedicle fracture.

Computed tomography imaging may be used for preoperative planning to assess pedicle size and location, and for postoperative screw placement.

### Special Instructions, Position, and Anesthesia

The patient is placed in the prone position on a well-padded radiolucent table. General anesthesia is administered. The arms are placed with the shoulders abducted 90 degrees and the elbows flexed 90 degrees. The neck should be placed in a neutral to slightly flexed position.

### Tips, Pearls, and Lessons Learned

Meticulous dissection with exposure of the transverse processes is mandatory. Facetectomies should be performed at each fusion level, and the cartilage should be removed. Fluoroscopy or intraoperative radiographs can be utilized to identify the pedicle shadow. The most important anatomic landmark is the midfacet, as the pedicle screw start point should always be lateral to this midpoint.

### Difficulties Encountered

Small pedicles may be particularly difficult to identify, and alternative fixation strategies should be considered at these levels if it is considered to be a critical level of fixation. Additionally, osteoporotic bone may be augmented with polymethylmethacrylate or other injectables such as hydroxyapatite cement, calcium phosphate, or carbonated apatite to enhance pedicle screw pullout; however, these techniques increase potential neurologic risk. Other strategies include supplemental wire or hook fixation to utilize the relatively preserved ventral lamina bone in osteoporotic vertebrae. Redirection of the pedicle probe can salvage screw placement after pedicle breach.

### Key Procedural Steps

After meticulous dissection, a high-speed burr is used to breach the dorsal cortex; see the pedicle screw start points in **Fig. 29.2**. A bleeding cancellous core is often visible, and is indicative of the pedicle channel. A pedicle probe, hand drill, or awl is used to prepare the screw channel. If a curved awl is used, the curve should initially be directed laterally. If resistance is encountered in the first 10 to 12 mm, then the trajectory is most likely too medial (encountering the dorsal spinal canal), or too lateral (encountering the lateral pedicle wall). Firm pressure is appropriate, and excessive force should be avoided. Slight inflection of direction will assist in finding the pedicle canal. In general, the transverse pedicle axis is approximately zero degrees at T12, increasing to approximately 30 degrees at T1.

After the pedicle channel is prepared, the channel is checked for potential breaches and the presence of a floor. A flexible feeler is used to determine channel depth for proper screw size selection. Tapping prior to insertion of the pedicle screw results in removal of material by the tap, thereby enlarging the hole volume. Undertapping the channel by 1.0 mm increases insertional torque and pullout strength. Monaxial screws have a lower profile than multiaxial screws, and for coronal deformities they provide superior derotation to that provided by multiaxial screws.

### Bailout, Rescue, Salvage Procedures

- For inadequate fixation, augmentation techniques can be utilized; however, these are not without risk, including extravasation through a fractured cortex, thermal damage, difficult removal in the event of infection or misplacement, and the potential for neurologic compromise.
- The anatomic trajectory can be used to salvage failure of a straightforward trajectory. In addition, screw salvage can be accomplished by using a larger diameter screw, a longer screw, or a screw both larger in diameter and longer.
- Intraoperative somatosensory and motor evoked potentials should be utilized throughout the procedure to detect potential spinal cord injury. In the case of significant evoked potential changes, or spinal cord injury, consideration should be given to screw removal, and initiation of the North American Spinal Cord Injury Study (NASCIS) III steroid protocol.

# 30

# Open Transthoracic Diskectomy

*Russel C. Huang, Patrick F. O'Leary, and Raja Taunk*

## Description

Open transthoracic diskectomy is performed to decompress symptomatic thoracic herniated nucleus pulposus (HNP) in patients with myelopathy or myeloradiculopathy.

## Key Principles

The reported radiographic prevalence of thoracic herniated disks in asymptomatic individuals is 37%. Therefore, radiographic findings must be well correlated with the history and physical examination findings before recommending surgery. Neural compression may result in myelopathy or radiculopathy. Myelopathy may manifest as motor, sensory, or reflex changes distal to the level of compression, gait disturbance, and bowel/bladder dysfunction. Radiculopathy may result in pain or sensory changes in a dermatomal distribution. The differential diagnosis includes cervical or lumbar stenosis, herpes zoster, infections or neoplasms, central nervous system disorders, and systemic or peripheral neuropathies. Thoracic axial pain from disk disease should be treated nonsurgically in most cases.

Selection of anterior or posterior approaches for thoracic decompression hinges upon the location and character of the herniation. Most authors agree that the transthoracic approach offers superior visualization of the disk and dura in the central zone of the spinal canal. Although lateral disk herniations can safely be decompressed via anterior or posterior approaches, the surgical morbidity of posterior approaches is lower than that of thoracotomy.

## Expectations

Surgery is performed to prevent progressive neurologic injury from ongoing cord compression. Despite adequate decompression, preexisting neurologic deficits may not resolve. Thoracic axial pain may not improve. The risk of postoperative paralysis is significantly higher than the risk of paralysis after cervical or lumbar decompressive surgery.

## Indications

- Absolute: Myelopathy with progressive neurologic deficits
- Relative: Painful radiculopathy from a thoracic HNP not amenable to posterior decompression

## Contraindications

Pulmonary disease prohibiting safe thoracotomy.

## Special Considerations

### Preoperative Planning

In addition to standard imaging, it is useful to obtain a continuous computed tomography (CT) or magnetic resonance imaging (MRI) scan that includes the entire thoracic and lumbosacral spine. The scans should be correlated with plain films and scrutinized for supernumerary vertebrae, rib abnormalities, or lumbosacral transitional anomalies that might generate confusion in the intraoperative identification of levels.

Measure the mediolateral width of the vertebral body at the level of the ventral floor of the spinal canal using CT or MRI. Knowing this width is helpful in ensuring that the mediolateral extent of disk removal is adequate.

## Tips, Pearls, and Lessons Learned

- We recommend intraoperative neural monitoring.
- Extensive calcification of the disk appears to raise the risk of intraoperative dural tears.
- A beanbag is useful to maintain true lateral decubitus positioning intraoperatively.
- Maintaining the patient in true lateral position keeps the surgeon oriented to the spinal canal and spinal cord.

- The rib, as the embryologic equivalent of the lumbar transverse process, leads to the identically numbered pedicle (e.g., tenth rib to T10 pedicle)
- Hypotensive anesthesia is not desirable. Blood pressure should be maintained normo- to hypertensive to maintain cord perfusion.

### Key Procedural Steps

The patient is placed in the lateral decubitus position. Above T6 a right-sided approach is preferred to avoid the heart and aortic arch. Below T6, left-sided approaches are preferred because the aorta is relatively safer to handle and mobilize. The break in the table is positioned at the level of interest and aids in exposure. The chest is usually entered one or two rib levels above the disk of interest. After entering the chest cavity, the ipsilateral lung is deflated using a double-lumen endotracheal tube. Preliminary identification of levels may be aided by intrathoracic palpation of the first rib and counting distally. Intraoperative radiographs are taken to confirm levels. In most cases, visualization of the 12th rib and corresponding vertebral body on anteroposterior radiographs provides the most reliable identification of levels.

Once the appropriate level has been identified, the rib head overlying the disk is resected. The neurovascular bundle caudal to the rib should be identified and protected. If necessary, the segmental artery should be ligated as distant from the foramen as possible to best preserve cord perfusion. Following rib head removal, dissecting and tracing the neurovascular bundle medially leads to the foramen, the pedicle, and the lateral margin of the disk and vertebral bodies.

The caudad pedicle is thinned with a burr and resected with a Kerrison rongeur, revealing the lateral aspect of the dural tube (ventral margin) of the spinal canal, and the disk itself (**Fig. 30.1**). Do not attempt to place any instruments between the disk and the cord at this time. A burr is used to perform partial corpectomies above and below the affected disk, leaving undisturbed the posterior shell of bone and disk material that is in direct contact with the dura (**Fig. 30.2**). Preoperative measurement of the width of the vertebral body is helpful in determining how "deep" to go with the burr to reach the other side of the spinal canal (right side of the canal in a left-sided approach).

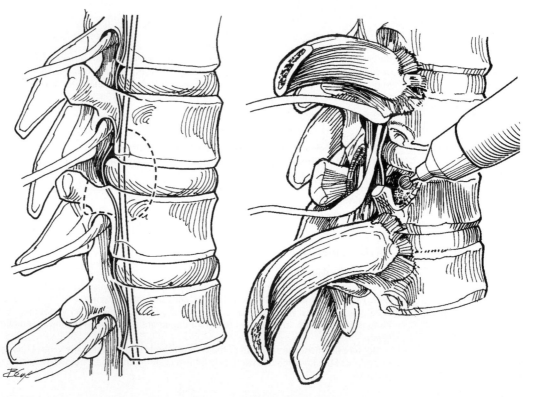

A                                                                                          B

**Fig. 30.1** *(A) Thinning of the caudal pedicle with a burr. (B) Resection of the pedicle reveals the lateral aspect of the dural tube, the ventral floor of the spinal canal, and the disk itself.*

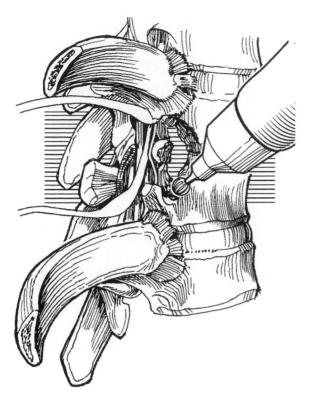

**Fig. 30.2** *Partial corpectomy of cephalad and caudal vertebrae is performed, leaving a thin shell of posterior bone and disk in contact with the dura.*

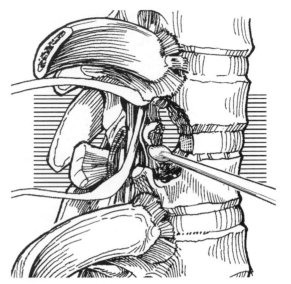

**Fig. 30.3** *Curettes are used to push the thin posterior shell of bone and disk away from the spinal cord.*

## PITFALLS

- Beware of the asymptomatic disk.
- Neurologic deterioration
- Wrong-level surgery
- Intercostal neuralgia
- Vascular injury
- Pulmonary morbidity
- Dural tears

Having created a void in the vertebral body anterior to the offending disk, the thin posterior shell of bone and the disk are pushed away from the cord using small curets (**Fig. 30.3**). Unnecessary contact with the dura, particularly near the zone of maximal compression, is avoided.

If significant bone resection is performed, or if the disk is at the thoracolumbar junction, fusion may be performed using rib autograft. Instrumentation is typically unnecessary. A thoracolumbar orthosis may help promote fusion.

Suture closure of the thoracotomy defect using drill holes through the ribs may reduce postoperative intercostal neuralgia. A chest tube is used postoperatively.

### Bailout, Rescue, Salvage Procedures

Irreparable dural tears may be partially sealed with fibrin glue. Placing a lumbar subarachnoid drain may be useful. Consider initiating a high-dose methylprednisolone spinal cord injury protocol in the event of postoperative neurologic deterioration.

# Open Thoracic Corpectomy via the Transthoracic Approach

*James D. Kang and Mustafa H. Khan*

### Description
Access to the anterior thoracic spine is used for decompression and fusion.

### Key Principles
Obtaining good exposure is the most important factor in performing adequate decompression of the neurologic elements of the thoracic spine. Depending on the level of thoracic spine, special consideration should be given to preserve vascular structures and thoracic/abdominal viscera.

### Expectations
The transthoracic approach offers excellent visualization of the anterior thoracic spine for decompression and fusion.

### Indications
Burst fractures with canal compromise and neurologic deficit, large extruded thoracic disks with cord impingement, intraspinal tumors, infections.

### Contraindications
Severe pulmonary disease, medical comorbidities such as severe cardiac disease, posterior spinal instability without intent to perform a posterior adjunctive procedure.

### Special Considerations
Preoperative workup should include imaging modalities (plain radiographs, magnetic resonance imaging [MRI], or computed tomography [CT] scan) to specifically define the area of decompression. If a tumor is being evaluated, CT angiography and embolization are helpful in preoperative planning. A thoracic surgery consultation for exposure and intraoperative assistance can be useful.

### Special Instructions, Position, and Anesthesia
Intraoperative somatosensory or motor evoked potentials should be used to monitor the cord. The patient is placed in a lateral decubitus position with the operative side (right or left, depending on the thoracic level) up (**Fig. 31.1**). The table is flexed to open up the intercostal intervals before beginning the approach. Magnifying loupes and head lights are helpful. We prefer to use a double-lumen endotracheal tube to deflate one lung. A nasogastric (NG) tube may be used for identifying the esophagus intraoperatively.

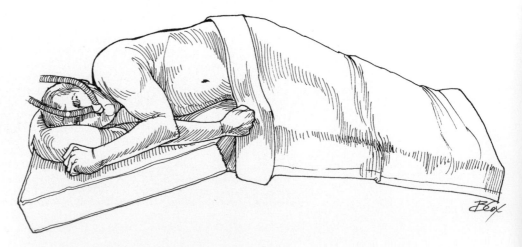

**Fig 31.1** The patient is placed in the lateral decubitus position.

**Tips, Pearls, and Lessons Learned**

In general, many surgeons prefer a left-sided approach. The level of entry between ribs depends on the level of pathology; it is better to err in the cephalad direction than in the caudad direction. A right-sided approach to T11-L1 may place the liver at risk. Access to the T2 and T3 vertebral bodies via a thoracic corpectomy is technically challenging; a sternal splitting approach may be easier. The other option is a very high periscapular thoracotomy, performed via excision of the fourth rib.

**Difficulties Encountered**

Ligation of segmental vessels is useful for maintaining good hemostasis. On the left side the artery of Adamkiewicz is at risk between T9 and T12. It is advisable not to tie off those vessels initially but rather to clamp them individually and watch for any somatosensory evoked potential (SSEP) signal changes. The blood supply to the spine via segmental vessels is highly variable. Also, exposing the wrong interspace and having to work cephalad for the appropriate exposure makes surgery more difficult. During left-sided approaches the thoracic duct is at risk for injury. The aorta and inferior vena cava are almost always visible in the surgical field. The hemiazygous and azygous systems are vulnerable to injury especially high in the thoracic spine. This is important because placement of anterior instrumentation under the aorta may lead to late aortic erosion and catastrophic aortic rupture. Some patients (especially those with severe lung disease) cannot tolerate unilateral lung deflation. Care must be taken not to puncture visceral pleura. Finally, inadequate decompression of the vertebral bodies may result if decompression is not carried all the way to the far pedicle.

**Key Procedural Steps**

A thoracotomy incision is made at the level corresponding to the vertebral level to which access is being sought. In large or obese patients, it may be difficult to identify the appropriate intercostal rib space to enter. Intraoperative plain radiographs with a spinal needle can help with the identification of the levels, but, in general, it is better to err on the more cephalad level because it is technically easier to perform the corpectomy working cephalad to caudad rather than vice versa. Care is taken to perform the dissection of the rib on its superior border to avoid damage to the intercostal nerve and vessels, which run along the inferior border. The dissection is carried down into the thoracic cavity by incising the pleura. A self-retaining rib-spreader is placed between the cephalad and caudad ribs. It is often necessary to resect the rib to allow for better retraction; otherwise, it is not uncommon to fracture the ribs with the rib spreading retractors. The lung is deflated via the double-lumen tube. Within the chest cavity, the rib that corresponds to the vertebral body that will be removed with the corpectomy is followed posteriorly to the spine where it articulates at the cranial border of the vertebral body and the intervertebral disk (e.g., the 8th rib articulates into the T7-8 disk space). It is strongly advisable at this time to obtain a confirmatory plain radiograph with a spinal needle to check that the levels have been counted correctly. The parietal pleura is resected, making a rectangular window over the vertebral body and the rib heads (**Fig. 31.2**). The segmental vessel is ligated to fully expose the lateral bony wall of the vertebral body, which is to be removed. The sympathetic chain is often encountered and may be ligated to enhance full exposure of the vertebral body and the adjacent disks. The rib head is now disarticulated to allow for exposure of the pedicle (the rib can be saved for use as bone graft). It is also important to remember that the rib head articulates with the transverse process (costotransverse articulation) as well as the vertebral body (costovertebral articulation), and good exposure of the pedicle requires complete resection of these structures.

Once this is done, the exiting intercostal nerve root can usually be visualized caudal to the pedicle. This anatomy allows the surgeon to clearly understand the posterior extent of the corpectomy (i.e., where the spinal canal begins) during the decompression phase of the operation. The pedicle is resected with a Kerrison rongeur, which allows for the exposure of the lateral border of the spinal canal (the lateral sleeve of the dura mater is now visualized along with the exiting nerve root). The cranial and the caudal disks are now resected with pituitary rongeurs. The vertebral body is then removed using a rongeur and a power burr (**Fig. 31.3**). Unless a tumor is being resected, it is not necessary to resect the anterior cortex of the vertebral body or the anterior longitudinal ligament. (These structures may provide a tension band during the reconstruction following the corpectomy and aids in keeping the bone graft encased within the corpectomy site.) The vertebral body should be burred toward the contralateral pedicle, and the posterior wall of the vertebral body adjacent to the spinal cord should not be removed until it is certain that corpectomy trough has reached the contralateral pedicle. It is advisable to use a diamond-tip abrasive burr to undercut the posterior cortex at the contralateral pedicle, which will make the posterior wall of the vertebral body (fracture fragments or tumor that is compressing the spinal cord) "float." Once this has been achieved, curettes are used to carefully pull the retropulsed bone fragments or tumor away from the spinal cord into the corpectomy trough. The posterior longitudinal ligament may be preserved or resected depending on the nature of the decompression that is being done (**Fig. 31.4**). The contralateral pedicle is palpated with a Penfield elevator to ensure that a complete decompression has been achieved.

Reconstruction of the corpectomy site can be achieved with a variety of different grafting options. Tricortical iliac crest bone graft, allograft humerus or femur, and titanium metallic cage devices, solid or expandable, can all be used effectively with or without anterior instrumentation. The authors' preference is to use an expandable cage device in elderly patients with tumors, and structural allograft in younger

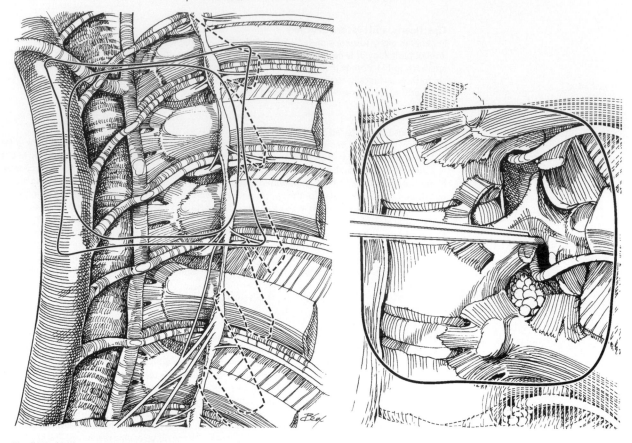

**Fig. 31.2  (A,B)** A window is made through the parietal pleura over the vertebral body.

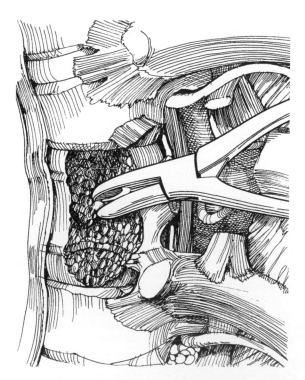

**Fig. 31.3** The corpectomy is performed all the way to the contralateral pedicle.

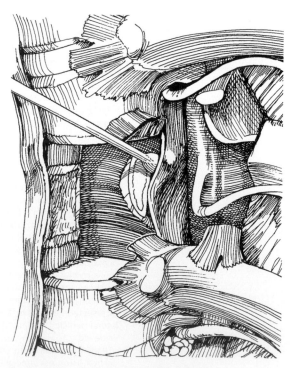

**Fig. 31.4** The spinal cord is fully decompressed.

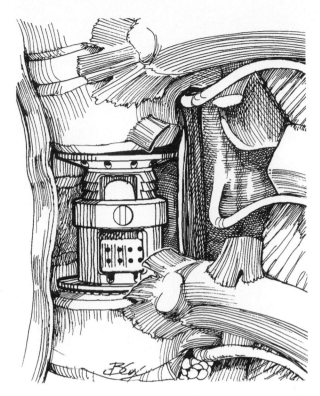

**Fig. 31.5** *An expandable cage is placed in the corpectomized vertebra.*

- If not properly ligated, segmental vessels can cause significant bleeding. Ligating more than two segmental vessels may compromise blood flow to the spinal cord. Bipolar electrocautery is useful in coagulating the small vessels. The vena cava and aorta are at risk with this approach when decompression is being performed with curettes or Kerrison rongeurs. If a double-lumen tube is used, the deflated lung should be inflated twice an hour to decrease the risk of postoperative atelectasis. Postoperative close and aggressive pulmonary support is needed to minimize respiratory complications.

patients with traumatic injuries (**Fig. 31.5**). Although anterior instrumentation is also available, many surgeons also prefer using posterior stabilization to obtain a more stable circumferential arthrodesis.

The thoracotomy is closed over a chest tube, and postoperative chest plain radiographs are taken to ensure normal lung reinflation.

### Bailout, Rescue, Salvage Procedures

If for technical reasons the anterior procedure cannot be completed, then a posterior decompression and fusion strategy may be adopted instead. Posterior surgery has limited usefulness, however, because the spinal cord does not tolerate any retraction.

# 32

# Anterior Thoracic Arthrodesis Following Corpectomy (Expandable Cage, Metallic Mesh Cages)

*D. Greg Anderson and Chadi Tannoury*

## Description

Various spine pathologies, such as fractures, destructive infections, and tumors, affect the vertebral body and lead to spinal instability. Surgical restoration of the anterior column, using metallic meshes or expandable cages, aims to decompress neural elements and provide biomechanical stabilization of the thoracolumbar spine following vertebrectomy.

## Key Principles

The use of autogenous tricortical iliac bone graft for vertebral body replacement has been a standard technique for vertebral body replacement in the past. However, problems with this approach including donor-site morbidities, pseudarthrosis, graft displacement, and graft collapse with kyphotic deformity have been reported. In recent years, a variety of surgical implants (cages) have been manufactured for vertebral body replacement in the thoracolumbar spine. First-generation cages for this purpose were made from titanium mesh or carbon fiber reinforced PEEK materials. More recently, complex cage designs have proliferated, including some cages that are "expandable," allowing the surgeon to place the cage into the spinal defect and lengthen or expand the cage to fill the defect or eliminate residual kyphosis at the corpectomy site (**Fig. 32.1**). Expandable cages offer several surgical advantages over nonexpandable metallic meshes; expandable implants can be inserted at a small volume through minimally invasive incisions, and the adaptation of the implant configuration to the exact defect height is possible by in vivo extension of the device, thereby avoiding further trimming of the nonexpendable cages. In general, cages are designed to support bone in-growth or facilitate fusion across the corpectomy site.

## Expectations

The use of a corpectomy cage is expected to reconstruct the anterior column of the thoracolumbar spine, restore normal alignment, provide stabilization, and achieve a solid fusion across the spinal defect. Clinically, this approach is designed to repair the spinal defect and provide a long-term stable solution to the underlying spinal disorder.

## Indications

Vertebral body replacement is indicated in various pathologic conditions affecting the anterior column integrity, including certain fractures, tumors, destructive lesions, infections, and deformities.

## Contraindications

Anterior column reconstruction should not be attempted as a primary or stand-alone treatment for severe spinal injuries with translation of the spine or rigid spinal deformities. Great care should be taken when anterior column bone quality is poor due to the risk of implant failure or subsidence. Also, many authors recommend avoiding prosthetic spinal implants in the settings of an active pyogenic infection.

## Special Considerations

To promote bone in-growth into and through the cage implant, bone graft or a bone substitute should be used. Depending on the clinical scenario, autogenous bone from the corpectomy site, morselized rib graft, iliac crest graft, allograft bone, ceramic bone substitutes, or even purified bone proteins have been used.

## Special Instructions, Position, and Anesthesia

The thoracic and thoracolumbar spine is approached with the patient placed in a lateral decubitus position. The ipsilateral lung may be deflated using double-lumen endotracheal tube ventilation, or ventilation pressures may be decreased allowing visualization of the spine. It is helpful to use neurophysiologic monitoring of the status of the neural elements, depending on the clinical scenario.

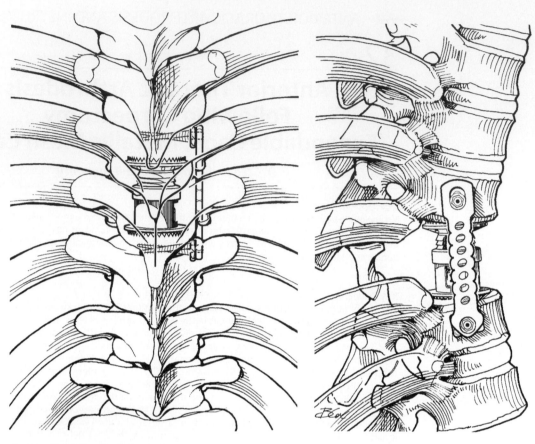

**Fig. 32.1** *(A) Anterior-posterior illustration of a thoracic arthrodesis construct using an expandable cage and a posterior instrumentation following corpectomy in a trauma patient. (B) Lateral illustration of a thoracic arthrodesis construct using an expandable cage and anterior instrumentation following corpectomy in a trauma patient.*

### Tips, Pearls, and Lessons Learned

A preoperative identification of the diseased vertebra is crucial prior to surgery. In cases where the vertebral abnormality is not clearly evident on plain films, a sagittal magnetic resonance imaging (MRI) that includes the lumbosacral junction and the lesion on the same film is useful, so that the operating surgeon can count the levels up from the sacrum to the lesion using fluoroscopy. A metallic marker placed over the spine may be used to identify the proper location for the skin incision prior to starting. Before starting the corpectomy, the rib heads should be removed to allow identification of the pedicle and posterior corner of the vertebral body. A wide exposure of the involved vertebrae is beneficial to ensure proper alignment of the implant following the corpectomy. Anterior exposure of the vertebra is facilitated by packing small sponges along the anterior aspect of the spine to retract the adjacent blood vessels. Maintenance of the bony end plates of the adjacent vertebrae is important to seat the cage and diminish the odds of subsidence of the cage.

### Difficulties Encountered

Poor localization of the incision or thoracotomy can make proper performance of the corpectomy and alignment of the cage difficult. Bleeding from the corpectomy or epidural vessels should be controlled with hemostatic agents. Ensure proper selection of cage length with the spine in a corrected position by manually applying force to the apex of the kyphotic deformity (push over the spine). This generally reduces the kyphosis at the corpectomy site and prevents undersizing of the cage implant.

### Key Procedural Steps

#### Approach

A thoracotomy or thoracoabdominal approach is performed in the lateral decubitus position. Segmental vessels are ligated and divided as needed to facilitate the procedure. Three to four cm of rib head are removed at the level of the corpectomy to expose the underlying pedicle and posterior region of the vertebral body. The exiting nerve root is protected during the procedure.

- Improper distraction of the spine prior to selection of the cage can lead to residual kyphosis and may predispose to construct failure or back pain. Destruction of the bony end plates increases the likelihood of implant subsidence in the postoperative period. Malplacement or migration of an unstable cage produces a risk or injury to adjacent vital structures. Additional stabilization with an anterior, posterior, or combined surgical construct should be performed to prevent cage migration, dislodgment, or pseudarthrosis (**Fig. 32.1**).

### Corpectomy

A Kerrison rongeur is first used to remove the pedicle and expose the lateral aspect of the spinal cord. A diskectomy of the adjacent intervertebral disks is then performed. The end plates of the adjacent vertebral bodies are carefully preserved to provide a solid support for the intervertebral cage implant. The anterior portion of the vertebral body is then removed with a rongeur or osteotome. The posterior wall of the vertebral body can be thinned with a high-speed burr and pushed away from the spinal cord with a small angled curette. The posterior longitudinal ligament can be removed to visualize the dura if indicated. In cases without infection or tumor, the bone from the corpectomy site is saved to use as graft to pack in and around the cage implant.

### Implant Placement

#### Nonexpandable Cages

Any deformity is manually corrected and the defect length is measured. An appropriate cage is selected and packed with bone graft or an appropriate substitute. The corpectomy site is distracted and gentle impaction of the cage is performed. If an expandable cage is chosen, the cage may be introduced into the defect in a collapsed state and lengthened to apply distraction to the spine at the corpectomy site (**Fig. 32.1**).

### Concerns

Ensure that proper placement of the cage is achieved with radiographs or fluoroscopy prior to the completion of the procedure.

### Bailout, Rescue, Salvage Procedures

If proper cage sizes are not available, use of either allograft bone (e.g., humerus, tibia, femur) or autogenous bone can be considered. If a stable anterior-only construct is not achievable, supplemental posterior instrumentation should be applied.

## 33

# Anterior Thoracic and Thoracolumbar Plating Techniques

*John T. Street and Marcel F. S. Dvorak*

### Description
Application of a low profile anterior/anterolateral plating system to the thoracic and thoracolumbar spine.

### Key Principles
Anterior thoracic and thoracolumbar plating systems provide additional stability by means of neutralization and load-sharing capacity when combined with reconstruction of the anterior and middle columns of the spine.

### Expectations
The primary function of anterior plating is to maintain the alignment of a short segment of the thoracic and thoracolumbar spine following direct anterior decompression of the neural elements. Secondary benefits include the stability provided to anterior interbody grafts, improved rates of surgical arthrodesis, minimizing the number of instrumented motion segments, and the avoidance of the need to augment with posterior instrumentation techniques.

### Indications
Thoracic and thoracolumbar segmental instability secondary to anterior and middle column incompetence. This instability is primarily the result of either complete diskectomy or corpectomy for fracture, tumor, infection, degeneration, iatrogenic injury, and failed previous stabilization surgery (either anterior or posterior) resulting in pseudarthrosis.

### Contraindications
The absolute contraindication to anterior plating techniques relates to the inability to obtain secure fixation of the implants in the adjacent vertebral bodies. This may be due to either disease involvement (infection, tumor) of adjacent vertebrae or to severe osteoporosis. Osteoporosis is known to disproportionately affect the cancellous bone of the vertebral bodies, and knowing this, the surgeon is advised to rely more on what cortical bone is preserved. In osteoporosis, posterior hook and wire fixation is preferred, whereas multisegment disease involvement by tumor or infection is optimally stabilized by adding posterior segmental fixation. Anterior plating techniques, functioning primarily as neutralization devices, require an intact posterior tension band (posterior spinal elements) and thus massive disruption of posterior elements by virtue of injury (flexion distraction fractures) or disease (tumor) make this technique less than ideal. The other major limitation of anterior plate fixation is the limited ability to correct deformity through this approach. Translational and rotational deformity cannot be corrected through anterior vertebral body manipulation, and thus these deformities are contraindications to this approach. Newly acquired kyphotic deformities, where there is "plasticity" in the posterior elements can be corrected through an anterior corpectomy, or release followed by the application of pure distraction through the anterior column. Stiff or long-standing kyphotic deformities require combined approaches and are not amenable to anterior plating alone. Relative contraindications include generalized or local osteopenia, pulmonary function prohibiting thoracotomy, and high risk of not being able to be weaned from the ventilator.

### Special Considerations
Detailed preoperative computed tomography (CT) and magnetic resonance imaging (MRI) is required for planning the surgical approach, decompression, reconstruction, and fixation. Preemptive estimation of plate size and bicortical screw lengths aids intraoperative decision making. Appreciation of three-dimensional anatomy, particularly that of the great vessels, is important. We have seen cases where plain radiographic images are initially interpreted to be vertebral osteomyelitis, which upon closer inspection of the CT scan images are clearly a mycotic aneurysm that has eroded into the vertebral bodies. Preoperative angiography may be indicated to identify the artery of Adamkiewicz. Thoracotomy allows access from T3 to T11. Right-sided thoracotomy is recommended due to the position of the aorta and the azygous vein. Rib resection should be performed one or two levels above the lesion. An extensile cervicothoracic approach should be considered for lesions cephalad to T5 (beware of the thoracic duct on left side and of the recurrent laryngeal nerve on the right). The 10th rib (Dwyer) thoracoabdominal approach, usually performed on the left side to avoid the liver, facilitates exposure cephalad to T11 and is extensile down to the L5 vertebral body.

### Special Instructions, Position, and Anesthesia

Surgery at the incorrect level is a major concern, often underestimated, in all anterior thoracic surgery. Advanced imaging such as CT and MRI often does not aid in the intraoperative determination of the correct level, where poor-quality intraoperative plain films do not facilitate rib visualization or counting up or down the spine. Plain anteroposterior (AP) and lateral scout films on CT or plain radiographs performed preoperatively are mandatory to determine the number of rib-bearing vertebrae, the number of lumbar vertebrae, and the levels of interest. Some techniques that have been used in particularly complex situations (e.g., the obese patient, or obscure anatomy) involve the placement of a needle under the skin, or contrast material in the vertebral body (similar to a vertebroplasty) at the desired operative level in the radiology suite prior to coming to the operating room. Double-lumen endobronchial intubation is required for thoracotomies to allow selective lung deflation. For thoracoabdominal approaches, the lung can simply be retracted and single lung ventilation is not required. Frequent, intermittent, intraoperative lung expansion reduces postoperative atelectasis. Intercostal nerve blocks should be administered under direct vision prior to any rib resection. Neurophysiologic monitoring is highly recommended for cases in which segmental arteries are to be sacrificed and decompressions performed.

Ensure that the patient is positioned in as true a lateral position as possible, to aid spatial orientation intraoperatively. An axillary roll should be used. The table may be flexed at the required thoracotomy level to aid access. When the patient is positioned, and prior to draping, an AP and cross-table lateral x-ray should be taken to aid in level identification and orientation. At this time the skin incision level corresponding to the required vertebral level should be clearly marked. These measures will help maintain orientation, optimize screw and plate position, and prevent iatrogenic segmental sagittal and coronal malalignment.

### Tips, Pearls, and Lessons Learned

During the approach, the segmental arteries can be temporarily clamped prior to ligation to determine if there is any alteration in motor evoked potential (MEP) or somatosensory evoked potential (SSEP) signals. The rib head inserts into the superior part of the corresponding vertebra and extends ventrally to obscure a significant portion of the dorsal disk space. The key to an adequate decompression is to resect the rib head, identify the neural foramen, and then proceed with decompression. Furthermore, resection of the rib heads facilitates true lateral positioning of the plate and screws. There is an inherent tendency to drift anteriorly and place the instrumentation in an anterolateral position, where it is more likely to contact the aorta. This is particularly risky in the more elderly patient with a tortuous aorta, which if it is adjacent to even smooth metal contours, can erode over time as it pulsates against a screw or plate. This has been known to cause fatal exsanguinations to occur in the early and late postoperative time frame. When rod-screw anterior fixation systems are used, great care must be exercised in cutting the rods and positioning them to avoid any sharp burrs or edges on the implants that may come in contact with vital intrathoracic structures. Bone graft may be obtained from the resected vertebral body or from the rib resected in the approach. This bone is often placed anteriorly under the anterior longitudinal ligament. In this position, it is visible on follow-up lateral radiographs as it consolidates into a fusion mass. The pleura may then be closed over the bone graft, plates, and screws to prevent intrathoracic migration of bits of bone graft.

### Difficulties Encountered

The most difficult screws to insert are often the screws in the most cephalad vertebra. The orientation of the end plate (following completion of the decompression) guides the screw trajectory and helps determine the screw length. In the presence of tumor, infection, or previous surgery, safe exposure of sufficient vertebral body may be challenging. If amenable, segmental vessels should be tied as well as clipped in case of inadvertent clip loss. During decompression and dissection in the neural foramen, Gelfoam, Avitene and other hemostatic agents should be available. Plate size constraints cephalad to T3 make an extended anterior cervical approach with sternal split and use of an anterior cervical plate preferable to high thoracotomies.

### Key Procedural Steps

Once exposure, decompression, and anterior and middle column reconstruction are complete, all bony protuberances (end-plate osteophytes, rib heads, etc.) should be removed to allow the fixation plate to sit easily on the flat surface of anterolateral vertebral body. Some plate designs, particularly those with "locking screws" do not facilitate lagging of the plate onto the lateral vertebral body cortex and thus positioning the plate along flat lateral cortical surfaces is critical to avoid a proud plate that sits off the bodies (**Fig. 33.1**). Many of the currently available anterior thoracic plating systems are gently curved to allow the best contour with the required thoracic kyphosis (**Fig. 33.2**). The holes to be used in the plate should now be identified and fixed with temporary fixation pins or Kirschner wires (K-wires). Intraoperative x-ray or fluoroscopy aids in ensuring optimum trajectory of the screws. Ensure that the screws are parallel to the end plates and angled to avoid inadvertent canal penetration. Most systems require the use of bicortical screws, and so care should be taken when passing probes or depth gauges to the far side of the vertebral body. Unicortical locking plate systems allowing ±5 degrees of screw insertion angulation are also available and are theoretically advantageous in situations of poorer bone quality. Screws should be placed in a convergent manner (anterior screws aimed slightly posterior and posterior screws aimed slightly anterior), to further enhance fixation (**Fig. 33.3**). As with all bridging plate systems, the plate should be fixed in

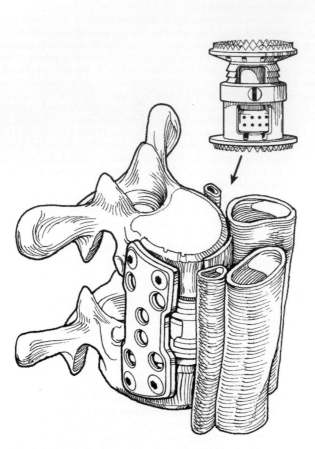

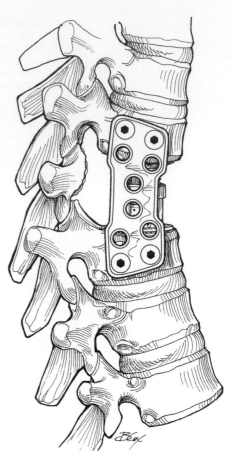

**Fig. 33.1** *Some plate designs do not facilitate lagging of the plate onto the lateral vertebral body cortex, and thus positioning the plate along flat lateral cortical surfaces is critical to avoid a prominent plate that sits off the bodies. Many of the currently available anterior thoracic plating systems are gently curved to allow the best contour with the required thoracic kyphosis.*

**Fig. 33.2** *Lateral view illustrating plate in-situ. Anterior thoracic or thoracolumbar plates provide neutralization and load-sharing capacity following vertebrectomy when combined with reconstruction of the anterior and middle columns of the spine.*

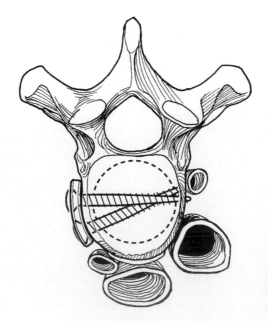

**Fig. 33.3** *Axial view illustrating how screws should be placed in a convergent manner (anterior screws aimed slightly posterior and posterior screws aimed slightly anterior), to further enhance fixation. Appreciation of three-dimensional anatomy, particularly that of the great vessels is important.*

## PITFALLS

- Intraoperative spatial orientation may be challenging and suboptimal screw fixation may result. Inadvertent fixation in excessive kyphosis must be avoided. Bicortical screw placement may result in inadvertent early or late vascular injury. Relative osteopenia must be recognized and adequate fixation achieved. The requirements to achieve biomechanical stability (adequate anterior and middle column reconstruction combined with adequate plate fixation) must be appreciated.

a compression mode across the interbody reconstruction. Prior to application of the plate, correct alignment must be achieved. Where the table has been aggressively flexed to facilitate exposure, this should be straightened. Furthermore, compression of the graft is often necessary and facilitated by some plate designs.

### Bailout, Rescue, Salvage Procedures

Remember: you can always abandon anterior fixation and reposition the patient for supplemental posterior fixation. If the deformity cannot be fully corrected from an anterior approach, if the end plates are significantly damaged, or if the biomechanical stability of the anterior construct is suspect, posterior fixation is always an option. By not inserting an anterior plate, further deformity correction can be achieved by means of a posterior osteotomy, but applying an anterior plate in poor alignment makes further posterior deformity correction impossible.

# 34

# Open Lumbar Microscopic Diskectomy

*David A. Wong*

### Description

The open posterior lumbar microscopic diskectomy provides a minimally invasive, often outpatient decompression of a nerve root compromised by a herniated nucleus pulposus. The operating microscope enhances illumination and visualization within the surgeon's visual field. This allows more precise identification of the pathology and other critical anatomic structures such as nerve roots and epidural veins. Superior orientation and careful handling of tissues minimizes the risks of intraoperative complications and postoperative problems such as scarring and instability. Integrating the fundamentals of anatomy, technology, and surgical technique in the open lumbar microscopic diskectomy establishes several critical skills. Mastery of these techniques opens the door to more advanced procedures such as the far lateral/ intertransverse diskectomy and the lumbar laminaplasty (bilateral decompression of the spinal canal via a unilateral surgical approach).

### Expectations

Most patients obtain significant relief of their radicular symptoms. If compression of neural structures is the dominant symptom generator, improvement may be seen in a matter of hours or days. However, inflammation in the nerve may take weeks to months to resolve, even once compression is removed. Axonal damage to the nerve already present at the time of surgery (usually correlating with a significant neural deficit on physical exam) may repair/regenerate over a year or more.

Diskectomy does not cure the patient's underlying degenerative changes. If mechanical back pain is part of the presenting symptom complex, the patient needs to be aware that this might persist and require long-term participation in a postoperative strengthening and stabilization program to optimize the surgical result. Rarely, mechanical factors of back pain or instability are sufficient so that fusion is a consideration.

Overall, a 50 to 75% reduction in symptoms, a 5 to 8% rate of recurrent disk herniation, and a 5% likelihood of future fusion are reasonable expectations for the patient and surgeon.

### Indications

Persistent radicular symptoms or signs despite 1 to 3 months of nonsurgical care are good clinical indications for surgery. Radicular findings should correlate to the pathology visualized on confirmatory imaging studies. More urgent surgical intervention may be considered in situations of severe, incapacitating symptoms, progressive neurologic deficit, or cauda equina syndrome. Back pain from a large central disk herniation is an indication for microdiskectomy.

### Contraindications

Conflicting symptoms and signs versus imaging studies is a situation for restraint. Significant nonorganic (Waddell's) findings, particularly in a scenario of minor radicular changes and minimal pathology on imaging, is a relative contraindication. Primary mechanical back pain is not likely to be significantly improved by diskectomy.

### Special Considerations

A key principle of successful microsurgery is the precise awareness of spinal anatomy. This bears on the preoperative analysis and localization of the patient's pathology as well as the intraoperative orientation of the surgeon. Pathology can be accurately localized by mentally mapping a grid to overlie the spinal canal **(Fig. 34.1)**. The horizontal lines of the grid corresponding to the inferior/superior direction are defined by McCulloch's first-, second-, and third-story house analogy. The first story is opposite the disk. The second story encompasses the lower half of the vertebral body with the foramen at its posterior aspect. The third story corresponds to the upper half of the vertebral body anteriorly with the solid, bony pedicle located posterior. Correlate the presence of disk fragments opposite the disk space versus foramen versus pedicle on the axial images to precisely locate pathology in a vertical orientation. The medial/lateral lines of the grid are laid out according to Macnab's system of central versus paramedial versus lateral recess versus foraminal versus far lateral location of disk herniation/root compression. The grid location L4-L5/R1P would thus describe a disk herniation at the L4-L5 segment, on the right side, first story vertically (opposite the disk space), and in the most common paramedial location. Pathology may encompass more than one grid area.

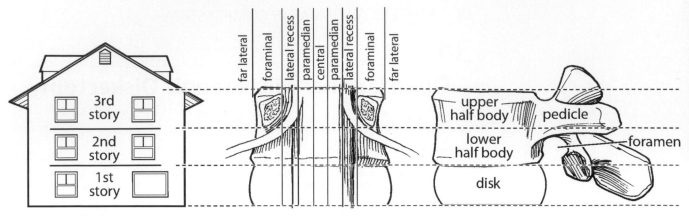

**Fig. 34.1** *Grid orientation to spine pathology.*

### Special Instructions, Position, and Anesthesia

Recognize that the first priority in any spinal procedure is to ensure that the proper surgical level is identified. The North American Spine Society (NASS) Sign, Mark, and X-Ray (SMaX) program outlines an appropriate protocol of patient identification, preoperative skin marking, and intraoperative x-ray confirmation of the pathologic segment.

### Tips, Pearls, and Lessons Learned

The ligamentum flavum is often hypertrophied as part of the pathologic process leading to a herniated disk. In the hypertrophied state, the ligamentum can be a visual barrier to precise identification of anatomic structures as well as a physical impediment to safe entry into the spinal canal. To obviate these problems, excise the superficial layers of the ligamentum separately. A plane of dissection can be found at the lower overflow attachment of the ligamentum to the top surface of the inferior lamina. The primary connection of the ligamentum is fixed to the leading surface of the inferior lamina. Hypertrophied ligamentum will generally expand posteriorly and mushroom up over the posterior, flat face of the lamina. Careful dissection with a small 2-0 or 3-0 curette with the blunt aspect against the flat of the inferior lamina usually defines the superficial layer for removal (**Fig. 34.2**). The remaining deep ligamentum can then be excised. Always release the attachment of the deep layer from the undersurface of the superior lamina first (with the ligamentum still under tension). A small cup curette is used to sweep under the lamina. This minimizes risk of dural tear. Releasing the inferior attachment first would slacken the ligament and require blind grasping under the superior lamina to remove the upper ligamentum. Blind use of a rongeur increases the risk of dural rents.

If the interlaminar space requires enlargement, this is best done with a side-cutting burr. Dural compromise is prevented by keeping the angle of the burr perpendicular to the dura so the noncutting tip is adjacent to vital structures (**Fig. 34.3**). A horizontal sweeping motion is used and an inward push is avoided. Take care to preserve the pars interarticularis. Bites from a Kerrison rongeur may produce stress fractures in the pars.

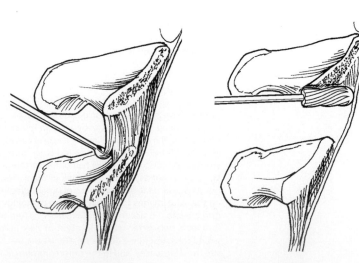

**Fig. 34.2** *Layered removal of hypertrophied ligamentum flavum.*

**Fig. 34.3** *Interlaminar space enlarged using a side-cutting burr.*

### Difficulties Encountered

Disorientation within the canal (e.g., struggles to identify the neural structures) and the disk is the problem with the most potential for catastrophe. Within the canal, orient yourself initially by identifying the pedicle (third story) immediately below the level of the herniated disk. The pedicle keys all the other principal anatomic landmarks (PALs). Recall that the traversing nerve root hugs the pedicle and then becomes the exiting root passing out the foramen below (**Fig. 34.4**). The root can be reliably found adjacent to the pedicle and additional neural structures dissected from this position. Be sure to adequately expose and identify the root and the lateral border of the dura both above the shoulder of the root and in the axilla of the root. One can be fooled by a medium to large disk herniation flattening the root over the apex of the herniation, making it look like an epidural vein and giving the mistaken impression that the lateral edge of the dura is the lateral border of the root. Cutting through that "vein" while attempting to incise the annulus does not "bleed" red blood but rather clear cerebrospinal fluid (CSF), leading to a permanent chronic neurologic deficit in the patient and an acute episode of heart failure in the surgeon. Once orientation is established and the neural structures identified, the preoperative grid outlining pathology can be mentally overlaid to ensure adequate decompression.

Epidural bleeding can first be avoided by early recognition of veins. Most of these can be swept out of the way superiorly, inferiorly, or laterally. Occasionally a vein traverses directly over the line of surgical dissection and will have to be isolated, bipolared, and cut. The use of even bipolar cautery is generally kept to a minimum to reduce the local inflammatory response, which might lead to postoperative scarring.

Dural tears can be avoided by using a small cup curette to carefully separate the dura and ligamentum flavum (often adherent or attached by vincula).

### Key Procedural Steps

In subligamentous disk herniations, a *T*-shaped incision into the annulus is preferred (**Fig. 34.5**). When inserting the pituitary into the disk space, visualize the tip of the pituitary passing below the top edge of the T on each pass. This ensures that the annulus is acting as a relative safety barrier against the posterior dura. A horizontal slit incision can be inadvertently extended medially, thus exposing the dura to potential harm (and illustrating Macnab's nickname for the up-biting pituitary: "the contralateral root nipper").

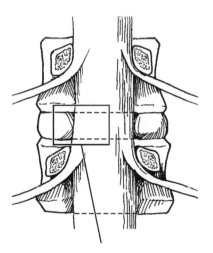
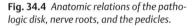

**Fig. 34.4** *Anatomic relations of the pathologic disk, nerve roots, and the pedicles.*

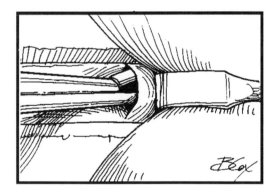

**Fig. 34.5** *T-incision in the annulus of the disk.*

### Bailout, Rescue, Salvage Procedures

The small microsurgical incision can be an impediment to resolution of several difficulties. The surgeon should have a low threshold for enlarging the incision if this enhances safety and effectiveness. For persistent epidural bleeding, a mix of powdered Gelfoam and thrombin can be injected into the wound. Be patient enough to wait a few minutes, by which time profuse bleeding usually has settled. The procedure-related life-threatening situation that, fortunately, is rarely encountered, is perforation of the great vessels by a deep bite with the pituitary during disk space evacuation. The same deterioration of the annulus that allows disk herniation into the canal can also affect the anterior annulus. One cannot rely on the annulus to be a stout physical barrier protecting the great vessels.

# 35

# Open Far Lateral Disk Herniation

*Ralph J. Mobbs and Charles G. Fisher*

### Description

A technique to access the nerve root and disk pathology lateral to the foramen for removal of a far lateral disk herniation.

### Key Principles

Midline or paramedian incision and an approach without entering the spinal canal to maintain the integrity of the facet joint and expose the nerve root (**Fig. 35.1** and **35.2**).

### Expectations

A hemilaminectomy and facetectomy may lead to poor long-term results for far lateral disk herniation surgery. Adapting a method to avoid issues of mechanical instability by approaching the impinged nerve root and disk lesion from lateral to the pars/facet joint will improve outcomes.

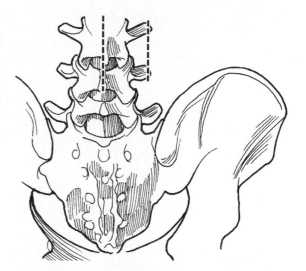

**Fig. 35.1** *Incision options include midline or paramedian. A midline approach requires a longer incision to expose far lateral to the TP and pars; however, it will be more "familiar" anatomy. A paramedian incision will be a shorter, muscle-splitting approach.*

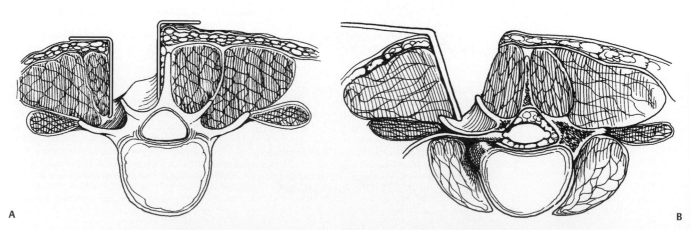

A                                                                                                                                        B

**Fig. 35.2** *(A,B) A midline incision results in a more painful muscle dissection and retraction combination. The paramedian incision is a more direct route to the pathology; however, it is an unfamiliar approach.*

## Indications
- Single-level radiculopathy secondary to far-lateral disk herniation
- Sensorimotor deficit or radicular pain—failure to improve with conservative care.

## Contraindications
- Pathology within the spinal canal
- L5-S1 far lateral disk lesion is difficult to approach from a lateral incision due to iliac crest; check with preoperative imaging first.
- Spondylolisthesis that requires fusion

## Special Considerations
If a far lateral disk herniation is suspected on computed tomography (CT), it can be confirmed with magnetic resonance imaging (MRI), including parasagittal views.

## Special Instructions, Position, and Anesthesia
Position the patient prone on a Wilson frame, Jackson spine table, or a 90/90 Andrews frame. Use x-ray or fluoroscopy to mark out the limits of the exposure *prior* to skin incision, and then reconfirm when landmarks are exposed. Illumination and magnification are paramount; use either a microscope or loupe/headlight combination. Endoscopy may be an option with tubular retraction devices.

## Tips, Pearls, and Lessons Learned
- The parasagittal T1 MRI reveals the extent of the foraminal pathology.
- If using a paramedian incision, find the plane between the multifidus and longissimus with finger dissection, and palpate the facet joints prior to retractor placement. The distance from the midline can be measured on the preoperative imaging.
- It is easy to "get lost" due to unfamiliarity with this exposure. Define bone landmarks in detail: transverse process (TP), pars, and facet joint.
- Elevate the intertransverse membrane from the inferior edge of the TP as it meets with the pars and then mobilize laterally and inferiorly.
- Always have a spine model in the operating room to orient yourself, as the anatomy can become confusing if you rarely perform a lateral exposure.

## Difficulties Encountered
- Bleeding down a deep hole: maintain strict hemostasis during initial exposure
- A consistent radicular vessel will be found lateral to the facet joint/pars: use bipolar cautery.
- The impinged nerve root may be effaced against the intertransverse membrane: care should be taken when elevating.
- If a large hypertrophied facet joint is overlying the nerve, be prepared to remove some lateral and superior joint for exposure.

## Key Procedural Steps
- Obtain x-ray *prior* to skin incision to define level.
- During muscle and bone dissection, preserve facet capsule.
- Key bone landmarks must be seen (**Fig. 35.3**): TP, pars, and facet joint. Reconfirm levels with x-ray when anatomic landmarks are exposed.

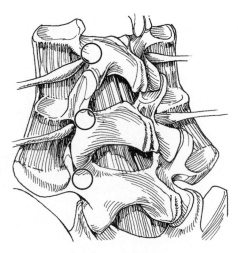

**Fig. 35.3** *After the initial exposure, the following landmarks must be seen before proceeding with nerve exploration. In this case, for a L3-L4 far lateral disk resulting in L3 nerve root impingement, the transverse process (TP) and pars of L3 must be clearly visualized. In addition, the L3-L4 facet joint and L4 TP should be seen to delineate the intertransverse membrane prior to incising this structure.*

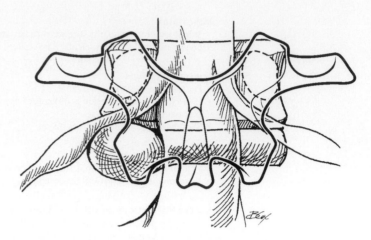

**Fig. 35.4** *Note the course of the L3 nerve root. Most far lateral disk herniations will push the nerve root superiorly against the L3 pedicle. Depending on the patients' individual anatomy, some bone from the pars and facet joint may require removal to clearly visualize the course of the L3 nerve root prior to disk removal.*

- Elevate the intertransverse membrane from the inferior aspect of the superior TP.
- Nerve location may be unpredictable and time consuming to dissect out (**Fig. 35.4**).
- Mobilize nerve superiorly to access disk herniation.

**Bailout, Rescue, Salvage Procedures**
If the anatomy is confusing, extend the incision to identify more normal anatomy especially medially, where you can work on either side of the pars and identify the root in a more familiar setting.

# 36

# Open Laminectomy, Medial Facetectomy, and Foraminotomy

*Mark A. Knaub and Jeffrey S. Fischgrund*

## Description
To safely perform decompression of the neural elements in the lumbar spine below the level of the conus medullaris without damage to the neurologic structures.

## Key Principles
Decompression of the spinal canal and foramen via laminectomy, partial facetectomy, and foraminotomy can be safely performed without injury to the neurologic structures and dural sac while maintaining the stability of the lumbar motion segments involved.

## Expectations
Decompressive laminectomy and facetectomy for spinal stenosis relieves symptoms of neurogenic claudication and radiculopathy in a vast majority of patients. Carefully performed surgery leads to few complications, a short hospital stay, and a rapid improvement in the patient's symptoms. Patients can expect to return to their activities of daily living in a relatively short period of time.

## Indications
Patients with neurogenic claudication or radiculopathy with confirmatory imaging studies documenting spinal stenosis.

## Contraindications
- Lack of neural element compromise on imaging studies
- Significant instability or deformity on imaging studies
- Local skin condition that would put patient at risk for postoperative wound infection (e.g., active eczema, burns, decubitus, or superficial infection)

## Special Considerations
Preoperative imaging studies must show evidence of neurologic compression that corresponds to the patient's symptoms and signs. A complete understanding of the local anatomy contributing to the patient's stenosis is mandatory to thoroughly decompress the neural elements. Elderly patients should have routine medical evaluation and optimization to lessen the likelihood of perioperative medical complications.

## Special Instructions, Position, and Anesthesia
Regional anesthesia via a spinal or general anesthesia can be utilized. The patient is placed in the prone position with the hips and knees flexed. Alternatively, the patient may be placed in a kneeling position. Flexion of the hips allows for straightening of the lumbar lordosis and opening of the interlaminar window, which will make decompression easier. For each of these positions the abdomen should hang free, which decreases the intraabdominal pressure and therefore the central venous pressure, leading to decreased engorgement of the epidural venous plexus. This decreases intraoperative blood loss. Careful positioning of the head and extremities should be employed to avoid iatrogenic neurologic injury or pressure-related problems. Special attention should be given to the eyes/orbits, especially when using general anesthesia.

If spinal anesthesia is employed the puncture must be cranial to the level of planned decompression if possible. A cerebrospinal fluid leak may develop postoperatively if the puncture site is uncovered by the decompression.

## Tips, Pearls, and Lessons Learned
Intraoperative imaging is mandatory to confirm the correct level of decompression. The use of anatomic landmarks can be helpful in many cases, but normal variants, such as sacralization of the lowest lumbar segment, may lead to confusion and ultimately to wrong-level surgery. Visualization can be enhanced with an operating microscope or with a combination of loupes and a fiber-optic head light.

If limited imaging studies are available, special care must be taken to avoid inadequate decompression. Computed tomography (CT) scans frequently only include from L3 to S1, so additional imaging may be necessary to ensure that the upper lumbar segments are not involved in the pathology. A double puncture technique may be necessary in patients with complete myelographic blocks to adequately assess the segments cranial to the block.

### Difficulties Encountered

Patients with severe stenosis or synovial cysts often have significant adhesions between the ligamentum flavum and the dural sac. Elderly patients tend to have a thinner, more fragile dural sac. Meticulous surgical technique should be employed to avoid an incidental durotomy.

### Key Procedural Steps

Once the levels to be included in the decompression have been identified with intraoperative imaging, the interspinous ligament of the involved segments is removed with a large Leksell rongeur. This rongeur is then used to remove half of the inferior spinous process and half of the most superior spinous process. After thinning the lamina with a rongeur or a high-speed burr, the central portion of the canal is decompressed (**Fig. 36.1**). Decompression is generally carried out from a caudal to cranial direction with Kerrison rongeurs. The ligamentum flavum may be temporarily left in place to protect the underlying dura. The location of the lateral edge of the pars interarticularis must be known to avoid iatrogenic pars removal or thinning of the pars, which may predispose the patient to a fracture.

Lateral recess decompression is performed by partial removal of the medial facets. This portion of the facet is removed with Kerrison rongeurs (**Fig. 36.2**). Alternatively, the medial aspect of the inferior articular facet may be removed with an osteotome or a high-speed burr. A portion of the underlying superior articular facet is then excised with a Kerrison. Lateral recess decompression is completed by removal of the ligamentum flavum and bone out to the level of the medial wall of the pedicle. Care must be taken to avoid violation of the pars interarticularis. Undercutting of the bone and, therefore, lateral recess decompression in general, is best accomplished by the surgeon operating from the opposite side of the table (**Fig. 36.3**).

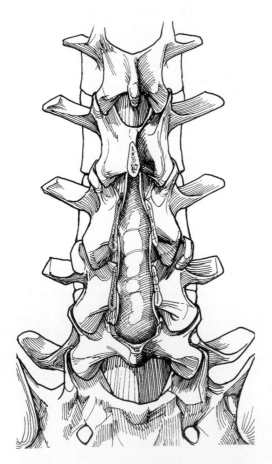

**Fig. 36.1** *A central laminectomy has been performed by removing the spinous process, central lamina, and the ligamentum flavum.*

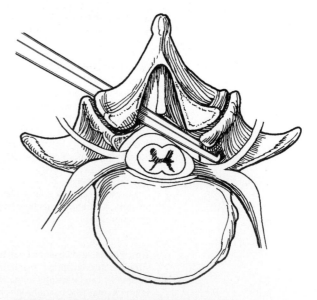

**Fig. 36.2** *Axial view of lateral recess decompression.*

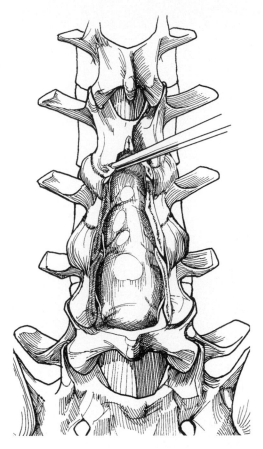

Fig. 36.3 *Lateral recess decompression is completed by removal of bone and ligamentum out to the level of the medial wall of the pedicle.*

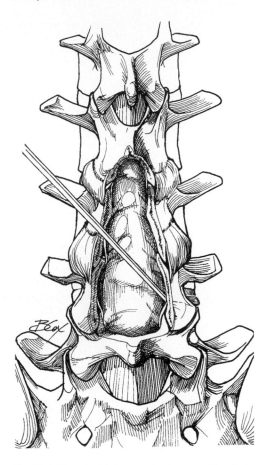

Fig. 36.4 *Foraminal decompression is assessed by placing a blunt dissector into the neural foramen.*

If foraminotomies are indicated, they, too, are best performed from the opposite side of the table. Identification of the adjacent pedicle will allow for visualization of the takeoff of the nerve root from the central dural sac. Once the nerve root is visualized the overlying osteophytes can be removed by placement of the Kerrison or curette dorsal to the exiting nerve root. A blunt dissector (i.e., a Woodson elevator) can be placed out into the foramen to confirm adequate decompression of the foramen (Fig. 36.4).

Hemostasis of the epidural venous plexus must be obtained prior to closure and may be accomplished with bipolar electrocautery or with various forms of collagen sponges with or without thrombin. These sponges are often removed before closure as they may expand and cause neurologic compression. Subfascial suction drains are not required for smaller procedures in which excellent hemostasis is obtained, but may be used in larger procedures or in patients with a history of bleeding problems.

### Bailout, Rescue, Salvage Procedures

If an incidental durotomy does occur, an attempt should be made to obtain a water-tight closure. We prefer primary closure of the dural defect with suture. If this is impossible, alternative techniques (e.g., synthetic collagen matrix or fibrin glue) must be employed.

# 37

# Lumbar Pedicle Screw Placement

*Robert W. Molinari*

## Description

To accurately place screws through the pedicles of the lumbar vertebrae with particular attention given to the avoidance of intraoperative and postoperative complications.

## Key Principles

Pedicles are short conical tubes with an oval cross section. The objective is to place the screws through the center of the pedicles and into the vertebral body. The screws should converge toward the midline to ensure that they do not penetrate the lateral wall of the vertebral body. Segmental instrumentation systems using lumbar pedicle screws are extremely effective in restoring and maintaining normal sagittal and coronal spinal alignment.

## Expectations

The goals of lumbosacral segmental instrumentation are to reduce deformity (such as that seen in scoliosis, spondylolisthesis, kyphosis, and trauma) and to provide stability. The pedicle is the strongest portion of the vertebra. Screws placed into the pedicles may provide rigid three-column fixation of the lumbar spine. Increasing construct rigidity enhances the chance for successful fusion and maintained spinal alignment.

## Indications

- Spondylolisthesis reduction
- Degenerative spondylolisthesis fusion
- Instability as a result of trauma or tumors
- Wide, destabilizing decompression
- Stabilization after osteotomy
- Posterior stabilization of degenerative disks
- Scoliosis correction and stabilization

## Contraindications

- Severe osteopenia
- Inadequate pedicle size or morphology
- Fractured or diseased pedicle

## Special Considerations

Patients with severe osteoporosis may not be suitable for lumbar pedicle screws. Bone density less than 0.45 g/cm$^2$ has been associated with pedicle screw loosening. Insertional torque will demonstrate the screw's degree of purchase in the bone. Undertapping, no tapping, and use of conical screws have been demonstrated to improve screw pullout strength. Approximately 75% of screw purchase is obtained in the pedicle. The screw should cross the midportion of the vertebral body in the lateral plane. Typically, 6-mm-diameter and 40- to 45-mm length screws are used. Screws that violate the anterior cortex of the vertebral body are not recommended due to the increased risk of vascular injury.

## Special Instructions, Position, and Anesthesia

A radiolucent table is imperative for proper anteroposterior (AP) and lateral intraoperative imaging during screw placement. Positioning the hips in extension improves lumbar lordosis. Fusing multiple segments of the lumbar spine with the hips positioned in flexion may cause iatrogenic flatback deformity. General anesthesia is used in patients for lumbar pedicle screw instrumentation.

## Tips, Pearls, and Lessons Learned

Appropriate positioning of the transpedicular screws in the lumbar spine is dependent on proper visualization of the posterior anatomic landmarks for insertion. Knowledge of the anatomy of the pedicle in relation to the neural structures is crucial. The nerve root is situated just medial and inferior to the pedicle as it exits into the intervertebral foramen. Violation of the pedicle cortex in this area may cause injury to the exiting nerve root.

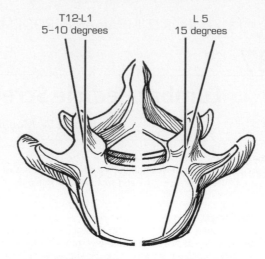

T12-L1
5–10 degrees

L 5
15 degrees

**Fig. 37.1** *Various entry points and inclinations have been described. A lateral converging approach spares the facets of the unfused levels.*

The entry point for the pedicle is at the intersection of a vertical line tangential to the lateral border of the superior articular process and a horizontal line passing through the middle of the insertion of the transverse process, or 1 mm below the joint line. The screws should be angled approximately 5 degrees medially at L1, 10 degrees at L2, and increasing to 15 degrees at L5 (**Fig. 37.1**). The amount of medial angulation of the pedicle varies depending on the level and on the surgeon's entry point location. Lateral entry points on the transverse process require greater medial angulation. Medially placed entry points on the superior facet may not require any medial angulation. Preoperative imaging studies should be used to determine the exact angulation, depth, and size of the pedicle. Intraoperative AP fluoroscopy will reliably identify the starting point's relation to the pedicle walls.

Continuous intraoperative fluoroscopy in the plane of the pedicle while simultaneously moving the ball tip feeler probe through the pedicle tract is a helpful technique to assess the accuracy of the screw trajectory. Electromyogram (EMG) monitoring is also of benefit in determining screw accuracy.

### Difficulties Encountered

Distortion of the posterior anatomy by the presence of a fusion mass, pseudarthrosis, or scar tissue may preclude the use of normal anatomic landmarks for screw insertion. The use of intraoperative fluoroscopy or a three-dimensional navigation imaging device may be helpful in these cases. Performing a laminotomy and feeling the medial, superior, and inferior borders of the pedicle is a technique that may enable accurate placement of pedicle screws in cases where imaging is compromised.

### Key Procedural Steps

Pedicle screw placement is analogous to intramedullary implant placement in a long bone. The point of entry to the pedicle is at the junction of the superior facet process, transverse process, and the pars interarticularis (**Fig. 37.2**). Placing a marker with AP imaging can be used to determine the location of the pedicle and its relation to the chosen starting point. The cortical bone overlying the entry point is removed with a burr, rongeur, or awl to expose the underlying cancellous bone. Next, the pedicle is probed with a gear shift–type pedicle probe having a tip similar to a dural elevator probe (**Fig. 37.3**). The passage is directed from lateral to medial to accommodate the transverse plane angulation of the pedicle. This is typically 15 degrees in the lower lumbar spine and 0 to 10 degrees in the upper lumbar spine. A lateral starting hole usually requires

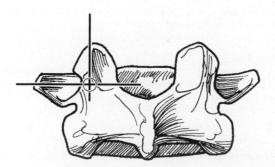

**Fig. 37.2** *The entry point for the pedicle is at the intersection of a vertical line tangential to the facets and a horizontal line bisecting the transverse process. Screw convergence increases as one moves caudally.*

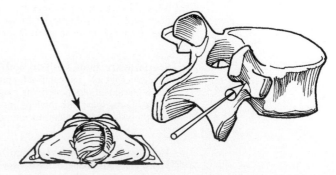

**Fig. 37.3** *After a blunt pedicle probe or curette is used to initiate the screw tract, the tract is tapped.*

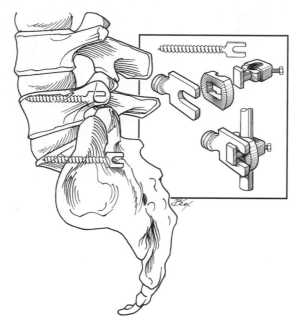

**Fig. 37.4** *Lateral view demonstrating proper placement of pedicle screws. Screws should parallel the end plate or angle slightly upward.*

## PITFALLS

- Malposition of the screw may cause injury to surrounding structures. Medial and inferior placement may injure the exiting nerve root. Excessive medial placement may cause dural tearing. Overpenetration may injure the vascular and visceral structures anteriorly. Pedicle fracture may occur with aggressive use of the pedicle probe or by placement of an oversized pedicle screw.

more medial angulation, and a medial starting point may not require any angulation of the pedicle probe. The pedicle is oval, with the larger diameter being vertical. This allows for variable angular positioning of the probe in the sagittal plane (**Fig. 37.4**). The motion of a swirl or a wiggle is used to advance the pedicle probe gently through the cancellous center of the pedicle and vertebral body. If resistance is suddenly lost during insertion, the probe has almost certainly violated the pedicle wall. The probe should be removed and the hole palpated with a semiflexible ball tip feeler probe to determine whether penetration has been medial, lateral, superior, or inferior. After this has been ascertained, the pedicle probe can be properly redirected into the pedicle isthmus. Probing the four walls and the floor of the hole with the ball tip probe is a good way to determine the accuracy of the screw tract. Placing a marker in the pedicle and obtaining AP and lateral radiographs also helps to determine tract position (**Fig. 37.5**). If screw tract tapping is desired, the isthmus of the hole should be tapped with a tap that has a slightly smaller diameter than the screw.

### Bailout, Rescue, Salvage Procedures

Placement of a larger-diameter screw sometimes will serve as an appropriate rescue technique. If a cortical breech has not occurred, a small amount of polymethylmethacrylate may be inserted into the screw tract to improve purchase. If the posterior elements are present, a laminar hook or sublaminar wires may be used in place of a pedicle screw. Other options include adding another level of fixation, or not using additional instrumentation and relying on the contralateral instrumentation. Lastly, removal of instrumentation and performing an uninstrumented fusion may be appropriate in some cases.

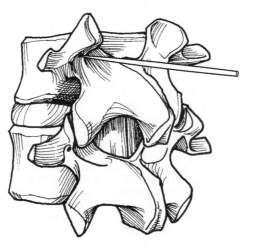

**Fig. 37.5** *If in doubt, a marker (such as a Kirschner wire) may be placed.*

# 38

# Transforaminal and Posterior Lumbar Interbody Fusion

*Todd J. Albert and Peter M. Fleischut*

## Description

The goal of transforaminal lumbar interfusion (TLIF) is to safely access the interbody area without significant dural retraction. This allows one to effectively fuse both anteriorly and posteriorly through a posterior only approach. Posterior lumbar interbody fusion (PLIF) achieves similar goals through a bilateral, more medial approach. PLIF requires more dural retraction than TLIF, which is essentially a far lateral PLIF.

## Key Principles

Anterior interbody support facilitates deformity correction, increased fusion rate, and disk space distraction, as well as at least unilateral if not bilateral direct foraminal decompression and traversing nerve root decompression.

## Expectations

An improved fusion rate compared with a posterior lateral intertransverse process fusion. A PLIF or TLIF at the end of a long fusion decreases the risk pseudarthrosis due to improved anterior column support.

## Indications

Isthmic spondylolisthesis (grades 1 to 4), junctional degeneration adjacent to a fusion mass, degenerative disk disease, recurrent disk herniation with significant back pain, the terminal end of long fusion requiring interbody fusion, short segment degenerative scoliosis, postlaminectomy spondylolisthesis.

## Contraindications

Severe osteopenia, bleeding disorders, and active infection.

## Special Considerations

Preoperative imaging studies including anterior/posterior and flexion/extension lumbosacral spine radiographs are necessary. Additionally, magnetic resonance imaging (MRI) or computed tomography (CT) myelography is necessary for understanding the anatomy and planning the surgical approach (left versus right or unilateral exposures). At times for discogenic back pain, diskography, though controversial, can be useful in determining the level of the pain generator.

## Special Instructions, Position, and Anesthesia

The patient should be placed prone with the abdomen decompressed. An Andrews frame is generally used for L4–sacrum exposures. For longer approaches such as adult deformity, a Jackson table is used. Triggered electromyography (EMG) recording can be used to test the accuracy of pedicle screw placement. Free-run EMG recording can be used during insertion of transforaminal lumbar interbody fusion grafts or cages to ensure that undue traction or injury is avoided to the exiting or traversing nerve roots.

## Tips, Pearls, and Lessons Learned

Complete radical diskectomy requires use of multiple interbody instruments including angled curettes and osteotomes (straight and angled and double-angled chondrotomes to scrape the end plates and remove the maximum amount of disk material from one side to the other if a unilateral approach is used [TLIF]). Special intervertebral distraction devices are helpful. In the TLIF procedure, the inferior articular process of the vertebra above is taken off to gain access to the transforaminal area and the superior articular process of the vertebra below is skeletonized to maximize the transforaminal opening. Bullet distractors are an optimal distraction instrument to obtain maximum annulotaxis. A large lamina spreader placed between the spinous processes also assists in disk space distraction, though this method risks a kyphosing force on the disk space. This technique of overdistraction is helpful when placing a banana-shaped cage through a unilateral TLIF approach and is often not necessary in a bilateral PLIF cage approach.

For interbody grafting, various approaches can be applied. Carbon fiber, metallic, or poly-ether-ether-ketone (PEEK) type cages in rectangular, bulleted, or banana shapes can be used. Maximum lordosization is achieved by placing the cage, especially a banana-shaped cage, in the anterior part of the disk space. Finally, with the anterior interbody device anteriorly situated, a compressive force is placed across the pedicle screw instrumentation to enhance lordotic alignment. Hemostasis is obtained by using bipolar cautery in the area just medial to the pedicle and in the axilla of the exiting nerve root where the majority of work is to be done.

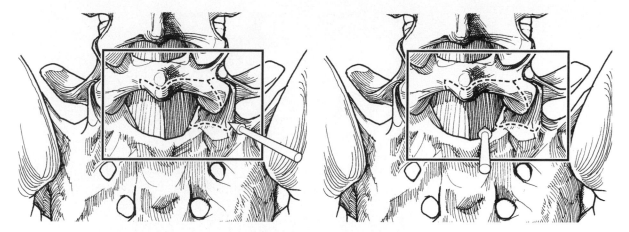

**Fig. 38.1** *Bony areas to be resected for transforaminal lumbar interfusion (TLIF) **(A)** and posterior lumbar interbody fusion (PLIF) **(B)**.*

### Difficulties Encountered

Significant bleeding can occur during these procedures, and there may at times be difficulty with interspace distraction. In cases with excessive bleeding, or with difficulty with interspace distraction, a nonstructural graft may be used.

### Key Procedural Steps

- For a TLIF procedure, a straight osteotome is used to create a laminotomy defect, removing a portion of the inferior lamina of the vertebra above and transecting the pars to remove the entire inferior articular process. In a PLIF procedure, the pars is preserved and a partial facetectomy is performed to allow for adequate clearance for bilateral cage or graft placement (**Fig. 38.1**).
- For a TLIF procedure the superior articular process of the vertebra below is removed with the straight osteotome or large rongeur and the pedicle skeletonized with a 4-mm Kerrison rongeur. For a PLIF procedure the lateral pars is protected and the medial border of the pedicles of the caudal vertebral body are exposed. Bipolar cautery is used again to maximally cauterize the epidural veins if necessary just medial to the pedicle of the vertebra below. Minimal retraction is performed at the shoulder of the traversing nerve root to give access to the annulus or transforaminal area in the TLIF procedure. With a PLIF, neural retraction is performed to the degree necessary to allow cage or graft placement (**Fig. 38.2**).

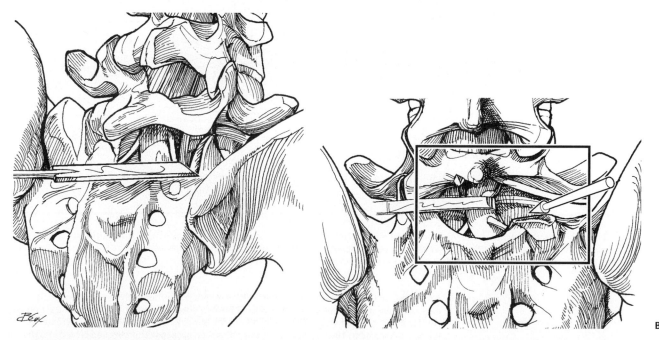

**Fig. 38.2** *Transforaminal area after bone resection. **(A)** The superior articular process of the vertebra below is removed with the straight osteotome or large rongeur. **(B)** Minimal retraction is performed at the shoulder of the traversing nerve root to give access to the annulus or transforaminal area in the TLIF procedure. (Continued on page 134)*

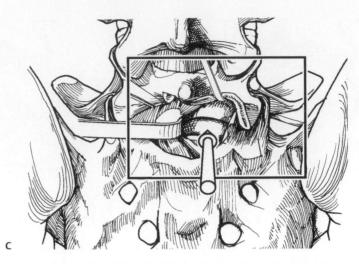

**Fig. 38.2** *Continued* **(C)** *With a PLIF, neural retraction is performed to the degree necessary to allow cage or graft placement.*

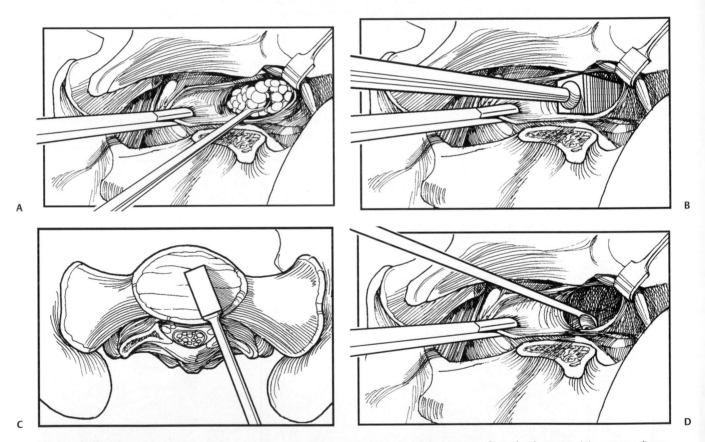

**Fig. 38.3** *Radical diskectomy with curette.* **(A)** *A sharp annulotomy is created and a radical diskectomy is performed with curettes.* **(B)** *Interspace distractors are used in a serial manner (6 to 12 mm) to obtain adequate disk space distraction between curettaging of the disk space.* **(C)** *Distractor in the TLIF approach.* **(D)** *The end plate may be punctured in several regions to create bleeding for fusion enhancement.*

- A sharp annulotomy is created and a radical diskectomy is performed with curettes (**Fig. 38.3**). Interspace distractors are used in a serial manner (6 to 12 mm) to obtain adequate disk space distraction between curettaging of the disk space. The end plate may be punctured in several regions to create bleeding for fusion enhancement. The interbody cage or graft is then packed with a filler and placed into the anterior disk space under either fluoroscopy or direct vision (**Fig. 38.4**).  Autogenous bone is then packed laterally and posterior to the cage or graft. Pedicle screws, previously placed or placed at this point, are then compressed and are fixed with longitudinal members. An intertransverse fusion is also often performed.

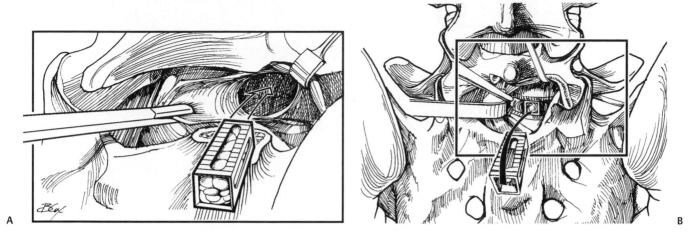

**Fig. 38.4** *(A) TLIF: autogenous bone is then packed laterally and posterior to the cage or graft. (B) PLIF: the cage is inserted from directly posterior and similarly packed with autogenous bone.*

PITFALLS

• Potential for excessive bleeding in the axilla of the exiting nerve root and medial to the pedicle, inability to distract the interspace adequately, violation of the end plate, and lack of parallel graft/cage placement to the disk space.

**Bailout, Rescue, Salvage Procedures**
If violation of the end plate occurs or the graft is placed into the body and not parallel to the interspace, the structural graft should be removed and autologous graft should be placed morselized and aggressively packed into the interspace.

# 39

# Facet Screw Placement

*Eeric Truumees*

## Description
To safely stabilize a lumbar motion segment by placing screws across the facet joint.

## Key Principles
Translaminar facet screw (TLFS) fixation passes cortical screws, 50 to 60 mm in length by 4.5 mm in diameter, through the lamina into the facet via a 4-cm percutaneous approach. TLFSs are the lowest profile and least expensive of all posterior lumbar implants. Thus, the additional cost, bulk, muscular irritation and stripping, superior segment facet injury, and neurologic risk engendered by transpedicular instrumentation are avoided.

## Expectations
Both anterior lumbar interbody (ALIF) and posterolateral lumbar (PLF) fusions are commonly utilized in the operative management of a wide variety of lumbosacral conditions. Given the high loads and limits of external immobilization, pseudarthrosis and clinical failure are common without instrumentation. As with other forms of lumbosacral fixation, TLFSs provide stability, thereby increasing the chance of successful fusion. These screws render the treated motion segment at least 2.4 times as stiff as an uninstrumented segment. In particular, TLFSs provide equal rotational and extension stability to transpedicular constructs. On the other hand, TLFSs are less strong in flexion. In that their mechanical strengths and weaknesses are exactly the opposite, they are ideally paired with cage reconstruction of the anterior column.

## Indications
Translaminar facet screws may be employed alone or as an adjunct to other forms of anterior or posterior instrumentation. Used alone, TLFSs are most commonly indicated for adjunctive fusion in stenosis patients with spondylolisthesis undergoing limited fenestration/laminotomy procedures. In some cases, the pedicles themselves are too small. Their use has been described in the stabilization of patients with pure ligamentous instability and in the management of pseudarthrosis in "stand-alone" ALIF patients.

Translaminar facet screws may also be used as an adjunct to a transpedicular construct. For example, in multilevel reconstructions to the sacrum, screws into the wide sacral "pedicle" may provide inadequate fixation and construct failure may result. TLFSs may be used, with or without other adjunctive measures (e.g., anterior column support or alar screws), to improve segmental fixation at the lumbosacral junction.

Most typically, TLFSs are used as an adjunct to cage fixation in patients undergoing ALIF (**Fig. 39.1**). While ring allografts and threaded, vertical mesh or horizontal interbody cages are ideal in resisting compressive, axial forces, they are inadequate in the neutralization of side bending, rotational, and extension forces. TLFSs function extremely well as an adjunct to these forms of anterior reconstruction by "locking in" the posterior elements.

## Contraindications
The most common contraindications include insufficient bone stock or excessive spinal instability. TLFSs rely on adequate purchase to the laminae, facets, and transverse processes. Marked osteopenia, lamina fracture, or excessive bone removal during decompression render the screws mechanically ineffective and are thus contraindications to their placement.

At this point, safety and efficacy data for TLFS are available for limited indications. In that each segment is immobilized individually, and there are no intersegmental connections, their effectiveness in fusions greater than two levels remains to be demonstrated.

In patients with significant instability or those who require reduction maneuvers, these implants are not indicated. For example, used alone, TLFSs do not provide adequate fixation in patients with isthmic or lytic spondylolisthesis, scoliosis, or in those with marked segmental kyphosis. TLFSs should not be used as stand-alone fixation in patients undergoing extension of a previous lumbar fusion.

## Special Considerations
With experience, these screws are easy to place safely and quickly. However, careful attention to operative technique leads to more satisfactory outcomes. Limit the midline exposure to protect the paraspinal muscles. In the exposed region, clear off the lamina in its entirety to delineate its superior and inferior extent. Particularly if a decompression is to be performed, close assessment of the bone available will assist in planning both the decompression and subsequent TLFS placement. Similarly, remove the entire facet capsule and resect facet osteophytes. Denude the facet cartilage while protecting the subchondral bone. This enables clear identification of the drill as it passes in a biomechanically favorable perpendicular direction through the center of the facets joint.

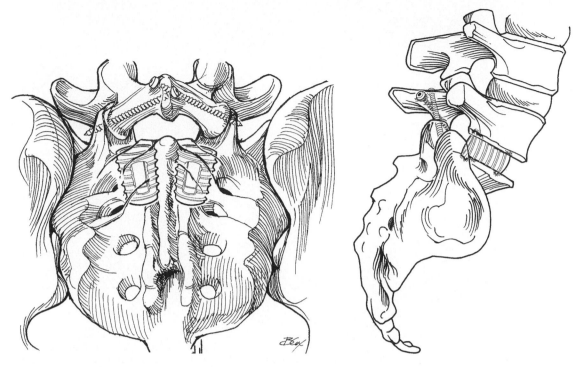

A                                                                                                                          B

**Fig. 39.1** *Anteroposterior (AP)* **(A)** *and lateral* **(B)** *images of a patient after an endoscopic ALIF performed with paired threaded fusion cages and a posterior TLFS placement using cannulated screws.*

Several implant systems are now Food and Drug Administration (FDA) approved for use as TLFS. While these systems are more expensive than the typical long-bone trauma screws, they are often available in titanium, which improves postoperative imaging.

### Special Instructions, Position, and Anesthesia
General anesthesia is used for most cases. In some cases, particularly when no posterolateral fusion is intended, spinal anesthesia may be recommended. Careful attention to positioning is critical. Failure to note hip flexion contractures and appropriate lordosis when positioning on the table may produce iatrogenic flatback deformity. TLFSs cannot be used in patients who require formal reduction maneuvers. On the other hand, some spinal flexion or extension may be introduced by compressing or distracting the spinous processes during drill passage.

### Tips, Pearls, and Lessons Learned
An oscillating drill has been recommended to decrease the possibility of wrapping up soft tissues. When placing the first screw, remember that another screw will be placed and space the entry point accordingly. That is, the first screw may have to be slightly more cranial than ideal and the second slightly more caudal. Because facet screws are placed essentially under direct vision, advanced imaging modalities are not required. Several manufacturers sell special guides for TLFS drill passage (**Fig. 39.2**). Most surgeons use these guides only for their first few cases and employ a "freehand" technique thereafter. Some surgeons place a feeler under the lamina during drill passage to act as a proprioceptive guide. Others have placed cannulated screws after drilling and tapping over a guide.

### Difficulties Encountered
Complications are uncommon. Lamina or facet fracture or other posterior element deficiency may be encountered, necessitating conversion to transpedicular instrumentation. Dural lacerations are repaired in the standard fashion.

### Key Procedural Steps
Fluoroscopic level localization allows minimization of the midline incision. Extend the subperiosteal dissection of the paraspinous muscles to base of the transverse processes. If no ALIF has been performed, extend the exposure to the tips of the transverse processes to create a trough for graft material. Protect the capsules of nonfused segments.

Resect the facet capsule and prepare the facet surface as above. Create a small depression in the base of the spinous process with a 3-0 bur. A guide-pin or a freehand technique may be used to estimate the

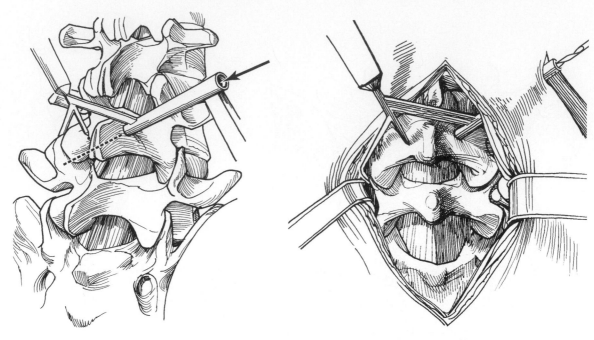

A                                                                                          B

**Fig. 39.2** *(A) The guide is positioned to allow the drill to pass from the base of the spinous process through the lamina, across the facet. The drill should emerge where the transverse process meets the pedicle. (B) Note the use of a second, more lateral stab incision to minimize the soft tissue stripping necessary for screw insertion.*

PITFALLS
- Dural tear
- Nerve root injury
- Vascular injury
- Spinous process or laminar fracture

required drill entry-point. A separate stab incision is made and blunt dissection is performed to allow passage of a 3.2-mm drill in its soft tissue protector to the base of the spinous process.

Drill through the base of the spinous process into the contralateral lamina aiming for the midpoint of the contralateral facet. Ultimately, a very flat trajectory is sought parallel to the lamina and nerve root. As depicted, guides are available, or a feeler may be used to palpate the transverse process and inferior laminar edge, thereby directing drill passage.

Next, palpate the tract with a depth gauge checking screw length and for cortical cut out. The appropriate 4.5-mm cortical screw is then inserted. At the L5-S1 level, a longer screw may be extended into the sacral ala. Tap the screw tract with a cortical tap. Do not attempt to "lag" the facet by overdrilling proximally. Lag technique will risk fracture of the posterior elements. A second screw is then inserted in the same manner from the opposite direction (**Fig. 39.3**). Surgeons working alone have to cross to the other side of the operating table.

**Bailout, Rescue, Salvage Procedures**
Any significant difficulty with placement or stability of facet screws should prompt early conversion to transpedicular instrumentation.

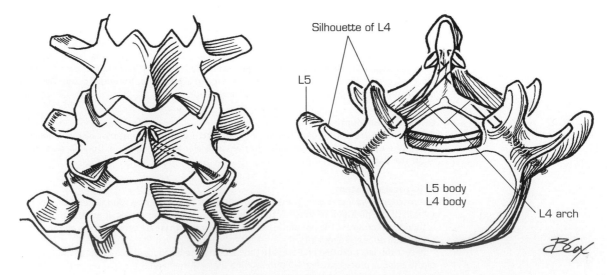

A                                                                                          B

**Fig. 39.3** *(A) Posterior view with both screws in place. (B) Axial view demonstrating proper screw placement.*

# 40

# Intra-Iliac Screw/Bolt Fixation

*James S. Harrop, Shiveindra Jeyamohan, and Alexander R. Vaccaro*

### Description

Intra-iliac screw placement entails a pelvic screw anchor used to fixate the lumbosacral spine to the pelvis for stability and deformity correction in long or multisegmental fusions, high-grade spondylolisthesis, of pelvic obliquity deformity correction.

### Key Principles

Posterior intra-iliac fixation provides a biomechanical advantage over sacral instrumentation through secure anchors in the pelvis. The screws cross anterior to the sagittal vertical axis or sagittal plumb line without violating the sacroiliac joints.

### Expectations

Intra-iliac fixation provides a solid distal foundation (pelvis) for the correction of spinal deformities, long spinal constructs, or high-grade spondylolisthesis.

### Indications

- Long thoracic and lumbar fusions extending to the pelvis (e.g., scoliosis, trauma, low lumbar osteotomy)
- Neuromuscular scoliosis correction with pelvic obliquity
- Reconstruction procedures after sacrectomies
- Fixation for unstable sacral fractures
- Adjunct posterior stabilization method for high-grade lumbar spondylolisthesis
- Salvage procedures for revision lumbosacral operations

### Contraindications

- Active spinal infection
- Pelvis insufficiency (i.e., extensive previous iliac crest bone graft harvesting)

### Special Considerations

Need for plain radiographs of the thoracolumbar spine including standing long cassette views (36-inch) to evaluate coronal and sagittal balance. Plain radiographs of the pelvis as well as dynamic lateral flexion and extension images of the lumbar spine. In revision cases, particularly ones where there was prior posterior iliac crest bone graft harvest, a computed tomography (CT) scan of the pelvis provides further information.

### Special Instructions, Position, and Anesthesia

- Patients are placed in the prone position on a Jackson-type frame, taking care to prevent excessive pressure on bony protuberances and the orbits.
- Operating table should maintain desired sagittal alignment with physiologic lumbar lordosis (e.g., four-post bed, Jackson table).
- A radiolucent operating table provides for the use of intraoperative fluoroscopy.

### Tips, Pearls, and Lessons Learned

Placement of the iliac screw from the contralateral side of the table provides for a more optimal sense of screw trajectory. An osteotomy or harvesting bone from the posterior iliac crest can result in weakening of the insertion site. Therefore, bone graft harvesting should be planned after iliac screw placement.

Intraoperative fluoroscopy or plain radiographs can evaluate the final position of screw placement:

- Sciatic notch: obturator oblique view
- Hip joint: pelvic inlet and outlet views
- Medial wall: iliac oblique view
- Lateral wall: difficult to detect by plain radiographs/fluoroscopy

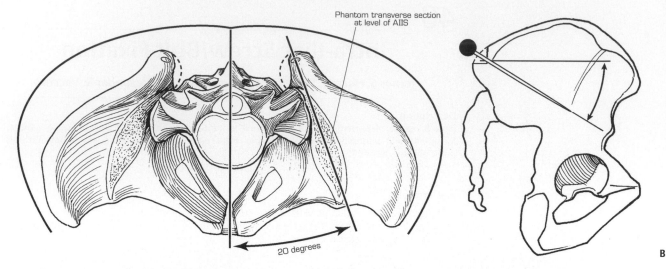

**Fig. 40.1** *Trajectories for canalization of the iliac screws.* **(A)** *Transverse plane. AIIS, anterior-inferior iliac spine.* **(B)** *Sagittal plane.*

- Screw length is typically less than 90 mm. A greater length may penetrate into the hip joint. Screw diameter:
  - Males: 8-mm implants
  - Females: 6- to 7-mm implants

Placement of S1 screws should be done prior to iliac screws placement. This provides for an accurate assessment of screw-to-screw distance and optimal iliac screw to facilitate construct assembly.

### Difficulties Encountered
- Breach of the cortical surfaces with the screw placement.
- Medial cortical wall penetration may result in injury to intrapelvis neurovascular structures, specifically the lumbosacral plexus.
- Violation of the sacral notch
  - May result in injury to the sciatic nerve
  - Injury to superior gluteal artery with subsequent retroperitoneal hematoma formation and blood loss
- Prominence of hardware with pressure ulceration formation and subsequent infection.

### Key Procedural Steps
Surgical exposure is performed with a posterior midline incision down to the spinous processes of the lumbosacral junction. The posterior superior iliac crest can be palpated and the erector spinae muscles are dissected from the midline in a medial to lateral direction in a subperiosteal manner to the medial border of the iliac crest, taking care not to disrupt its distal insertion to maintain muscle viability and prevent the formation of a dead space. The soft tissues (gluteal muscle attachments) on the lateral iliac crest wall are dissected off the ilium in a subperiosteal manner to allow finger palpation of the sciatic notch. The starting point for iliac screw placement is often the distal prominence of the posterior superior iliac crest, which is anatomically located directly lateral to the S2 pedicle (**Fig. 40.1** and **40.2**). Precise screw starting point, however, is guided by the location of the sciatic notch, which is felt during screw path development.

A modification of this method of screw insertion, as developed by Vaccaro, begins the screw starting point along the medial border of the posterior iliac crest using a 5-mm burr to expose the intra-iliac cancellous bone (**Fig. 40.3**). This allows the polyaxial screw head of the iliac bolt to project medially over the sacrum, which obviates the need for a lateral connector rod to mate the longitudinal component (spinal rod) with the iliac screw. Once the starting point is chosen and developed, a blunt joystick is used to develop a screw path in a general trajectory of 20 degrees lateral to midsagittal plane and 30 to 35 degrees caudal to the transverse plane toward the anterior superior iliac spine (**Fig. 40.1**). Actual screw insertion trajectory is guided through tactile finger palpation of the sciatic notch with the goal of screw passage within 1.5 to 2 cm above the sciatic notch. The sciatic notch is made of thick cortical bone above which a narrow isthmus exists for screw passage. Therefore, if resistance is met to probe or screw placement, then the trajectory must be modified. The intended screw path is confirmed with a ball probe to detect any cortical breaches. The iliac screw is then inserted. The head of the polyaxial screw is assessed in relationship to the surrounding posterior iliac crest bone and soft tissues to make sure it is not prominent. Fluoroscopy can be utilized to further assess and adjust screw placement.

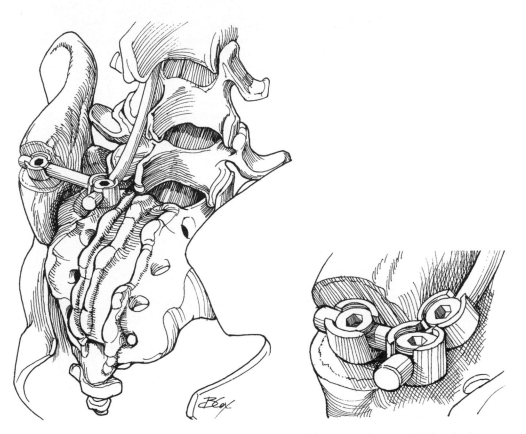

**Fig. 40.2** *(A)* *Traditional iliac screw placement.* *(B)* *Note the removal of the posterior iliac spine, which makes for a more lateral connection to the lumbar pedicle screw system.*

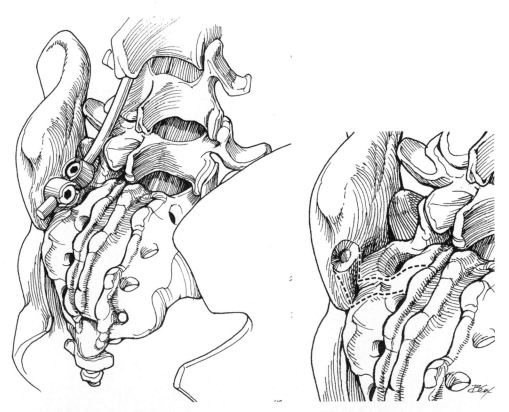

**Fig. 40.3** *(A)* *Medial iliac screw placement.* *(B)* *The utilization of a starting point that is located at the S2 pedicle provides for a straight connection to the lumbar pedicle screws, making the construct assembly easier.*

PITFALLS
- Violation of the cortical boundaries
- Inability to advance probe
- Placement of screws into the hip joint

**Bailout, Rescue, Salvage Procedures**

A cortical breach can be detected by a change in the joystick or pelvic probe resistance. This defect can be confirmed with a ball probe or sound. The defects are typically in the lateral wall prior to entering the sciatic notch. If the sciatic notch was not initially palpated, then subsequent dissection and palpation will further define the correct screw trajectory. The utilization of fluoroscopy may be of further assistance.

Inability to pass the probe can occur with contact with the thick cortical bone margins typically around the sciatic notch. Reconfirming and modifying the trajectory of the approach typically resolves this issue. Again fluoroscopy may be of further assistance.

Passage of the probe into the hip joint is detected with a void at the distal end of the hollowed intended screw path. This typically does not occur with placement of an iliac screw shorter than 8 cm in a male and 6 cm in a child or women. Fluoroscopy with pelvic inlet and outlet views demonstrates this region and can confirm screw location in relation to the hip joint.

# 41

# Iliosacral Screw Fixation Techniques

*Paul T. Rubery and John T. Gorczyca*

## Transiliac Rod Placement

### Description
A bar or rod placed transversely through the posterior iliac tubercles, posterior to the sacrum, can serve as a safe and reliable distal anchor for complex instrumentation constructs across the lumbosacral junction.

### Key Principles
Force concentration at the junction of the relatively mobile lumbar spine with the relatively immobile pelvis is a significant cause of spinal instrumentation failures. The relatively poor bone stock of the sacrum compromises pedicle screw fixation. Additional anchor points enhance fixation and may decrease the incidence of instrumentation failure and pseudarthrosis.

### Expectations
This technique provides additional, extraspinal fixation into relatively strong bone.

### Indications
Instrumentation constructs extending proximal to L2 and crossing the lumbosacral junction. The technique can be applied in clinical situations involving particularly high-grade instability at L5-S1, as well as pseudarthroses of previous L5-S1 fusions.

### Contraindications
Deficiency or absence of posterior iliac bone precludes rod placement.

### Special Considerations
A preoperative computed tomography (CT) scan of the pelvis is useful to assess the adequacy of the ilium for passing the transiliac rod. Specially manufactured connectors may be required to join the transversely oriented transiliac rod to the longitudinal member of the spinal instrumentation.

### Special Instructions, Position, and Anesthesia
The surgeon should carefully position the patient's hips to preserve or reconstruct the normal sagittal contours of the spine.

### Tips, Pearls, and Lessons Learned
- It is occasionally necessary to remove the medial portion of the bony posterior ridge of the sacrum to pass the transverse rod from side to side.
- Connection of the transverse rod to the longitudinal member of the construct is challenging, and may require specially ordered or custom-manufactured components. This is especially true in revision surgery. Furthermore, this process requires generous elevation of the gluteus maximus origin from the crista glutei to preserve its fascia for repair over the hardware.
- Structural interbody support placed in the L5-S1 disk will reduce strain on the posterior instrumentation.
- Iatrogenic sagittal plane deformity (flatback) is an inherent risk of this instrumentation technique, and surgeons must be especially cognizant of the sagittal plane.

### Difficulties Encountered
- Locating the transverse bar too proximally hinders connection to the L5 and S1 screws.
- Inadequate bone posterior in the posterior ilium may lead to iliac channel fracture.
- Prominent hardware with thin overlying tissues places the patient at risk for wound problems and for symptomatic hardware.

### Key Procedural Steps
With the patient in the prone position, using a midline skin incision, the sacrum is exposed out to the ala bilaterally. Separate vertical incisions are made lateral to the palpable posterior-superior iliac spines (PSISs), and their lateral aspects are exposed. A rod insertion site is identified. This is approximately 2 cm anterior to the PSIS, and positioned to allow transverse rod placement dorsal to the sacrum. An appropriate trocar-tipped threaded rod is chosen, mounted on a hand drill, and using an additional laterally placed stab incision, the rod is driven through the ilium, and toward the contralateral side (**Fig. 41.1**). The surgeon must take care to ensure that the advancing rod remains dorsal to the sacroiliac (SI) joint and the sacrum, and also ensure that any connectors are placed on the transverse rod before engaging the opposite ilium. As the rod emerges at the opposite ilium, it can be cut to length with a rod cutter, and nuts or locking washers applied to prevent disengagement from the bone. Coupling the rod to the longitudinal members completes the construct (**Fig. 41.2**).

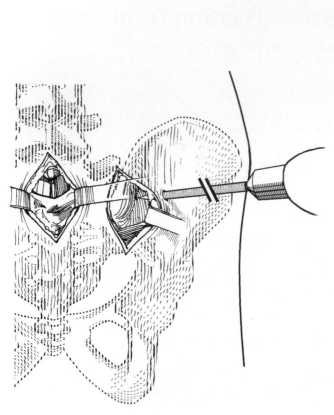

**Fig. 41.1** *A hand drill is used to pass the bar through the iliac wing posterior to the sacroiliac (SI) joint and dorsal cortex of the sacrum.*

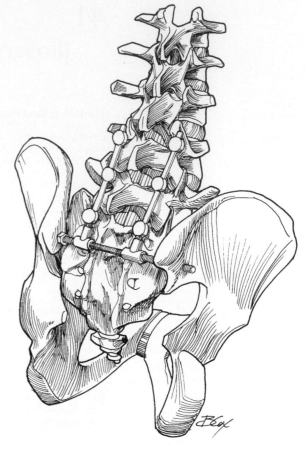

**Fig. 41.2** *Longitudinal rods are connected to the transverse bar by T-connectors or hooks, and the construct is completed by introducing the rods into the proximal spinal anchor sites.*

---

PITFALLS
• Intraoperative fracture of the PSIS during rod placement results in failed fixation.

**Bailout, Rescue, Salvage Procedures**

If PSIS fracture occurs, pedicle screws can be placed between the tables of the pelvis, somewhat similarly to the Galveston technique. The transverse rod can then be anchored to the pelvis via the screws. Polyaxial screws may facilitate connection to the transverse rod.

## Percutaneous Iliosacral Screw Fixation

### Description

Percutaneous placement of screws across the SI joint is a minimally invasive technique of reestablishing the mechanical integrity of this articulation. Severe trauma may cause disruption of the SI joint. Occasionally, degenerative changes of this articulation can result in painful hypermobility.

### Expectations

Surgeons can achieve excellent stability of the SI joint with screws placed through small skin incisions. This technique minimizes soft tissue dissection and intraoperative bleeding, and thus is associated with very low rates of soft tissue complications.

### Indications

This technique is indicated in patients who have suffered vertically unstable disruptions of the pelvic ring, whose posterior pelvis injury can be acceptably reduced by closed or percutaneous reduction, and whose pelvis can be successfully imaged with fluoroscopy in surgery, thereby allowing safe screw placement. Screw fixation may be indicated to immobilize SI joints being fused for degenerative disease. This technique is indicated in patients with soft tissue injuries that preclude open reduction and internal fixation.

### Contraindications

This technique relies on fluoroscopy. Patients whose habitus or injuries preclude the use of fluoroscopy are contraindicated. Complex fractures of the ilium or sacrum may compromise screw fixation. Multifragmentary sacral fractures may be at risk for nerve injury by fracture displacement during screw placement or tightening. Inadequate closed reduction of the posterior pelvic injury compromises the stability achieved and increases the risk of complications with this procedure. Sacral and pelvic dysmorphism may prevent use of this technique.

### Special Considerations

Preoperative computed tomography (CT) scanning should be performed to ascertain the exact fracture anatomy. X-rays should be carefully analyzed after closed reduction maneuvers to ensure adequate alignment. Intraoperative fluoroscopic visualization is critical: inlet, outlet, iliac, and obturator oblique views and a true lateral of the sacrum must be obtainable during the procedure. Supplemental intraoperative fluoroscopic views, as dictated by the patient's individual anatomy, will be necessary to evaluate reduction of the pelvis and to ensure safe screw placement. Surgeons should consider the use of neuromonitoring techniques such as free running electromyography (EMG) during the procedure.

### Tips, Pearls, and Lessons Learned

- Preoperative analysis of CT scans and plain x-rays of the sacrum help to identify sacral dysmorphisms.
- While screws can be placed with the patient in the prone, supine, or lateral position, the supine position proves most practical for the polytraumatized patient.
- Intraoperative fluoroscopic evaluation is critical, and relies on multiple views of the pelvis to ensure safe and strong screw fixation.
- Cannulated screws should be used as they allow for radiographic confirmation of wire position prior to screw placement.
- Screw placement into the S1 vertebra is safer than placement into the S2 vertebra because the SI vertebra is larger and more easily visualized by fluoroscope.

### Key Procedural Steps

Patients are positioned on a radiolucent operating table. Prone, lateral, and supine positioning is possible, although supine positioning is most practical in most patients, and is safest in polytraumatized patients. Anteroposterior (AP) pelvis, inlet, and outlet views confirm reduction of the SI joint. The inlet view should be modified so that it is tangential to the anterior S1 body, and the outlet view should be modified so that it is tangential to the L5-S1 interspace, to visualize the anterior and superior ends of the S1 vertebral body (**Fig. 41.3**). By angling the C-arm beam around the axis of the body toward the affected side, one can obtain the "obturator-inlet" view that provides optimal visualization of the SI joint. The true lateral assists in selecting trajectory. Using fluoroscopy, the surgeon should select a starting point that will allow the screw to pass from lateral to medial, across the SI articulation, perpendicular to the joint line (or fracture line), and

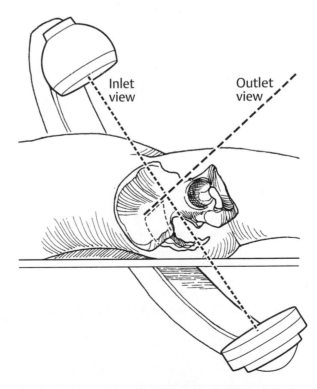

**Fig. 41.3** *Intraoperative angles for obtaining (modified) inlet and outlet views of the pelvis with the patient in the supine position.*

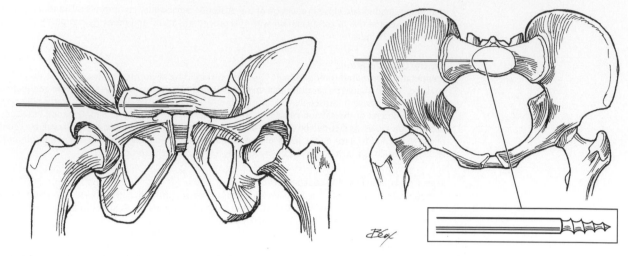

**Fig. 41.4** *(A) Illustration of the pelvis from the outlet view, with guidewire positioned across sacroiliac joint and into first sacral vertebal body. (B) Illustration of pelvis from the outlet view, with guidewire positioned across sacroiliac joint and into first sacral vertebal body. (C) Note threaded tip of guidewire.*

• The osseous and neural anatomy of the pelvis is very complicated. Understanding the three-dimensional anatomy from two-dimensional imaging requires experience. Screw malposition can cause nerve injury to the L5 and sacral roots.

into the center of the S1 body (**Fig. 41.4**). A lateral stab incision is made, and the guidewire is passed using fluoroscopic modified inlet and outlet views to ensure a safe trajectory. After confirming that the wire remains in bone and does not violate the canal or foramina on inlet and outlet views, the cannulated screw is positioned (**Fig. 41.5**).

### Bail Out, Rescue, Salvage Procedures
Open reduction and internal fixation with plate and screw devices or transiliac bars, and application of a pelvic external fixator are alternative methods of stabilizing the SI joint.

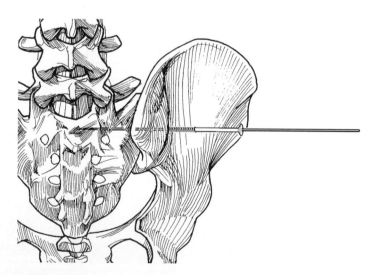

**Fig. 41.5** *Posterior view of pelvis depicts appropriate position of guidewire in first sacral vertebral body, and cannulated screw passing over guidewire. Tightening an appropriately-positioned lag screw will stabilize the sacroiliac joint.*

# 42

# Intrasacral (Jackson) and Galveston Rod Contouring and Placement Techniques

*Roger P. Jackson and Douglas C. Burton*

## Description

The intrasacral (Jackson) screw and rod fixation technique involves the safe insertion of intrasacral screws and rods into the best bone possible with avoidance of injuring the surrounding neurovascular structures. The Galveston technique of intra-iliac anchorage utilizes careful osseous placement of a three-dimensionally contoured rod, taking into account spinopelvic deformity and allowing for connection to other lumbosacral anchors.

## Key Principles

### Intrasacral (Jackson) Technique

Insertion of the S1 screw head into the lateral sacral mass where the head is much closer to the back of the L5-S1 disk, as well as the L5 and S1 vertebral bodies, thereby significantly reducing bending loads on the screw/rod construct at the L5-S1 level and increasing the stiffness of the fixation. The low- to no-profile rod/screw construct provides an interlocked, "sacroiliac buttress" type of fixation that allows for application of in-situ rod contouring principles to create lumbopelvic lordosis and better balance.

### Galveston Technique

Intra-iliac anchorage provides a strong sacropelvic foundation for long spinal constructs crossing the lumbosacral junction while maintaining a low profile in a patient population where implant prominence is often a significant concern.

## Expectations

### Intrasacral (Jackson) Technique

- Increased sacropelvic fixation in three planes without bridging the sacroiliac (SI) joints or compromising the iliac crests
- Posterior lumbosacral instrumentation that provides for improved biomechanics and increased lordosis in the distal lumbar spine with essentially no profile on the back of the sacrum

### Galveston Technique

The bilateral placement of carefully contoured rods in the supra-acetabular intra-iliac passageway provides a strong sacropelvic foundation for the correction of rigid spinopelvic deformity and resists the flexion-extension and rotation forces that exist. This strong and stable foundation facilitates the establishment of a solid arthrodesis across the lumbosacral junction in long spinal constructs.

## Indications

Long spinal deformity fusions to the sacrum, spondylolisthesis, L5 burst fractures, lumbar flatback, osteopenia or osteoporosis, and revisions including L5-S1 pseudarthrosis.

## Contraindications

### Intrasacral (Jackson) Technique

Congenital abnormalities, tumors, or infections involving the proximal sacrum.

### Galveston Technique

Abnormalities of iliac anatomy that preclude the placement of anchorage and severe osteopenia are situations that may not allow this technique.

## Special Considerations

Computed tomography (CT) scan to better delineate the sacral anatomy preoperatively. CT also is helpful in the setting of a previous or planned pelvic osteotomy, or prior bone graft harvest that has altered the normal iliac orientation for the Galveston technique.

### Special Instructions, Position, and Anesthesia

Prone positioning on a surgical table or frame that provides for improved pulmonary compliance, reduced blood loss, unrestricted fluoroscopic imaging, and that preserves or creates increased lumbopelvic lordosis, such as the Jackson surgery table. Severe hip flexion contractures and lumbar hyperlordosis are critical to recognize and account for in patient positioning. If using a standard four-poster frame, the posts must be built up to allow for the hip flexion contractures and keep undue pressure off of the knees. Hyperlordosis should be recognized preoperatively, and anterior releases performed, if needed. Positioning out of a hyperlordotic position can be aided with the use of two additional posts placed between the usual two. This eliminates, as much as possible, the sag that occurs between the posts, which accentuates lordosis.

In situations with severe fixed pelvic deformity, a single femoral traction pin placed on the "high pelvis" side with 20 pounds of traction (depending on patient size) can aid in the reduction of spinopelvic deformity.

### Tips, Pearls, and Lessons Learned

#### Intrasacral (Jackson) Technique

Intraoperative anteroposterior (AP), lateral, and angled fluoroscopic images, by tilting of the C-arm in the sagittal plane to get a tangential view of the S1 endplate, are critical. Good AP fluoroscopic imaging of the sacrum is necessary for insertion of the intrasacral rods after the S1 screws have been deeply buried in the bone. The end of the rods should perforate the anterolateral cortex of the sacrum and not extend more than 5 to 10 mm beyond the distal aspect of the inferior SI joint.

#### Galveston Technique

Careful preoperative planning of types and locations of anchors, particularly if S1 pedicle screws are going to be used, is paramount. If S1 screws are planned, they should be placed prior to exposure of the iliac anchor, as this will help to show how far distally the iliac anchor must be placed. If using a pedicle bolt/connector system, short post screws are recommended, and often an open slotted connector is necessary, though not always. Transverse connection is important, and preferably performed between the S1 screws and iliac post, though anatomic considerations preclude this at times. Utilization of three- and four-rod constructs, depending on sagittal profile and coronal curve position, may facilitate Galveston rod placement. The use of a short Galveston rod on the concavity of the curve (high pelvis side) allows for ease of placement and the ability to distract against the longer, more proximally placed rod. This connection may make an S1 screw on the ipsilateral side unworkable due to bunching of connectors.

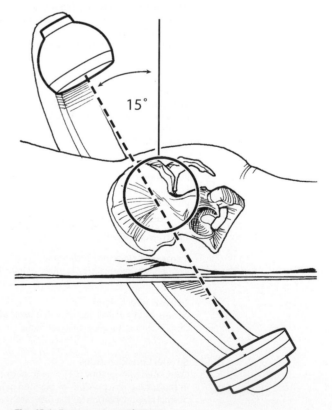

**Fig. 42.1** *Ferguson view with C-arm.*

**Difficulties Encountered**

*Intrasacral (Jackson) Technique*

A transitional lumbosacral vertebra is not a contraindication, but may make insertion of the implants more difficult, especially with partial sacralization of L5. Closely spaced iliac crests can also make the procedure more difficult.

*Galveston Technique*

The neuromuscular patient population will frequently have severe, fixed pelvic obliquity in all three planes that makes contouring a challenge. The use of multiple rods improves, but does not eliminate, this problem. Myelomeningocele, due to its dysraphic posterior elements, widens the rod position, thereby making the connection to S1 screws and rod contouring more difficult.

**Key Procedural Steps**

*Intrasacral (Jackson) Technique*

A good intraoperative Ferguson view of the proximal sacrum with the C-arm is needed (**Fig. 42.1**). A reduced-volume closed S1 screw head is deeply countersunk into the lateral sacral mass (**Fig. 42.2**). A special angled sacral curette is then inserted through the screw head and used to open up and sound

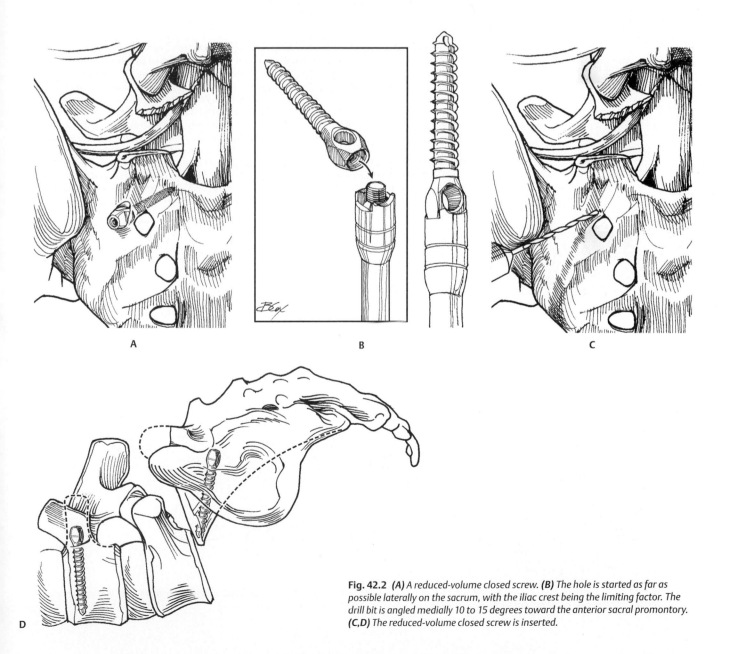

**Fig. 42.2** *(A) A reduced-volume closed screw. (B) The hole is started as far as possible laterally on the sacrum, with the iliac crest being the limiting factor. The drill bit is angled medially 10 to 15 degrees toward the anterior sacral promontory. (C,D) The reduced-volume closed screw is inserted.*

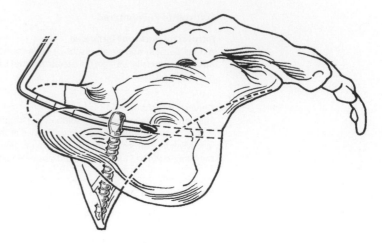

**Fig. 42.3** *A special angled sacral curette is inserted through the screw head and used to open up and sound the lateral sacral mass.*

the lateral sacral mass (**Fig. 42.3**). The length of intrasacral rod required can then be determined. A rod is cut to length, contoured, and directed distally into and through the closed canal of the S1 screw. Under fluoroscopic control, the rod is then worked caudally into the lateral sacral mass. The distal end of the rod is directed toward the inferior SI joint. The rod must be contoured properly and guided out laterally to get better fixation in the distal sacral mass adjacent to the SI joint. Rolling the curved rod to direct its distal end more laterally and anteriorly in the sacrum is helpful. The safest and strongest area is in the distal lateral sacrum adjacent to the SI joint. At no time is the rod intentionally driven across the sacroiliac joint. The pelvic anatomy in this area can provide considerable fixation and support for the end of the rod. This is especially so for resisting flexural bending moments. After the distal end of the rod has been driven caudally into the lateral sacral mass and out through the cortex, the proximal end is manipulated down and up into the other screw(s), then the set screw is tightened down in the S1 screw head. The second rod is implanted in the same way. **Fig. 42.4** shows a typical multilevel construct with insertion of the intrasacral rods. The rod is positioned as closely to the back of the L5-S1 disk space as possible.

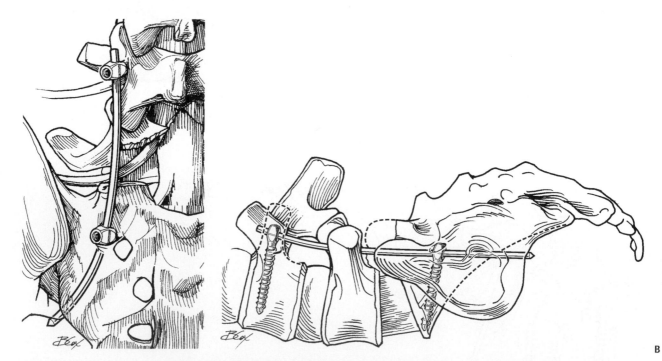

A                                                                                                      B

**Fig. 42.4 (A)** *The sharp end of the rod penetrates the anterolateral sacral cortex. **(B)** A typical multilevel construct with insertion of the intrasacral rods distally and adjacent to the inferior sacroiliac (SI) joints.*

### Galveston Technique

The successful placement of Galveston rods requires two equally important steps: establishment of the iliac passageway, and bending and insertion of the rod. The ilium is approached through a separate fascial incision made along the posterior-superior iliac spine (PSIS). The outer table is exposed in a subperiosteal manner and the sciatic notch is identified and marked with placement of an elongated Freer elevator (Slim Jim; Sklar Instrument Corp., West Chester, PA) into the cephalad portion of the notch. This provides constant visual feedback to the surgeon (who stands on the opposite side of the table) during probing of the passageway. The very distal portion of the PSIS is removed with a rongeur down to the level of the sacrum. This improves the profile by keeping the host bone more dorsal than the implant and places the rod directly on the sacrum, also improving profile.

A standard blunt pedicle finder is used to probe the ilium. The starting point should be just medial to the lateral cortex, with the curved tip of the pedicle finder directed medially. Drilling is not recommended, particularly in osteopenic bone, as it increases the likelihood of a cortical breach. The orientation should be to a point 1.0 to 1.5 cm above the notch and along the lateral cortex. A medial starting point or directing the probe too proximally will potentially shorten the passageway. Most adults can accommodate 8 to 10 cm of a ¼-inch rod, whereas children have between 6 and 8 cm of length and thus accommodate ¼- or 3/16-inch-diameter rods. A fine ball-tipped probe is used to search for any breaches of the cortical bone. The passageway is then widened with a dilator prior to final rod placement, as this decreases the chance of cutout during insertion.

Proper bending of a Galveston post requires four measurements and is facilitated by the use of variable radius benders (two flat and two tube benders). The measurements required are (1) the length of the intrailiac segment (**Fig. 42.5A**); (2) the transverse plane angle of the iliac fixation site to the midsagittal plane (**Fig. 42.5B**); (3) the mediolateral distance from the iliac entry site to the intended line of longitudinal passage along the spine (**Fig. 42.5C**); and (4) the length of rod from the sacrum to the most cephalad level of instrumentation (**Fig. 42.5D**).

The initial bend is a right-angle bend using the tube benders. The short length is the sum of measurements 1 and 3 (the length of the intrailiac segment and the mediolateral distance from the iliac entry site to the intended line of longitudinal passage along the spine) and represents the sacroiliac portion of the rod. The next bend separates the short end of the rod into its iliac and sacral portions. The bend point is measured from the midportion of the right-angle bend and equal to measurement 3 (the mediolateral distance from the iliac entry site to the intended line of longitudinal passage along the spine) minus 3.0 mm (to account for the length of the bend). The plane of this bend is perpendicular to the plane of the right-angle bend and equal to measurement 2 (the transverse plane angle of the iliac fixation site to the midsagittal plane). The right-left orientation must be accounted for, and this bend is made with the tube bender on the iliac portion and the flat bender on the sacral portion of the rod. The sagittal plane contour is then achieved with the flat benders. It is important to allow for the length of the sacrum before beginning lordotic bending and to remember that L4–S1 lordosis is much greater (usually) than L1–L4. The final sagittal plane orientation of the iliac segment can be adjusted, if needed, with the flat benders, but is often not necessary.

The iliac rod segment is tunneled under the multifidus and inserted into the ilium with the spinal segment of the rod directed away from the back. The rod is then rotated toward the spine and the iliac segment impacted into the ilium.

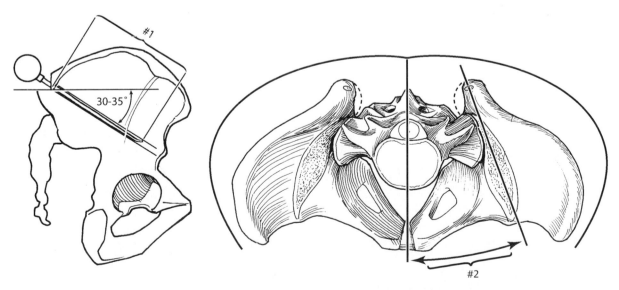

**Fig. 42.5** *Graphic representation of the four measurements needed to calculate bend angle and rod length when preparing a Galveston bend. (A) Measurement 1: rod length and sagittal angle (to the midaxial plane) of the intra-iliac segment. (B) Measurement 2: the transverse plane angle of the iliac fixation site to the midsagittal plane.* *(Continued on page 152)*

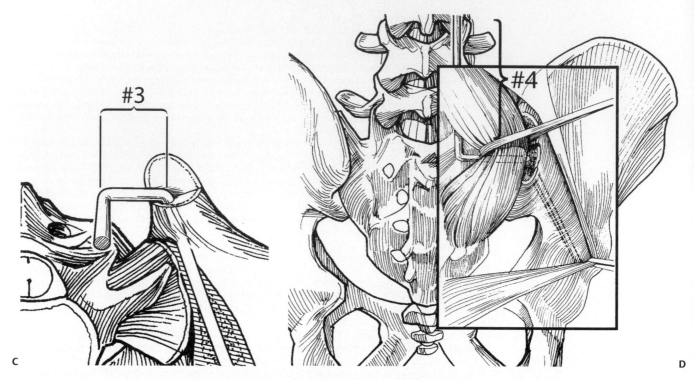

**Fig. 42.5** *Continued* **(C)** *Measurement 3: the mediolateral distance from the iliac entry site to the intended line of longitudinal passage along the spine.* **(D)** *Measurement 4: the length of rod from the sacrum to the most cephalad level of instrumentation.*

PITFALLS

*Intrasacral (Jackson) Technique*
- Contouring can cause indentations on the rod that can reduce the fatigue life of the implant; therefore, 6.35-mm stainless steel rods should be used. The use of polyaxial screws at L5, and perhaps L4, can facilitate the procedure (**Fig. 42.4B**).

*Galveston Technique*
- Cutout of the iliac portion duration preparation or placement of the rod is the main complication encountered intraoperatively.

**Bailout, Rescue, Salvage Procedures**

**Intrasacral (Jackson) Technique**
If the implants fail or loosen, a more traditional approach for insertion of the S1 screw, tangential to the sacral end plate, is still possible. The Galveston technique and other methods for more distal pelvosacral fixation can also be used at the time of revision. If significant manipulation of the lumbopelvic junction is performed, structural interbody support at L5-S1 is needed. The most likely mode of failure with intrasacral fixation is rod breakage proximal to the S1 screws. Sacral screw loosening or breakage is reduced (rarely) when the technique is performed properly. Structural interbody fusion at L5-S1 minimizes rod breakage and helps maintain lumbopelvic lordosis.

**Galveston Technique**
If iliac breach occurs during preparation, it is usually recognized with the ball probe. The most common reason for breach during preparation is an incorrect starting position or orientation. Typically the probe is oriented too proximally. Intraoperative posterior-anterior and lateral radiographs with a probe in the passageway can help to identify this, and the passageway can be probed again in the proper orientation. If the cutout occurs during rod placement, salvage is more difficult. Conversion to the Dunn-McCarthy technique of sacral ala S rod may be an option. Other options are S1 and S2 screws, iliosacral screws, or a modified sacral bar technique.

# 43

# Sacral Screw Fixation Techniques

*Daniel E. Gelb*

## Description

Mechanical stabilization of the distal lumbar spine to the pelvis (lumbosacral joint) may be achieved with the use of screws inserted into the proximal sacrum incorporated into mechanical constructs that span the lumbosacral joint. This method of fixation is widely adaptable, more rigid than hook-based constructs, and more effectively maintains anatomic alignment (lordosis).

## Key Principles

Pedicle screw–based segmental fixation systems provide rigid fixation with control of all three columns of the spine. However, anatomic considerations limit options for screw placement because placement of screws outside the anatomic boundaries of the pedicle may result in iatrogenic neurovascular injury. The sacral spinal canal contains the distal elements of the cauda equina (S1 to S5). The iliac vessels lie immediately anterior to the lumbosacral disk, whereas the L5 nerve root lies anterior to the ala of the sacrum, medial to the sacroiliac joint **(Fig. 43.1)**. Although the S1 pedicle is broad, the bone density of the proximal sacrum is poor. This deficiency necessitates bicortical purchase of S1 screws to ensure optimal screw purchase and may require supplemental fixation techniques to obtain adequate mechanical stability.

## Expectations

Adequate surgical exposure and thorough understanding of sacral pelvic anatomy allows safe placement of screws within the sacrum. Medially directed bicortical S1 screws are the preferred technique. Laterally directed screws into the sacral ala can be used as an adjunct or as a substitute for medially directed screws when standard implantation is unfeasible. S2 pedicle screws are used to supplement proximal sacral fixation sites for enhanced mechanical stability.

## Indications

- Posterior stabilization of painful degenerated disks
- Fusion of lumbosacral spondylolisthesis
- Correction of scoliosis with pelvic obliquity
- Posterolateral fusion pseudarthrosis revision
- Stabilization following wide posterior decompressions of the lumbosacral spine
- Traumatic lumbosacral instability
- Extension of a previous fusion to the sacropelvis (flatback syndrome)

## Contraindications

- Inadequate pedicle size for screw
- Inadequate anterior column support (associated with late fatigue failure of the implants)
- Pedicle fracture
- Metal allergy
- Severe osteopenia

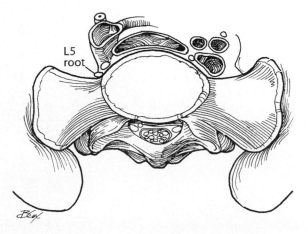

L5
root

**Fig. 43.1** *The common iliac vessels and L5 nerve roots travel immediately anterior to the lumbosacral disk and S1 body lateral to the midline, making bicortical screw fixation possible.*

## Special Considerations

Medially directed S1 pedicle screws are the preferred technique. Large-diameter S1 pedicles and poor bone quality in the body of S1 make bicortical screw insertion a more rigid option than unicortical fixation. Anterior cortical penetration may put the viscera, iliac vessels, or L5 nerve root at risk. Graduated punches with stops are available to safely perforate the anterior sacral cortex and measure appropriate screw length. Screws should penetrate the anterior cortex medial to the iliac vessels. Screws should be placed parallel to the superior sacral end plate or toward the promontory. In muscular patients with a narrow pelvis, it may be difficult to achieve the appropriate angulation to the midline. Retraction of the paraspinal muscles is blocked by the iliac wings.

## Special Instructions, Position, and Anesthesia

The patient is positioned prone on a spinal frame with care taken to avoid pressure on the abdomen. General anesthesia is employed. Hips should be placed in maximal extension to enhance lumbar lordosis and prevent iatrogenic postoperative flatback syndrome.

## Tips, Pearls, and Lessons Learned

The sacral pedicle is large, and use of a large-diameter (7-mm) screw is generally necessary to obtain adequate pedicle fill. Adequate exposure of the sacral ala may be difficult. Brisk bleeding may occur lateral to the superior sacral facet in the depth of the lateral gutter. Lumbosacral lordosis may require extreme rod contouring.

A high rate of failure of stand-alone S1 pedicle screws has been reported in long constructs. Consideration should be given to supplementary pelvic fixation anchor points or rigid structural anterior column support to protect the S1 screws in these situations.

## Difficulties Encountered

Adequate exposure of the correct starting point may be difficult in heavyset muscular patients. A narrow pelvis with tall posterior iliac wings may prevent appropriate medial screw trajectory.

## Key Procedural Steps

Exposure of the posterior elements of the lumbosacral junction is completed through either a midline or paramedian approach. In particular, the soft tissues adjacent to the lumbosacral facets and ala must be stripped for adequate visualization of bony landmarks. The starting point for the medially directed S1 screw is the confluence of the base of the superior sacral facet and the ala of the sacrum (**Fig. 43.2**). The posterior cortex is opened with either a burr or an awl. A blunt pedicle probe or curette is passed through the sacral pedicle perpendicular to the posterior sacral cortex aiming 20 to 30 degrees medially (**Fig. 43.3**). Directing the probe in a slightly more vertical orientation allows the tip of the screw to abut the superior end plate of the sacrum or into the promontory, the area of greatest bone density (**Fig. 43.4**).

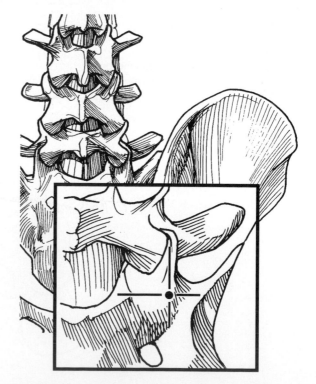

**Fig. 43.2** *The starting point of the medially directed S1 screw is at the confluence of the base of the S1 superior facet and the sacral ala.*

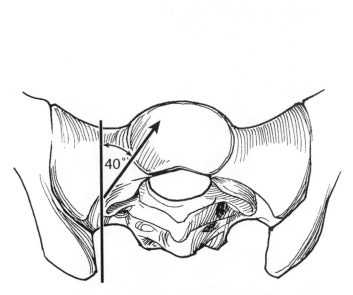

**Fig. 43.3** *Axial view of the proximal sacrum showing the appropriate medial angulation of the S1 and S2 screws 40 degrees medial from the posterior starting point. The screw tip should protrude no more than 2 mm anterior to the anterior sacral cortex, medial to the iliac vessels.*

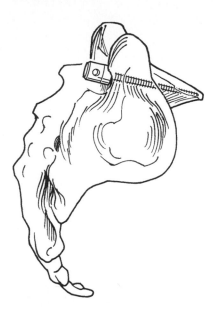

**Fig. 43.4** *Sagittal plane angulation for medially directed S1 pedicle screws. The tip of the screw should engage the sacral promontory where the sacral bone of greatest density is found.*

A ball-tipped probe or depth gauge is used to palpate the pedicle walls for penetration. Free-running EMG monitoring of the lower extremity muscles may be used to monitor for nerve root irritation. The pedicle probe is gently advanced until the anterior cortex is perforated. Alternatively, a graduated punch with stop can be used to safely penetrate the anterior sacrum. Image intensifier guidance is generally not necessary. The pedicle is tapped, if desired, and screws of appropriate length and diameter (based on measurement with a depth gauge) are placed. Screw position is assessed by radiographic criteria. Direct visualization of the medial border of the sacral pedicle or triggered EMG can also be used to assess screw placement. Perforation of the sacral end plate with penetration of the screw tip into the lumbosacral disk is considered acceptable (**Fig. 43.5**).

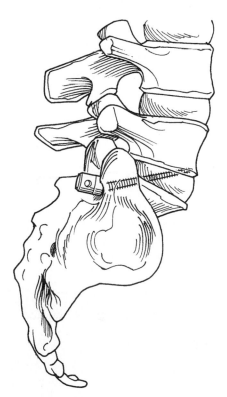

**Fig. 43.5** *Lateral view of the lumbosacral joint demonstrating screw placement through the S1 end plate into the L5-S1 disk. Screw placement into the inferior end plate of L5 can supplement fixation of L5-S1 such as in cases of spondylolisthesis.*

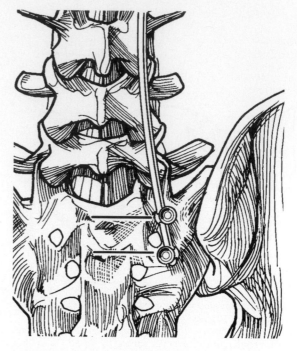

**Fig. 43.6** *The starting point of an S2 screw is halfway between the dorsal foramina of S1 and S2, in line with the starting point of the S1 screw.*

S2 pedicle screws are placed in a similar fashion. The appropriate starting point is midway between the posterior S1 and S2 foramina, in line with the S1 screw starting point (**Fig. 43.6**).

### Bailout, Rescue, Salvage Procedures

In revision situations, adequate screw purchase may be difficult to achieve. Screw purchase can be improved by using expansile tipped screws or supplementing screw purchase with polymethylmethacrylate (PMMA) in the pedicle. Alternative pelvic anchor points are available and include the Galveston technique, iliosacral screws, and transverse iliac bars.

# 44

# Sacral Plating Techniques (Chopin)

*Jeff S. Silber*

## Description
The Chopin plate, also known as the Colorado II sacral plate, combines an S1 screw and a laterally placed sacral alar screw. It was introduced by Chopin in France and has been used in clinical practice since the early 1990s. The two-hole plate, or three-hole plate if pelvic fixation is also required, is placed on the dorsal aspect of the sacrum in a longitudinal direction (**Fig. 44.1**). The superior hole is for placement of an S1 pedicle screw angled medially (10 to 15 degrees) toward the sacral promontory, and the inferior hole is for placement of a sacral alar screw angled laterally (30 degrees). With the three-hole plate an additional hole located laterally can be utilized for fixation into the pelvis (**Fig. 44.2**). Located midway between the superior and inferior holes is a post that allows connection of the plate to the longitudinal component extending down from the lumbar spine.

## Expectations
Spinal pathology involving the lumbar-sacral junction may be due to trauma, infection, tumor, or congenital or degenerative disease. Commonly, fusion procedures need to include this junction to obtain stability and improve the overall biomechanics of the spine. Increased fusion rates have been reported with the use of instrumentation, and although posterior sacral pedicle screws are widely used, cases of fixation failure have been reported with their use. Screw failure is most commonly due to inadequate purchase, incorrect direction or depth of screw placement, and osteoporotic bone, especially in the setting of long fusion procedures that place high bending loads across this junction. Overall, based on biomechanical testing, S1 screws placed anteromedially into the sacral promontory with bicortical purchase tend to have the highest pullout and bending strength. Furthermore, the Chopin (Colorado II plate) may add additionally needed fixation points across the lumbosacral junction in various clinical scenarios.

## Indications
Biomechanical studies have demonstrated improved strength using this divergent two-screw construct compared with a single pedicle screw construct alone. This technique is especially useful in cases of high-grade (III–V) spondylolisthesis, long fusions to the sacrum, revision procedures, pseudarthrosis at the L5-S1

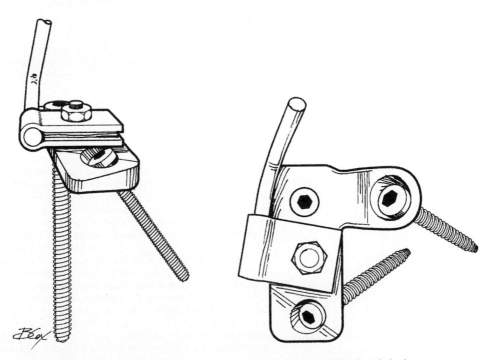

**Fig. 44.1** *Side view of the two-hole plate.*　　　**Fig. 44.2** *Axial view of the three-hole plate.*

157

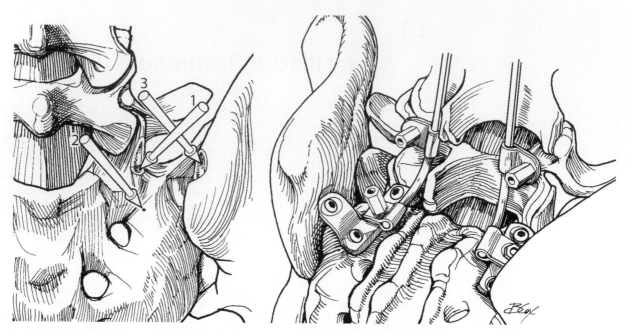

**Fig. 44.3** *(A)* *Cadaveric specimen showing starting points of S1 pedicle screw (1), sacral alar screw (2), and iliac screw (3). (B) After placement.*

level, significant osteoporosis, sacral trauma, and scoliosis (neuromuscular) with pelvic obliquity requiring sacral and pelvic fixation.

### Contraindications
This technique should not be used if fusion to the pelvis and sacrum is not indicated or needed.

### Special Considerations
The posterior-superior iliac spine may need to be removed or at least flattened with a rongeur or burr to make the plate seat flush against the pelvis.

### Tips, Pearls, and Lessons Learned
Unicortical versus bicortical screw placement is based on surgeon preference, as the increased pullout strength provided by the technique is due to the divergent placement of the two screws. If further pelvic fixation is needed, a three-hole plate utilizing a pelvic screw placed through the posterior-superior iliac spin may be utilized.

Upon completion, intraoperative fluoroscopy or plain radiographs are obtained to confirm adequate screw placement and appropriate spinal alignment.

### Key Procedural Steps
In the prone position the lumbar spine and the sacrum are exposed inferior to the L5-S1 facet joints. The inferior articular process of the L5-S1 facet is removed to expose the superior facet of S1. Once exposed, the superior S1 articular facet is then removed to provide a flat surface for the Chopin plate. The plate is placed longitudinally along the flattened S1 superior articular process, with the top hole over the starting point of the S1 pedicle. The pedicle of S1 is cannulated, probed, and tapped prior to placement of the plate. The starting hole is about 4 to 5 mm lateral to the inferior aspect of the S1 superior articular process **(Figs. 44.3** and **44.4)**. The S1 pedicle screw is not tightened all the way to allow rotation of the plate to the ideal location for placement of the alar screw. With the plate flat on the sacrum, an awl or burr is used to create a starting hole for the alar screw, which is cannulated with a pedicle finder followed by probing and taping. The screw is placed anterolaterally and parallel to the slope of the SI joint, being careful not to penetrate the joint that is located lateral to the screw placement **(Figs. 44.3** and **44.5)**. Once the alar screw is placed and tightened, the S1 pedicle screw is tightened, bringing the plate flush to the dorsum of the sacrum. The screw is placed within the outer and inner cortices of the ileum **(Figs. 44.3** and **44.6)**. Once the screws are placed, locking screws are then placed to prevent screw backout; they may be inserted in holes adjacent to the S1 and alar screws. Once the plate is placed, a connector is then attached to the post on the plate, which is then connected to either a 5.5-mm or 6.25-mm rod.

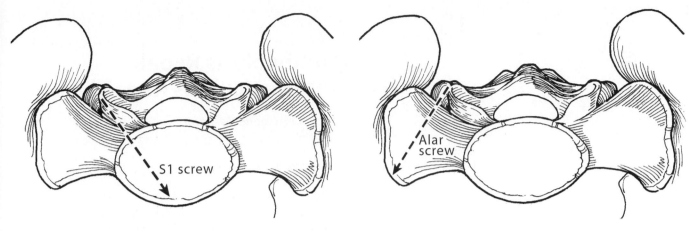

**Fig. 44.4** *Starting hole and direction of the S1 pedicle screw.*

**Fig. 44.5** *Starting hole and direction of the sacral alar screw.*

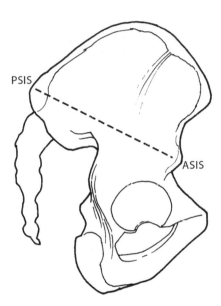

**Fig. 44.6** *Starting hole and direction of the iliac screw. ASIS, anterior superior iliac spine; PSIS, posterior superior iliac spine.*

PITFALLS

• Increased fusion rates across the lumbosacral junction have been reported with the use of instrumentation. Sacral screw failure is most commonly due to inadequate purchase, direction, or depth of screw placement, and to osteoporotic bone in long fusion procedures.

**Bailout, Rescue, Salvage Procedures**

The Chopin (Colorado II plate) technique may add additionally needed fixation points in cases of high-grade (III–V) spondylolisthesis, degenerative disorders with long fusion constructs to the sacrum, revision cases, and pseudarthrosis at the L5-S1 level, as well as in osteoporotic patients and in sacral trauma and scoliosis (neuromuscular) with pelvic obliquity requiring sacrum and pelvic fixation. This posterior technique provides additional fixation points into the sacrum and pelvis and can be used as a salvage procedure in revision cases. Lastly, if this technique does not provide sufficient areas for either instrumentation fixation or an adequate fusion surface, one would have to consider an anterior approach.

# 45

# Spondylolysis Repair
# (Pars Interarticularis Repair)

*Christopher M. Bono*

## Description
Direct bone grafting and stabilization of spondylolytic (pars) lesions.

## Key Principles
Unhealed fractures of the pars interarticularis, also known as isthmic spondylolysis, can be chronically painful despite appropriate nonoperative treatments. Although patients with slippage (i.e., isthmic spondylolisthesis) are usually treated with fusion, direct repair of the nonunion without intersegmental lumbar fusion may be effective in some cases of spondylolysis without spondylolisthesis. Several techniques have been described, which generally involve bone grafting (usually autogenous) of the defect followed by some form of stabilization of the posterior elements. Methods of stabilization have varied from wire loop fixation, to interfragmentary compression screw, to pedicle screw-hook constructs. Though a clear clinical advantage of one technique over another has yet to be demonstrated, biomechanical studies suggest that a pedicle screw-hook construct offers the greatest stability at the nonunion site. As a basic tenet of nonunited fracture treatment, greater stability is usually desirable for better healing.

## Expectations
To decrease low back pain from an unhealed spondylolytic (pars) defect by maintaining motion and avoiding intervertebral fusion.

## Indications
- Direct pars repair is indicated for those patients with a clearly identified, painful spondylolytic defect.
- Clinically, the patient should have low back pain that is localized to the lumbosacral (L5 pars is most common) or lower lumbar region (L4 pars is second most common) without lower extremity radiation.
- The neurologic exam should be normal.
- Symptoms are typically exacerbated by extension and relieved by flexion.
- Ideally, physical examination should reveal tenderness with palpation of the spinous process of the level in question, though paraspinal tenderness over the defects themselves is not uncommon.

## Contraindications

### Relative
- Grade I slips: It is often not desirable to perform a direct pars repair in patients with spondylolisthesis, though some have described good results in select patients with mild (grade I) slips.
- Mild to moderate disk degeneration

### Absolute
- Slips of grade II or higher
- Advanced, painful disk degeneration (pain more with flexion than extension)

## Special Considerations
- Flexion-extension radiographs can be obtained to rule out dynamic subluxation, which is another contraindication to the procedure.
- A magnetic resonance imaging (MRI) study should demonstrate minimal to no evidence of degeneration, desiccation, or height loss at the involved disk space.
- Temporary pain relief from an intralesional anesthetic injection may be a prognostic indicator of a good response to pars repair.

## Special Instructions, Position, and Anesthesia
The patient is positioned prone on a radiolucent operating table. Using a lateral view, the proximal and distal extents of the incision are marked, with the former being the level of the cranial facet joint (usually L4-L5 for a planned L5 repair), and the latter being the superior aspect of the S1 lamina. In addition, a separate incision is marked over the iliac crest bone-graft harvest site. Alternatively, bone graft may be harvested through the same midline lumbar incision.

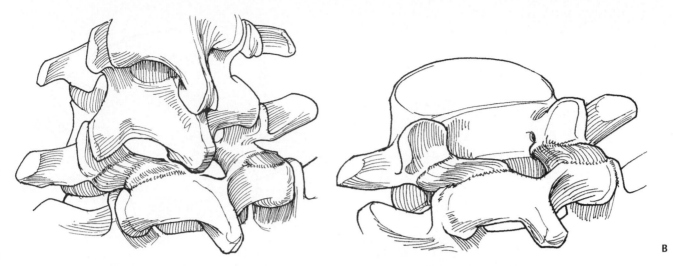

A                                                                                                    B

**Fig. 45.1** *(A,B) A pseudocapsule forms around pars defect, a response of the continued motion through the unhealed fracture.*

### Tips, Pearls, and Lessons Learned

It is important to understand the anatomy of the two fragments of the affected vertebra. The superior fragment consists of the superior articular processes, which are connected to the pedicles and transverse processes by a small portion of the pars (above the lesion). The proximal fragment is in continuity with the vertebral body. The distal fragment consists of the majority of the pars interarticularis (distal to the lesion), the laminae, the spinous process, and the distal articular processes.

### Difficulties Encountered

Adequately seating the hook at the lower border of the lamina.

### Key Procedural Steps

#### General Technique and Bone Grafting

- After sterile prepping and draping, a midline incision is made.
- The lumbosacral fascia is incised on either side of the spinous processes; take care to preserve the midline interspinous and supraspinous process ligaments.
- Next the bilateral laminae are subperiosteally exposed, being careful to avoid injury to the facet joints. The transverse processes at the level of the lesion are also exposed with electrocautery.
- Next, a large curette is used to clearly delineate the entire pars interarticularis and its defect.
- A pseudocapsule is usually present over the unhealed pars lesion (**Fig. 45.1**). This is carefully opened with small and medium-sized curettes (**Fig. 45.2**). The anterior and medial portions of the pseudocapsule are left intact to protect the neural elements and help avoid extrusion of bone graft into the spinal canal. Once the proximal and distal surfaces of the pars nonunion are clearly identified, a high-speed burr can

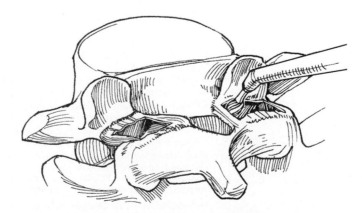

**Fig. 45.2** *The pseudocapsule is opened to allow the bony ends to be prepared to accept the bone graft.*

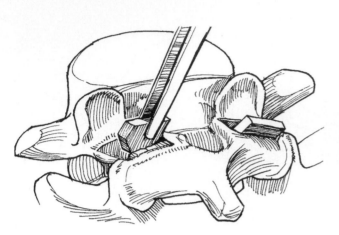

**Fig. 45.3** *The contoured piece of bone graft is tamped into the prepared defect site.*

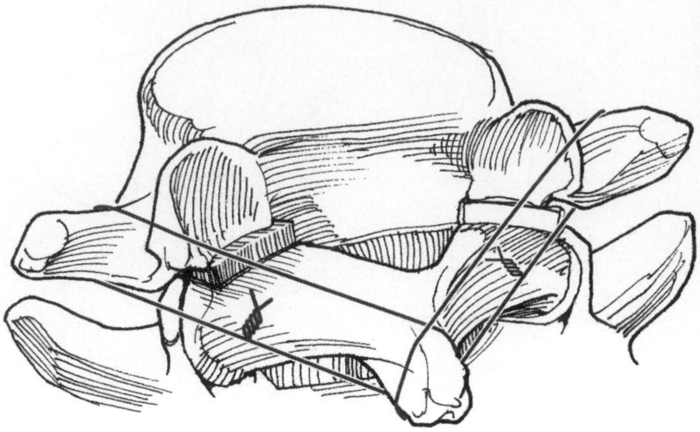

**Fig. 45.4** *Scott's wire fixation technique.*

be used to shape them into flat, transverse surfaces. In addition, burring should expose viable bleeding bone on either side of the lesion.

- Next, two small cube-shaped pieces of autologous iliac crest bone should be harvested. The exact size of the graft can depend on the size of the defect, though a 1 cm by 1 cm piece is usually adequate. The defect site should be prepared with the burr to accept the dimension of the graft. The graft is then tamped gently into place to span the defect (**Fig. 45.3**). Even without fixation applied, the graft should have some degree of stability from an interference fit.

### Fixation Techniques

#### Wire Fixation (Scott's Technique)
Wires or cables are carefully looped around the transverse processes bilaterally. These are subsequently passed around the inferior aspect of the spinous process. The wires or cables are tensioned to place a compressive force across the grafted defect (**Fig. 45.4**).

#### Interfragmentary Screw (Buck's Technique)
A compression screw (i.e., lag screw) can be placed across the defect. The starting point is just inferior and medial to the pars defect. The drill is directed superior and slightly lateral to cross the defect. The screw path ends in the dense bone of the pedicle. The screw is then inserted and tightened to compress the bone graft into place (**Fig. 45.5**).

#### Pedicle Screw-Infraspinous Process Rod
See Bailout, Rescue, Salvage Procedures, below.

#### Pedicle Screw-Infralaminar Hook (Author's Preferred Technique)
With the graft in place, attention is directed toward placement of the pedicle screw. For an L5 lesion, an L5 pedicle screw is placed. To avoid injury to the suprajacent facet joint, the entry site should be placed as lateral as possible (at the junction of the pars and the transverse process), with the screw angled medial toward the vertebral body. It is the author's preference to use a polyaxial screw, though a fixed screw can also be inserted.

After releasing the ligamentum flavum from the inferior aspect of the L5 lamina, an up-going lamina hook is inserted close to the spinous process. Because the hook by itself has little stability (and tends to dislodge), it is my preference to loosely fix the short rod to the hook head with a locking cap. Holding the hook in place with the inserter, the proximal end of the rod can then be directed into the pedicle screw head. The locking cap is then placed loosely into the head of the pedicle screw (**Fig. 45.6**).

Next, the rod is finally tightened to the lamina hook. Using a compressor placed below the hook and above the pedicle screw, the graft is compressed in its position (**Fig. 45.7**). The pedicle screw is then finally tightened. An anteroposterior and lateral fluoroscopic view is then obtained to confirm positioning of the implants.

The wounds are then copiously irrigated and closed in layers using absorbable suture. The skin is closed with staples, and a sterile dressing is applied. Postoperatively, the patient remains on prophylactic antibiotics for 24 hours. Ambulation is encouraged on postoperative day one. No brace is applied. In follow-up,

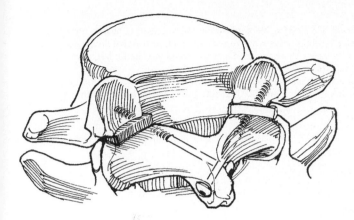

**Fig. 45.5** *Buck's compression screw technique.*

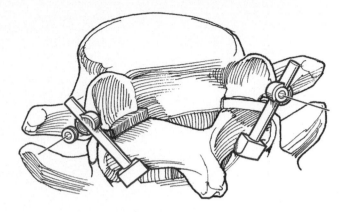

**Fig. 45.6** *Pedicle screw-hook technique. Trick: The hook is first attached to the short rod prior to insertion. With the hook in position, the rod is then levered into the pedicle screw head.*

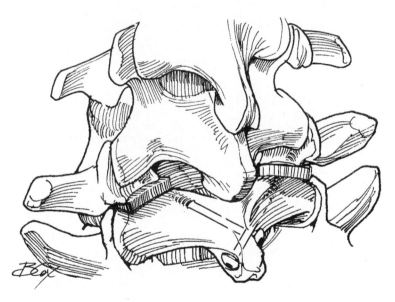

**Fig. 45.7** *Prior to final tightening, the construct is longitudinally compressed.*

radiographs are obtained at 6 weeks, 3 months, 6 months, and 1 year to monitor healing of the defect as well as positioning of the implants.

### Bailout, Rescue, Salvage Procedures

#### Intraoperative
- Depending on the extent of inadvertent facet injury, the surgeon may consider performing a facet fusion. In my experience, this is rarely necessary. If the facet joint has been badly injured, a fusion is recommended.
- The most cumbersome portion of the operation is securing the rod to the hook and screw. Because the rod is so short and the hook unstable by itself, I recommend fixing the hook to the rod prior to insertion. Depending on the angulation of the posterior lamina surface, the rod can preclude the necessary angle for hook insertion. In these cases, the rod can be lordotically bent to avoid this obstruction. If the hook is still too difficult to place, a single rod may be bent into a V shape, passed beneath the spinous process of L5, and connected to both screws. The rod can be advanced cranially prior to final tightening to effect compression across the pars defect and graft.

---

**PITFALLS**

*Intraoperative*
- Injury to the facet joints
- Inability to adequately seat the hook

*Late postoperative*
- Late hook dislodgment
- Nonunion

### Late Postoperative

- If late hook dislodgment occurs, and interfragmentary compression appears to be lost, revision surgery to replace the hook can be elected. Alternatively, a different construct, such as that described above with a V-shaped rod can be used. However, this has a tendency to extend the inferior fragment (apex anterior), and it is not my first option for fixation.
- If symptomatic nonunion is evident, a second attempt at direct pars repair may be attempted; however a posterior/posterolateral fusion with instrumentation and autograft is the preferred treatment.

# 46

# Anterior Lumbar Surgical Exposure Techniques

*Rick B. Delamarter, Salvador A. Brau, and Ben B. Pradhan*

### Description

Anterior approaches have been developed for easier and more direct access to the anterior and middle columns of the lumbar spine. Easier access for the spine surgeon implies that a more thorough and complete diskectomy or corpectomy can be performed with increased efficiency. Today this often involves collaboration with a vascular-trained access surgeon. Depending on the circumstance, a left-sided or right-sided (for L5-S1 only) retroperitoneal approach, can be performed. A direct transperitoneal (transabdominal) approach is usually reserved for revision cases.

### Key Principles

The location, orientation, and size of the incision and the approach can vary according to the location and extent of the pathology, the size of the patient, prior anterior abdominopelvic surgeries, the nature of the spinal procedure to be performed, and the experience of the access surgeon (**Fig. 46.1**).

### Expectations

The expectation is not only that the area of pathology be well visualized, but also that all the abdominal and pelvic structures be safely retracted, and that they remain well retracted during the extent of the surgical procedure (**Fig. 46.2**). Furthermore, it is desirable that adequate lighting be available because the overhead

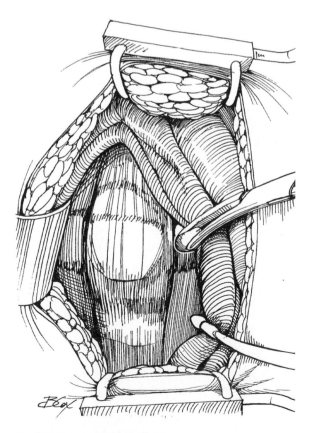

**Fig. 46.1** *Exposure of the L5-S1 disk.*

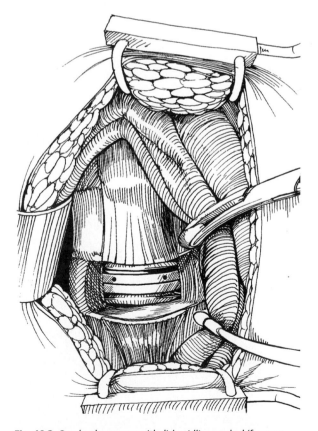

**Fig. 46.2** *One-level exposure with disk midline marked (for prosthetic disk placement).*

lights are often blocked by the surgeon during the procedure; adequate lighting can be provided by self-illuminating retractors or by head lights. With some of the modern interbody or corpectomy devices, and artificial disk replacements, it is also necessary for the surgical segment(s) to be visualized radiographically with the retractors in place, which is made possible by radiolucent retractors.

### Indications
Any procedure involving anterior lumbar interbody fusion or anterior lumbar corpectomy and fusion, which are usually performed for intractably symptomatic degenerative disk disease, deformity, instability, trauma, tumor, or infection.

### Contraindications
An active abdominal or pelvic infection is a contraindication to anterior lumbar surgery in the same vicinity, unless the target of the surgery is an infection in the spine itself. Relative contraindications include previous anterior surgery at the operative level, morbid obesity, severe atherosclerosis of the anterior blood vessels, and severe endometriosis or other pelvic inflammatory disorders.

### Special Considerations
Because the exposure is only as good as how well it can be maintained, having a good retractor system is key. We favor a table-held retractor system, because it keeps a steady pressure (as determined to be safe by the access surgeon) on the abdominal contents, minimizes readjustments of the retractors on the tissues, and frees up the hands for performing the procedure. Our experience is that the anterior lumbar surgery (ALS) radiolucent retractor blades with reverse lips at the tips (Thompson Surgical Instruments, Inc., Traverse City, MI) stay anchored onto the sides (anterolateral gutters) of the lumbar spine very well, minimizing slipping and springing out. These retractors come with adaptable handles for use with any of the existing table-held retractor systems currently available. These retractors come in both rigid and malleable versions and are strong enough to hold back the tissues once deployed. This is especially helpful during artificial disk replacement surgery, where a wider anterior exposure of the disk is necessary to identify the midline of the disk, perform a thorough diskectomy, restore disk height symmetrically, and elevate a contracted posterior longitudinal ligament if necessary (**Fig. 46.3**).

We caution against the use of Hohman retractors and Steinmann pins drilled into the vertebral bodies for retraction, as they may structurally damage the vertebra if knocked loose, and by virtue of their sharp tips can damage nearby tissues during placement or removal.

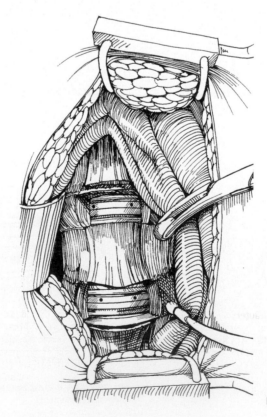

**Fig. 46.3** *Final view with prosthetic disk in position.*

Some of the modern interbody or corpectomy devices, and all of the artificial disks, require fluoroscopic visualization during instrumentation. To this end, a radiolucent Jackson table may be used. Proper lighting is essential when working in confined spaces such as the anterior lumbar spine, which necessitates either multiple overhead lights (to avoid blockage by the working surgeon) or head lights. Local visualization can be greatly facilitated by self-illuminating retractor blades as well. Some surgical field illuminators are available as sleeves that fit over existing retractor blades.

It is generally a good idea to have cell saver machinery set up during the surgery, as bleeding can be brisk from a vascular laceration in this area, although this is fortunately a rare occurrence with experienced access surgeons. Rarely, a clot can form or an atherosclerotic plaque may break off inside a vessel at the retracted site, which may require additional vascular surgery, and the cell saver will be necessary.

A pulse oximetry setup on the patient's left big or second toe can provide valuable information about blood flow and pulses across the vessels in the operative area. A warning tone tells the access surgeon when blood flow to the extremity is compromised, and thus the amount of ischemia time can be monitored. If the procedure causes ischemia for 45 to 50 minutes, the pressure on the vessels can be released for 30 seconds and the retractors reapplied for another 30 minutes. Pulse oximetry can also be invaluable in assessing pulse and blood flow at the end of the procedure. If the saturation does not return to preoperative levels, left iliac artery thrombosis is diagnosed unless proven otherwise. In our experience, cases of arterial thrombosis have been detected with the help of this technique.

Antiemetics, such as Reglan, and gastric decompression are recommended during the procedure. Nasogastric or orogastric tubes may be inserted after the patient is under anesthesia and removed at the completion of the procedure. They help reduce the incidence of ileus.

### Special Instructions, Position, and Anesthesia

It is good practice to examine the preoperative radiographs to assess the location of the surgical level against palpable landmarks such as the iliac crests or pubis. Inspection of the lateral radiograph also reveals whether the bottom disk spaces are easily accessible with a good line-of-sight over the pubis, and where the incision should be made for ideal visualization of the angled disk spaces.

The exact procedure planned and the type of instrumentation to be performed should be relayed to the access surgeon (e.g., fusion versus artificial disk replacement), because the optimal type, extent, and orientation of the approach may vary. For example, for an artificial disk replacement, a symmetric anterior exposure of the disk space is needed to properly center the device, whereas for a fusion, a limited anterolateral exposure may be sufficient.

The patient is positioned supine on a radiolucent (e.g., Jackson) table that will accommodate a fluoroscopy machine positioned under and across it for anteroposterior and lateral image intensification. If a regular operating table is used, it may have to be reversed head-to-toe to make this possible. The arms should be abducted at approximately right angles to the body to allow plenty of room for fluoroscopy machine positioning. Although not used at our center, a Trendelenburg position is reported to be helpful sometimes as it allows the abdominal structures to move in a cephalad direction.

A small bump may be placed under the back to lordose the spine for access into the disk space. However, too large a bump can cause the anterior vessels to drape against the anterior of the spine, making them difficult to mobilize. An inflatable pneumatic bladder and pump make it easy to adjust the lordosis intraoperatively.

Anesthesia should provide complete muscle relaxation throughout the procedure because the retractors are under tension, and loss of relaxation can cause them to become dislodged.

### Tips, Pearls, and Lessons Learned

At times, optimal retraction cannot be maintained by self-retaining retractors, and a hand-held malleable retractor may need to be held in place by an assistant. The surgeon must always keep an eye out for tissues, such as vessels or the ureter, that may be exposed or may protrude between the retractor blades. We recommend holding an instrument (e.g., suction tip or surgical sponge) in the nondominant hand to protect tissues from the working field where the dominant hand is performing the diskectomy. If the protrusion is large or increasing, or if the retractors are unstable, it is better to adjust them early or to call this to the attention of the access surgeon sooner than later. If a burr or drill has to be used, it should be turned on only after the working end (bit) is totally inside the disk space, and should be turned off and the bit should be still before removing it from the disk space.

Retrograde ejaculation is a possible complication with this approach in males, with a reported incidence ranging from less than 2 to 10%. This is a risk that must be discussed with patients, especially if they are planning on fathering children in the future. If so, some may choose to exercise the option of donating sperm to a sperm bank.

Cautery around the anterior spine should be minimized. It has been reported that the incidence of retrograde ejaculation in males may be higher with the use of cautery in this area (bipolar cautery is probably safer, with less electrical arcing). To reduce retrograde ejaculation, elevate the peritoneum away from the promontory with a Kittner. The fibers of the superior hypogastric plexus run adherent to the peritoneum, much as the ureter does. Mobilize this peritoneum to the right, if working from the left at L5-S1, and then the fibers will be protected once the retractor is deployed on the right side of the spine. Other means of maintaining hemostasis (e.g., ties, clips, Gelfoam, thrombin, other hemostatic agents), and blunt dissection (peanuts, laps) are also recommended.

When obtaining intraoperative radiographs, it is helpful to fill the exposed area with irrigation so as to avoid the "whiteout" effect seen with air on fluoroscopic imaging. This is especially true when trying to determine precise locations for artificial disk reconstruction.

Oval-shaped, sturdy suction tips may be useful to enter narrow disk spaces, and can also be used to lever open tight disk spaces during diskectomy.

Specially designed disk space distractors can be used to sequentially distract the disk space, making it easier to progress along with the diskectomy with good visualization. Distractors also allow visualization of the posterior vertebral edges, which is necessary for complete diskectomy and if posterior longitudinal ligament (PLL) elevation is needed. We prefer the ProDisc-L distractor (Synthes Spine, Paoli, PA) because it can be confined in one half of the disk space while the surgeon works in the other half, and then can be switched to the other side once the first half is finished. It is key, however, not to distract the distractor with its tips in the central weaker part of the end plate, as this may cause fractures and increase the risk of subsidence of the interbody device (which is especially undesirable for an artificial disk). The distractor tips should reach across to the posterior apophyseal ring before expansion (fluoroscopy may be needed to ensure this).

It may be advisable to instrument the tightest disk level first if operating on multiple levels; otherwise the surgeon may find it difficult to get a decent-sized device in after the other levels have been instrumented. Sometimes it may even be necessary to perform diskectomies at the other levels, and then to begin instrumentation at the tightest disk space. However, one has to minimize the number of times the retractors have to be moved. One solution would be to perform diskectomies from the taller disk to the tightest one, and then instrument from the tightest disk to the taller one.

### Difficulties Encountered

The greatest difficulty is encountered during mobilization of the great vessels, especially at the L4-L5 level, where over 90% of all vascular injuries have been shown to occur. At the L5-S1 level, this is not as serious a problem because it is usually below the bifurcation of the vessels.

Scarring produced by a previous surgery or inflammatory process can certainly increase the difficulty of the dissection. Meticulous attention must be paid to identifying all the important anterior structures such as the bowel, vessels, and ureters. Stents may be placed in the ureters by an urologist prior to the surgery to aid in identifying and protecting them. The stents can be removed after surgery.

### Key Procedural Steps

The patient should be positioned as mentioned above (**Fig. 46.4**). If autologous iliac crest bone graft is to be harvested, this can be done during the approach, but prior to deployment of the table-held, self-retaining retractors. Additional risk is possible if the retractors are removed for graft harvest, and then placed in again.

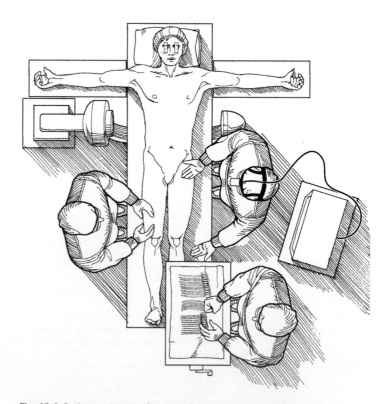

**Fig. 46.4** *Patient positioning, location of surgeon (with head light), assistant (across the surgeon), scrub tech, and fluoroscopy machine.*

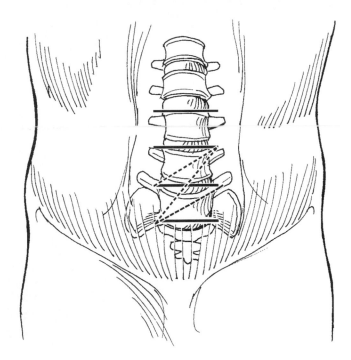

**Fig. 46.5** *Mapping the incisions for approaches to various levels.*

Incision location: Fluoroscopically localized and placed transverse incisions are best for single-level cases. Oblique or vertical midline incisions are acceptable for multiple levels. Vertical, paramedian incisions are to be avoided because a larger incision for the same amount of exposure is required and there is more disruption of the retroperitoneal planes above and below the target levels, thus making revision surgery in the future that much more difficult (**Fig. 46.5**).

It is recommended that retraction and exposure for more than one level at a time not be pursued unless it is easily accomplished, and only at L4-L5 or above, as excessive traction or stretch may be imparted on the vessels and the abdominal structures. It is better to have the retractors moved as the procedure is completed a level at a time.

To reduce the incidence of venous injury, we recommend that the ileolumbar vein always be ligated and transected when approaching L4-L5. With experience, the surgeon sometimes may decide not to take it, but initially it is a good habit to get into. Remember also that the lumbosacral plexus is very close to where the ileolumbar vein dips posteriorly, so be careful if clips are used for its distal control (**Fig. 46.6**).

To help reduce the incidence of left iliac artery thrombosis, make sure that the distal external iliac artery is mobilized as distally as possible. This is very easy to do with a Kittner because this artery has no branches except for a very occasional muscular branch to the psoas that can be easily clipped and transected. This reduces stretch when mobilizing the vessels far to the right and placing the retractors. Stretch is not well tolerated, as it may lead to microintimal tears that release cytokines and create a thrombogenic situation.

### Bailout, Rescue, Salvage Procedures

The approach surgeon should be comfortable in converting the approach type. If a retroperitoneal approach is difficult and dangerous, especially in revisions, then the approach can be converted to a transabdominal transperitoneal approach.

If it is discovered that only some of the planned levels are accessible, or if an unforeseen event precludes performing the entire surgery, alternate means of treating the spine should be planned (e.g., posterior procedures).

The approach surgeon should be comfortable handling any vascular complication or event. This can range from repairing lacerations to performing thrombectomies. If an iliac vein tear needs to be repaired with sutures, then the patient may need to be anticoagulated because the incidence of ileofemoral venous thrombosis is higher after these repairs. Careful deep vein thrombosis (DVT) monitoring is also mandatory in these patients.

Patients undergoing thrombectomy or arterial repair may need to be anticoagulated during the procedure, but the heparin should be reversed after the arterial procedure and then the patient placed on an antiplatelet medication such as Plavix.

In cases of massive disruption of a major vein, especially in an inaccessible area, an attempted repair may result in too much blood loss and significant morbidity or fatality. It may be prudent in such situations to obtain control of the injured area with pressure and then go above and below and ligate the vessel, even if it means ligating the inferior vena cava and both common iliac veins. This is relatively well tolerated and may be an appropriate salvage procedure.

**PITFALLS**

- Improper incision placement can result in significant struggling during the approach or the spinal procedure. A retroperitoneal approach in the setting of prior abdominal procedures may be difficult due to scarring, granulation tissue, and difficulty in identifying and preserving the peritoneum and its contents. Wrong-level surgery is easily avoided by good radiographic/fluoroscopic visualization. The approach surgeon may find this useful intraoperatively to confirm surgical level.

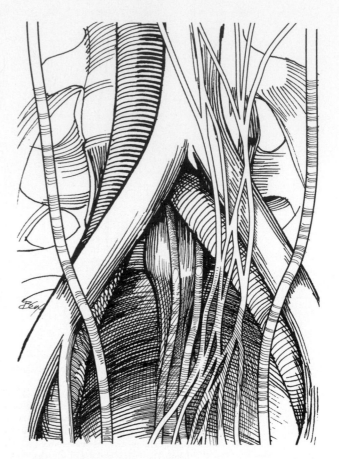

**Fig. 46.6** *Retroperitoneal anatomy at the anterior lumbosacral region.*

Revision surgery should be performed only by very experienced access surgeons, as it requires thorough knowledge of how tissues react to prior surgery in the area. Knowledge of what was done before is also crucial to plan the revision approach. Within a week to 14 days it may be acceptable to return via the same incision and approach path. Beyond 14 days we recommend that an alternate route be mapped.

Imaging studies, such as venograms (or MRI venograms), may be necessary, especially for an anteriorly dislocated prosthesis at L4-L5 that may be impinging on the left common iliac vein. If clots are present, a vena cava filter must be inserted prior to the revision.

In general, revisions at L5-S1 should be attempted from the opposite side of the prior approach or via a transabdominal route. Revisions of L4-L5 are best approached either via a more lateral approach or a transabdominal approach that goes lateral to the sigmoid colon along the peritoneal reflection. For L3-L4 and L2-L3, it is prudent to go lateral above or below the prior approach to try to find undisturbed retroperitoneal planes.

Do not try revision approaches from the right side except for L5-S1. The location of the vena cava makes the risk prohibitive when going from the right, even in primary cases.

# 47

# Anterior Lumbar Diskectomy

*Matías G. Petracchi, Federico P. Girardi, and Frank P. Cammisa, Jr.*

## Description
Disk resection by an approach that provides direct visualization of the anterior or lateral aspect of the lumbar spine.

## Key Principles
Good exposure, retraction of the great vessels when necessary, especially in gaining anterior access to the disk.

## Expectations
Complete diskectomy permits insertion of an interbody spacer to allow either motion preservation with a device such as a disk arthroplasty or insertion of an allograft, autograft, or cage to aid fusion. Direct debridement of a diskitis is also possible via this approach. Finally, anterior release as part of the correction of a spinal deformity can be undertaken.

## Indications
Interbody fusion, release for correction of spinal deformities, debridement in spondylodiskitis, open biopsy, corpectomy, disk replacement, nucleoplasty.

## Contraindications
Related to the approach: abdominal or pelvic infection.

## Special Considerations
The interbody space can be accessed by anterior, anterolateral, or lateral windows, depending on the indication for the diskectomy and interbody reconstruction. If the procedure requires the insertion of an interbody device such as a strut graft, cage, arthroplasty, or nucleoplasty, recommendations of the manufacturer should be followed. There are various interbody spreaders that help to open the disk space when performing diskectomy. Usually a wide resection of the disk and precise preparation of the end plate is necessary. This permits accurate contact of the interbody device with the vertebral end plates' surfaces and better release. Some devices require resection of posterior osteophytes or the longitudinal ligament.

Special care should be taken to preserve or restore the size of the disk space. Frontal and sagittal alignment evaluation is crucial to avoid iatrogenic imbalance. Also, it is important to preserve or restore the disk height, which can be evaluated with the preoperative studies, measuring the adjacent normal levels. In general, fusion or motion preservation implants are designed with different size options, which can help to reconstruct the alignment and height of the disk space.

## Special Instructions, Position, and Anesthesia
Patient positioning on the operating table can greatly facilitate diskectomy. Ideally the operative level should be positioned over the "break" in the table so that the disk space can be opened up by changing the angulation of the table at the level of the break. This can be very helpful, both in preparing the disk space and inserting the interbody device. A radiolucent table should be used to allow intraoperative imaging. The arms of the patient can be strapped in by the side, around the chest, or abducted, but special attention should be paid to avoid distraction of the brachial plexus and ensure adequate intraoperative radiographic quality. After the approach and before starting the diskectomy lateral and anteroposterior images, confirm the level and locate the midline of the disk space. During the diskectomy, tilting the table toward the surgeon, proper illumination, and magnification loupes are essential to visualize the space and work comfortably. If an interbody rigid device is to be used, the table should be replaced in a neutral position after its insertion, and the position of the device checked with x-ray or fluoroscopy. Be sure that the device is well aligned in the frontal and sagittal plane, maintains or restores the lumbar lordosis, and does not create an iatrogenic imbalance (**Fig. 47.1**).

## Tips, Pearls, and Lessons Learned
Patient positioning is crucial and permits good intraoperative visualization of both the disk space and end plates in addition to adequate radiographic imaging. Visualization of the disk space is further aided by the use of a combination of self-retaining and hand-held retractors. Long curettes and rongeurs are useful to perform the diskectomy. Interbody spreaders help to distract the space during the diskectomy.

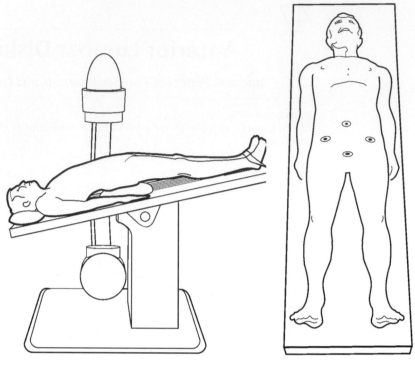

A                                                                                    B

**Fig. 47.1  (A)** *The patient is positioned supine with a bolster under the pelvis to allow for proper visualization. The steep Trendelenburg position is desirable and beneficial. The patient must be stabilized to avoid migration during the procedure. **(B)** The same patient as seen from above.*

### Difficulties Encountered

If the level to be treated has osteophytes, they can complicate the localization and initial disk resection. A spinal needle is utilized to confirm the level. A large rongeur or osteotome is useful to remove the osteophytes and identify the disk space. After resecting the majority of the disk, it is important to evaluate the residual disk located on the opposite side of the approach. Interbody spreaders help to distract the space during the diskectomy and permit a better evaluation of the remnant disk. Small curettes, Woodson or dental elevators, and nerve hook or ball-tip palpators are valuable to evaluate the opposite surface.

### Key Procedural Steps

After exposing the levels, good visualization of the disk space is necessary. Retraction of the paraspinal structures is required prior to diskectomy. The presacral plexus of nerves, the genitofemoral nerve, and the sympathetic chain should be preserved. The presacral plexus runs vertically across the L5-S1 disk space, superficially to the middle sacral artery and veins (**Fig. 47.2**). The genitofemoral nerve lies on the psoas and exits the muscle belly at the L3 level. The sympathetic chains are closely applied to the vertebral bodies medial to the psoas muscle. They can be mobilized by blunt dissection. Avoid dissecting directly over them, cutting transversely across them, or using cautery (especially unipolar). If the disk has to be resected through an anterior window, proximal to the great vessels bifurcation, the vascular structures should be mobilized laterally to the opposite side of the approach (**Fig. 47.3**). Distal to the great vessel bifurcation each vessel can be mobilized to its own side. Sometimes it is necessary to ligate and divide the adjacent segmental vessels, the iliolumbar vein (L4-5 disk space), or the middle sacral artery and veins (L5-S1 disk space) to permit the mobilization of the great vessels. The retraction of the vessels can be done with a retractor blade, protected pin or combination of both.

If small perforating veins are present in the disk space, they can be cauterized with a bipolar coagulator and divided.

The extent of disk resection and which ligaments should be divided depends on several variables including the approach utilized, indications for surgery, and the specific interbody implant or graft utilized. The anterior longitudinal ligament (ALL) and the anterior annulus can be preserved or minimally resected in the anterolateral approach to the disk but it should be divided, elevated, and restored later if a direct anterior approach is utilized. If the indication is an arthrodesis, the goal should be to remove the complete disk and cartilage to increase the area available for fusion. Deformity correction requires a release of structures including the ALL and the complete annulus. Also the size, design, and purpose of the interbody device are a guide to deciding how much intervertebral soft tissue must be removed. For example, for most cylindrical cage systems and nucleoplasty, partial diskectomies can be undertaken. On the other hand, some disk arthroplasties require extensive detachment of the surrounding soft tissue prior to inserting the device.

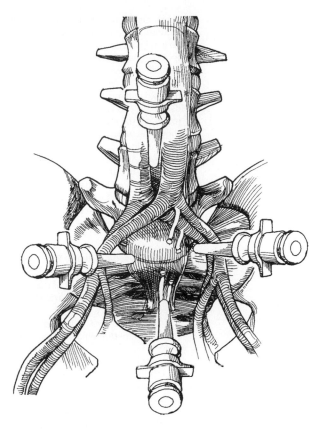

**Fig. 47.2** *The exposure and pin or blade retractors used for L5-S1 within the bifurcation of the iliac vessels.*

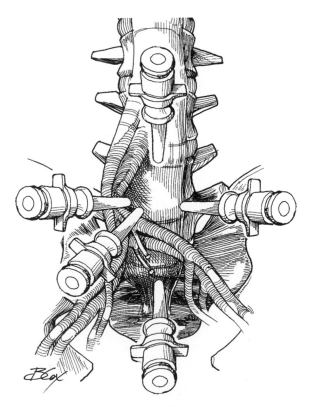

**Fig. 47.3** *The position of the pin or blade retractors and retraction for L4–5 and above, with the aorta and the vena cava retracted laterally.*

**PITFALLS**
- Related to the approach: great vessel injuries, anterior spinal artery ischemic syndrome, urogenital complications, injury to the sympathetic nerves, superior hypogastric plexus lesions, and genitofemoral or ilioinguinal nerves injuries. Complications during the diskectomy include wrong-level surgery, retropulsed remnant disk material, neurologic injury, dural tear, epidural bleeding. During the postoperative period: epidural hematoma, spondylodiskitis.

The diskectomy starts with the annulotomy. Long instruments are helpful during the disk resection. The annulus is incised parallel to the end plates with electrocautery or a small blade (No. 15). The unipolar cautery helps to detach the annulus from the external edge of the adjacent end plates, and the blade is used to disconnect the disk. A window or flaps of the annulus can be performed. The flaps of the annulus can then be utilized to protect the paraspinal structures. A narrow and sharp Cobb elevator continues with the separation of the disk from the end plate and should be directed from the external to the internal surface to avoid damage of vital structures. Angle and straight pituitary rongeurs are utilized to continue with the diskectomy as far back as the posterior annulus. Later on, different curettes (straight, curve, ring) help to detach the remnant disk and cartilage from the end plates and the annulus, but the subchondral bone should remain intact to support the interbody device and prevent its subsidence.

Initial distraction can be done with wide Cobb elevators, followed by a laminar spreader or by specially designed interbody spreaders. When the disk space is collapsed, disk space distracters can be utilized to permit better access. To monitor the distraction, lateral fluoroscopy or x-ray and handheld disk space distractors are essential.

The end plates can be partially decorticated with a burr to enhance the fusion or make a plane surface if it is required by the implant. Burring the end plate enhances vascular ingrowth and is recommended if sclerotic bone is present or when nonthreaded cages will be implanted.

### Bailout, Rescue, Salvage Procedures

Epidural bleeding and dural tear are difficult to control because of the lack of visualization and limited exposure of the dorsal aspect of the interbody space. Direct coagulation with bipolar is difficult, and unipolar cautery should be avoided. Irrigation, time, and thrombin-soaked sponges such as Gelfoam help to stop the bleeding.

A dural tear is very difficult to repair by direct suture, and free muscle, fascia graft, fibrin glue, or a combination of them should be attempted. On rare occasions it is necessary to implant a lumbar subarachnoid drain.

If a radiculopathy occurs after the procedure, consider a possible epidural hematoma, malposition of the interbody prosthesis, or retropulsed disk material because of the pushing effect of the prosthesis on a remnant disk. After confirming the diagnosis with an appropriate image and if the motor function has deteriorated, a revision surgery to reposition the implant or a posterior approach to resect the disk herniation or the epidural hematoma should be attempted.

In the case of a postoperative infection, prolonged antibiotic treatment has to be initiated promptly, and a surgical debridement should be considered, especially if there is no response to the conservative treatment or if an abscess has formed.

# 48

# Anterior Lumbar Interbody Fusion (ALIF): Cylinder Cages, Femoral Ring Allograft, Trapezoidal Synthetic Implants

*Arya Nick Shamie*

## Description

Using the anterior retroperitoneal, transperitoneal, or lateral trans-psoas approach, the disk space is exposed. A complete diskectomy is performed and an implant is used to distract the end plates, create annular tension, and accomplish a fusion of the disk space. Autogenous bone graft, bone marrow, biologics, or bone morphogenetic protein (BMP) is used to increase the fusion rate.

## Expectations

Anterior lumbar interbody fusion (ALIF) exposure allows for a near-complete diskectomy. This anterior exposure allows for a larger implant with a greater area of contact with the end plates as compared with smaller, posteriorly placed interbody implants. Therefore, less risk of subsidence and higher fusion rates are expected. BMP implantation not only increases the fusion rates as comparable to autogenous bone graft but also avoids the morbidity associated with the bone graft harvest site. ALIF avoids the exposure through the posterior musculature and the "fusion disease" associated with it.

## Indications

Discogenic back pain with positive diskogram, instability, or grade one spondylolisthesis, pseudarthrosis, or continued back pain following a posterolateral fusion. Relative indication includes revision of failed spine arthroplasty.

## Contraindications

Multilevel discogenic back pain, spinal canal pathology, osteoporotic bone, bone-on-bone degenerative disk disease, instability with greater than 25% listhesis in any direction. Relative contraindications include prior retroperitoneal surgery with adhesions, and a young male patient.

## Special Considerations

Anterior lumbar interbody fusion in osteoporotic patients should be avoided. Complete diskectomy and exposure of the underlying bleeding end plates improve fusion rates. Fixation with an anterior plate or pedicle screw fixation can also improve fusion rates. The use of BMP in cages is indicated for improved fusion rates.

Preoperative planning with templating of the operative level and the adjacent disk space is helpful to restore the appropriate disk height. Bifurcation of the great vessels can be visualized on magnetic resonance imaging (MRI), and hence the surgical approach can be individualized. Calcified great vessels visualized on preoperative radiographs should be retracted carefully to minimize the risk of a thrombotic event, which could compromise lower extremity perfusion.

The extreme lateral trans-psoas approach (XLIF) has its own unique considerations. Electromyograph (EMG) monitoring of the tubular dilators, as they are advanced through the psoas down to the disk space, is a requirement to avoid nerve root injury. XLIF is not generally possible at the L5-S1 level due to obstruction by the iliac wing. In rare cases, the XLIF procedure may need to be converted to an ALIF procedure due to anatomic limitations; patients should sign consent forms for both procedures when an XLIF is planned.

## Tips, Pearls, and Lessons Learned

Lateral fluoroscopy versus spot radiography is helpful in identifying the disk space margins as the implant is seated in its ideal position. This ideal position is a few millimeters recessed deep to the anterior margin of the adjacent end plates. The osteophytes should be rongeured off the anterior end plates prior to the diskectomy as they may obscure normal anatomy and result in improper placement of the interbody implant. Once the anterior annulus is incised with a scalpel, a Cobb elevator can be used to detach the Sharpey's fibers from the superior and inferior end plates, and then the disk can be removed in one piece. Overly sclerotic end plates can be burred in the center to expose the bleeding end plates. Sequential

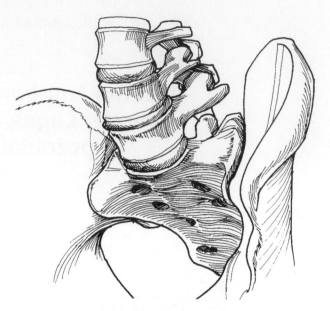

**Fig. 48.1** *Anterior view of the lumbosacral spine and the intervening disks.*

dilation of the disk space with sizers is an important step to adequately distract the end plates and insert a press-fit implant. An AO cancellous screw with a washer can be placed at the anterior corner of the inferior end plate to minimize the risk of anteropulsion of the implant.

### Key Procedural Steps

#### *Direct Anterior Approach* (Figs. 48.1 and 48.2)
This approach is typically used for the L5-S1 level, which is below the bifurcation of the great vessels. A Pfannenstiel incision is made, and the retroperitoneal approach to the disk space is accomplished. The middle sacral artery, which typically crosses the field, is dissected and ligated. The diskectomy and end-plate curetting to bleeding bone is performed and distractors followed by sizers are used for proper implant size selection. The implant is then packed with bone graft or BMP and is impacted into the disk space using fluoroscopy guidance. The implant can also be inserted while the patient's lumbar spine is in hyperlordosis, created by patient positioning. The patient needs to be returned to neutral alignment after the implant is positioned to check for stability.

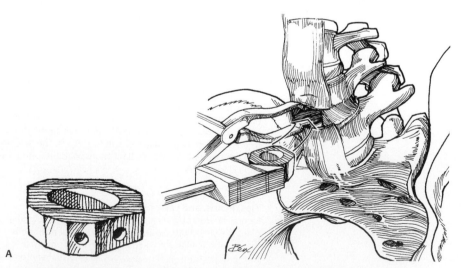

A                                                             B

**Fig. 48.2** *(A) Femoral ring alloimplant spacer. (B) Direct anterior approach of the L4-5 disk space.*

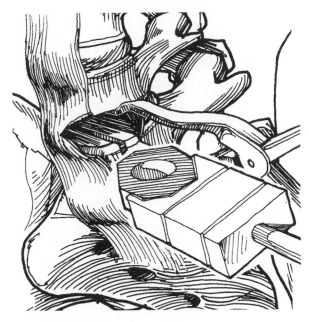

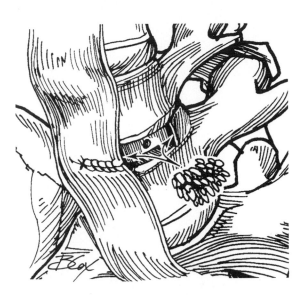

**Fig. 48.3** *Anterolateral approach using the 30-degree offset femoral ring alloimplant spacer.*

**Fig. 48.4** *Packing bone graft around the anterior space of the implant.*

### Anterolateral Approach (Figs. 48.3 and 48.4)

This approach is used for L2–L5 levels and is approximately 30 degrees lateral to the direct anterior approach. This approach allows for retraction of the vessels to the right side for proper visualization of the disk space. The left iliolumbar vein needs to be ligated when the L4-L5 level is being exposed. This approach does not require the takedown of the anterior longitudinal ligament, which helps maintain the vertebral segment's stability. The diskectomy and end-plate preparation is the same as the direct anterior approach. Anteroposterior and lateral fluoroscopy should be used throughout the procedure for proper placement of the implant.

### Lateral Trans-Psoas Approach (XLIF)

This is also a minimally invasive approach requiring one lateral flank incision overlying the disk space and another incision at the same level but just lateral to the paraspinal muscles. Through the paraspinal incision the retroperitoneal space is digitally expanded and the dilators are placed through the lateral incision. The trans-psoas dilation is performed with constant EMG monitoring to avoid nerve injury. The ribs and the pelvis limit the levels that can be exposed to L3-L4 and L4-L5 using this approach. The anterior longitudinal and the posterior longitudinal ligaments are preserved in this approach, and the implant is placed through a left annular window and across to the right edge of the end plates.

### Bailout, Rescue, Salvage Procedures

If the fracture of the implant is noted during implantation, reinsertion of a new implant is recommended. If the implant is not easily removed, hyperlordosis of the patient on the surgical table may aid the safe removal of the implant. Burring of a femoral ring allograft (FRA) is possible to help with safe removal. If the implant is not secure despite appropriate sizing, anterior or posterior fixation is used. Percutaneous pedicle screws can be used to avoid "fusion disease."

# Anterior and Anterolateral Lumbar Fixation Plating

*Thomas N. Scioscia and Jeffrey C. Wang*

## Description

Recent advances in plating systems have made anterior fixation possible after anterior lumbar interbody placement. Following a supine retroperitoneal or transperitoneal approach, diskectomy is performed and end plates are prepared to bleeding bone. The anterior lumbar interbody fusion (ALIF) graft of choice is then press-fit into the interspace, and fixation is achieved with a low-profile conventional or locking plate. After meticulous hemostasis, abdominal closure is performed. Anterolateral plating is performed through a lateral retroperitoneal approach. After exposure and corpectomy, a structural graft or cage is placed to re-create lordosis. A low-profile conventional or locking contoured plate is then applied laterally with two screws in the superior and inferior vertebral bodies.

## Expectations

Fusion rates of stand-alone ALIF have been extensively studied, and pseudarthrosis rates have been reported up to 35%. This may be due to the loss of the anterior longitudinal ligament, which increases instability in the flexion/extension plane. The advent of BMP has also raised the concern of remodeling and weakening of femoral ring allografts. These problems have prompted surgeons to back up ALIF procedures with either standard or percutaneous pedicle screws. Anterior plates have been studied in vitro, and they restore the anterior tension band and sagittal stability. The risk of vascular injury tempered the early excitement about anterior lumbar plating, but newer designs have rekindled interest. The Pyramid plate (Medtronic, Memphis, TN) is specially shaped to fit below the bifurcation of the great vessels and has a cover plate to prevent screw back-out (**Fig. 49.1**). The anterior tension band (ATB) plate (Synthes Inc, West Chester, PA) is a very low profile plate (3.5 mm), and the screws lock into the plate, minimizing the risk of vascular erosion (**Fig. 49.2**).

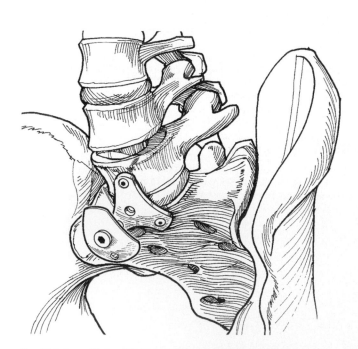

**Fig. 49.1** *Pyramid plate (Medtronic) placed at the L5-S1 interspace.*

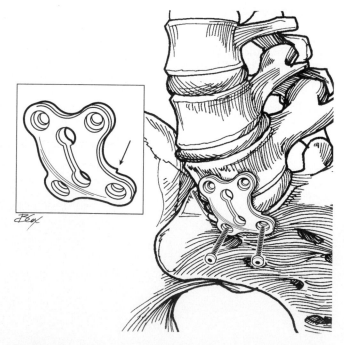

**Fig. 49.2** *The anterior tension band (ATB) plate (Synthes Inc.) placed at the L5-S1 interspace.*

## Indications

Supplemental fixation after ALIF for discogenic back pain with positive diskogram, instability or grade one spondylolisthesis, and pseudarthrosis after failed posterior surgery. The Pyramid plate is indicated only at the L5-S1 disk level. The plate is indicated from L1 to S1, though it should be placed anterolaterally above L5-S1 and used with extreme caution at these higher levels.

### Relative Indications

Supplemental fixation after ALIF for revision of failed spine arthroplasty.

## Contraindications

Instability with greater than 25% listhesis in any direction. Low-lying bifurcation of the great vessels.

### Relative Contraindications

- Prior retroperitoneal surgery with adhesions
- Calcification of the aorta and iliac arteries
- Osteoporosis

## Special Considerations

Great vessel anatomy must be visualized on magnetic resonance imaging (MRI). The bifurcation should be located superior to the L5 vertebral body when plating the L5-S1 interspace. If this is not the case, consent for posterior instrumentation should be obtained. Calcified great vessels visualized on preoperative radiographs should be retracted carefully to minimize the risk of a thrombotic event with catastrophic consequence. Pulse oximetry placed on the left second toe can alert the surgeon to the need for emergent thrombectomy of the left lower extremity vessels. A retroperitoneal approach is favored over a transperitoneal approach. The transperitoneal approach is associated with a five- to 10-fold increase in retrograde ejaculation as a complication. Placement of the conventional Pyramid plate needs to be flush on both vertebral bodies because it relies on friction with the screw/plate/bone interface for fixation. This implies that all osteophytes must be removed and the plate may not be ideal with spondylolisthesis. The locking plate is a fixed angle device and it still affords stability even if the plate is not fully seated on bone. When placing the ATB plate at all levels above L5-S1, careful attention must be paid to the great vessels.

## Tips, Pearls, and Lessons Learned

An experienced vascular surgeon minimizes the risk of vascular injury during the approach. The placement of the interbody graft should be recessed a few millimeters in the disk space. Lateral fluoroscopy is helpful in identifying the disk space margins as the implant is seated and is useful to guide plate and screw placement. The osteophytes should be rongeured before plate placement to ensure maximum bony contact. The smallest plate possible should be used to minimize the risk of vascular erosion. Placement of the plate should be away from the vessels, avoiding direct placement under venous structures.

## Key Procedural Steps

### Direct Anterior Approach with the ATB Plate

A Pfannenstiel incision or a small left-side oblique incision is made, and the retroperitoneal approach is utilized to access the L5-S1 disk space. The middle sacral artery located in the midline is ligated. The diskectomy includes all of the nucleus, end plates, the anterior annulus, and the ALL. Trial spacers are then impacted to a press-fit position. The implant is then packed with bone graft or bone morphogenetic protein (BMP) and is impacted into the disk space a few millimeters deep to the anterior vertebral body. The plates are sized using the smallest plate that will gain screw purchase into L5 and the sacral promontory. The L5-S1 plate has a cutout for the promontory, which is located on the inferior aspect of the plate. The correct-size plate is then placed on the interspace with all four threaded screw guides attached to the plate. Temporary fixation pins are placed in the contralateral screw holes, and fluoroscopy is used to confirm the correct plate position (**Fig. 49.3**). The awl is used to prepare the remaining two screw holes through the threaded drill guide. The thread drill guides are removed, the depth gauge is then pushed through the cancellous bone, and the unicortical depth is measured. The screws are then placed and locked into the plate. The temporary pins are removed and the remaining screws are placed in a similar manner. For levels above L5-S1, the plate may need to be placed anterolaterally for better fit around the vessels. An alternative approach for compression may be performed by placing the two inferior screws first. A Schanz pin is placed in L5, and compression forceps are applied to the plate and the pin (**Fig. 49.4**). The superior screws are then inserted in the previously described manner.

### Anterior Approach Using the Pyramid Plate

Using the same surgical exposure, the interbody graft is placed in the L5-S1 interspace. The plate is placed with the narrow end over L5. The correct-size plate is then attached to the plate holder and placed in the

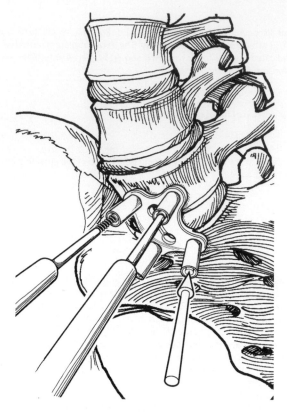

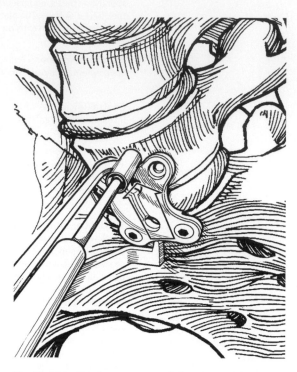

**Fig. 49.3** *The ATB plate is provisionally fixed using the detachable fixation pins.*

**Fig. 49.4** *The ATB plate is compressed after placing the inferior locking screws.*

proper position. The corresponding drill guide is then fastened to the plate using the screw-in mechanism. The awl is then used to create pilot holes for screw placement. The correctly measured screws are placed through the guide into the plate. The guide is then disengaged from the plate and removed from the wound. The corresponding cover plate and holder are then introduced, and the post in the cover is fitted into the inferior opening of the Pyramid plate. The *T*-handle of the holder is then rotated clockwise seating the cover plate onto the Pyramid plate (**Fig. 49.5**).

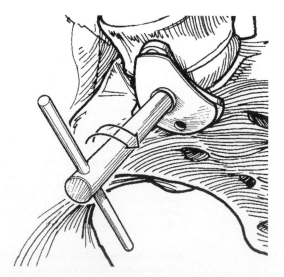

**Fig. 49.5** *The T-handle of the holder is then rotated clockwise seating the cover plate onto the Pyramid plate.*

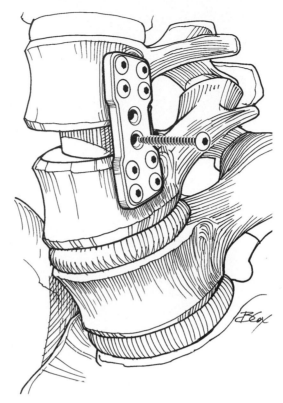

**Fig. 49.6** *The TLSP plate is placed laterally and fixed with optional bone graft screw.*

- The biggest pitfall of the procedure is symptomatic pseudarthrosis. Great vessel injury can be catastrophic either during the approach or because of chronic venous erosion. Screw back-out causing injury is minimized by the locking technology and the low profile of the plate. Thrombosis in the left lower extremity is also a concern. Retrograde ejaculation and sterility is possible, especially when the transperitoneal approach is utilized. Fracture of the L5 vertebrae or sacrum has also been described. Hernia and bowel injury have also been reported. Sympathetic injury could cause unilateral leg symptoms.

### *Anterolateral Approach with the Locking Thoracolumbar Spine Locking Plate (TSLP)*

The left-sided approach is favored due to the position of the liver. The patient is placed in the lateral position, and a flank incision is made through the abdominal muscles. The peritoneum is reflected anteriorly, exposing the psoas muscle. The psoas muscle is dissected off the vertebral body to access the vertebral body for a corpectomy. An abdominal retractor set is utilized for complete exposure from the 12th rib to the iliac crest. After corpectomy, diskectomy, and placement of a cage or structural allograft, the plate is then trialed similar to the anterior ATB plating technique. The rest of the technique is identical to that for the ATB technique, with the exception that the plate is of different configuration and placed laterally. After application, a screw can be placed in the center hole through a structural allograft if desired (**Fig. 49.6**).

### Bailout, Rescue, Salvage Procedures

Percutaneous or conventional pedicle screws can be used if the plate cannot be safely placed. Posterior fusion can also be added for pseudarthrosis or fracture of the L5 vertebral body. Bed rest combined with a thigh extension thoracolumbar spinal orthosis (TLSO) may also be reasonable for vertebral body fracture until healing occurs. Pulse oximetry can alert the surgeon to lower extremity thrombosis and the need for emergent thrombectomy. Direct repair of the great vessels and the consideration for anticoagulation is the treatment of choice for great vessel injury.

# 50

# Reduction of High-Grade Spondylolisthesis

*Charles C. Edwards and Charles C. Edwards II*

### Description
Full correction of high-grade spondylolisthesis (**Fig. 50.1**) is achieved through an entirely posterior approach, with or without sacral dome osteotomy, by using graduated instrumented distraction, posterior translation of the proximal spine, and flexion of the sacrum.

### Expectations
Careful preoperative planning, complete neural decompression, and the gradual application of corrective forces over time with effective instrumentation consistently yields anatomic reduction of the spine and a high rate of successful fusion without the need for anterior surgical approaches. For spondyloptosis, sacral dome osteotomy or a second stage of surgery may be necessary to limit lumbar root stretch.

### Indications
High-grade spondylolisthesis and spondyloptosis.

### Contraindications

#### Lack of Patience or Surgical Experience
This is a technically difficult and demanding undertaking even for the most experienced spinal surgeon. The surgeon cannot force reduction ahead of stress-relaxation and nerve accommodation. Hands-on training, experience with lesser slips, and a long learning curve are necessary to master the planning and reduction techniques for consistently excellent results.

#### Older or Frail Patients
This surgery is rarely indicated in patients over 40 or 50 years of age.

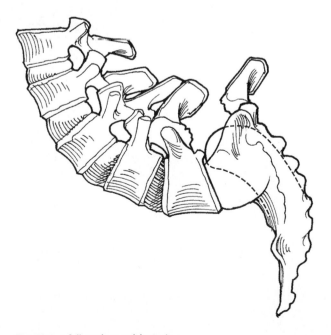

**Fig. 50.1** *A full-grade spondyloptosis.*

### Special Considerations

Preoperative planning is essential. Standing lateral and supine flexion/extension radiographs are needed to determine the "root-lengthening limit" and for planning surgery. First, make two tracings of the flexion lateral film: sacrum and L1–L5. To simulate complete reduction, the sacrum is flexed with its long axis oriented 35 degrees from vertical. The L1–L5 tracing is then positioned with L5 reduced, L3 horizontal, and L1 vertically centered over the anterior body of S1 (**Fig. 50.2**). To determine how much L5 nerve root lengthening will occur with full reduction, measure the distance from the L4 pedicle (root origin) to the sciatic notch (root exit) on the pre-reduction standing lateral and postreduction lateral tracings. The difference represents expected root lengthening.

The root-lengthening limit without deficit for one stage of surgery varies between 2 and 5 cm depending on several factors. The lengthening limit is reduced (from 5 toward 2 cm) when (1) the patient is older than 20; (2) the duration of optosis exceeds 2 years; (3) the L5/S1 slip angle is greater than 50 degrees; (4) bending films demonstrate a rather fixed panlumbar lordosis; (5) there have been prior lumbosacral (LS) fusion attempts or; (6) preoperative lumbar radiculitis/radiculopathy is present. If all six predictors are negative, only about 2 cm of lengthening is safe in one day, whereas if there are no negative predictors, 5 cm of lengthening is generally possible without deficit. If reduction exceeds the root lengthening limit, there are two alternatives: (1) the reduction may be divided between two procedures a week apart, or (2) the spine is shortened by removing 0.5 to 1.5 cm from the proximal sacrum through the posterior approach.

### Special Instructions, Position, and Anesthesia

Before surgery the patient practices ankle dorsiflexion for the wake-up test. An overhead traction frame is assembled over the head of the table. The patient is positioned prone with hips initially flexed 30 degrees to facilitate LS visualization and knees flexed 70–90 degrees to relax the sciatic nerve. Hips are extended later to facilitate reduction.

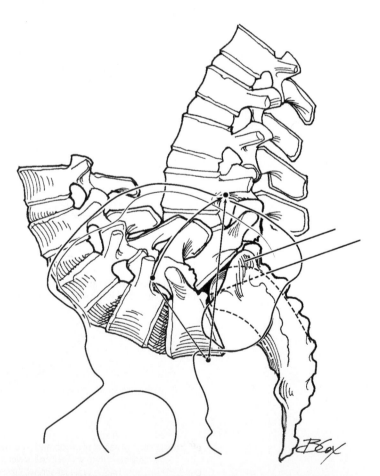

**Fig. 50.2** *Preoperative planning demonstrating the corrected position of the spine, the location of the sacral osteotomy, and measurement of the anticipated change in the L5 nerve length.*

**Tips, Pearls, and Lessons Learned**

The Spondylo Construct of the Edwards Modular Spine System (EMSS) (Scientific Spinal, Baltimore, MD) is specifically designed to facilitate this operation. It allows the surgeon to move and stabilize the spine simultaneously with 6 degrees of freedom. Controlled incremental change in spine position is made possible with ratcheted rods and threaded connectors.

**Difficulties Encountered**

The relationship of L5 to the sacral ala and L5 transverse process changes during the reduction sequence. The L5 roots need to be checked often during reduction to ensure no compression. Reduction lengthens the L5 root, which must also be checked for excessive tightness in addition to somatosensory evoked potential (SSEP)/electromyogram (EMG) monitoring. Reduction must be stopped if there is depression of the SSEP or EMG response or excess nerve tightness to palpation. Additional sacral shortening, root decompression as it crosses the ala, or an additional stage may be needed to safely complete the reduction.

**Key Procedural Steps**

- *Exposure:* Expose the spine from L3 to S2. Identify and protect the L3-L4 and L4-L5 facet capsules. L5 may sit anterior to the sacrum and be difficult to see. Partial reduction is therefore needed to safely decompress the L5 roots. This is accomplished with concurrent alar rod distraction and posterior traction.
- *Alar rods:* Insert EMSS combination connectors (reduction screws) into the L4 pedicles without injuring the facet capsules. Combination connectors consist of a pedicle screw–swivel joint-threaded rod and adjustable ring body. Next, insert the shoe of high (10 mm) anatomic hooks into holes burred in the top of the sacral ala. A short ratcheted universal rod is inserted into the hook distally and into the ring body of the L4 combination connector proximally. The ring bodies are ratcheted up these "alar rods" in small gradation to gradually raise L5 out of the pelvis.
- *Overhead traction:* Initial reduction to achieve L5 visualization requires both distraction and posterior translation of the lumbar spine. The posterior vector is provided by 18-gauge wires attached to the ring bodies of the L4 connectors or proximal end of the alar rods. The two sterile wires are passed to the anesthesiologist who ties them to traction rope. The rope passes over a pulley attached to the trapeze erected over the head of the bed; 20 to 30 lb are added to the end of each rope to create the cephalodorsal vector. Sequential distraction of the alar rods combined with the constant pull of dorsal traction yields stress-relaxation of the contracted anterior tissues. The L5 vertebra gradually rises out of the pelvis and around the sacral dome.
- *L5 root decompression:* Remove the L5 arch as a single block using the Gill technique. The L5 roots are covered by the medial edge of the superior facet of L5 and pars nonunion fibrocartilage. Place a small angled Kerrison punch into the canal just proximal to the L4-L5 facet joint and resect redundant ligamentum flavum, the osteophytic medial projection from the L5 superior facet, and various arrays of fibrocartilage all covering the L5 roots. Continue the decompression laterally with a 3- to 4-mm narrow-shoe Kerrison punch across the iliolumbar ligaments until the L5 roots pass anterior to the sacral ala. To prevent root injury, the L5 root must be continuously observed.
- *Sacral osteotomy:* If the preoperative planning radiographs indicate the need for proximal sacral osteotomy, the L5 and S1 roots and dural sac are fully mobilized to expose the sacral dome. The epidural venous plexus overlying the annulus is cauterized with a bipolar electrode. A ¼-inch osteotome is tamped into the sacral dome and adjusted under C-arm visualization until it matches the position planned for the osteotomy on the preoperative radiograph. The osteotomy is completed with ½-inch osteotomes from one side and then the other side of the dura extending to the lateral ala. The posterior annulus is then resected from its origin on the posteriorly projecting osteophytes at the base of the L5 vertebral body using curved osteotomes and large pituitary rongeurs. The resected sacral dome is cut into sections and removed in pieces together with the lumbosacral disk. If more than 1 cm is removed from the sacral dome, it is necessary to fashion posteromedial to anterolateral channels (pseudo-foramen) into the superior ala for the L5 roots to exit between the L5 transverse processes and the ala.
- *The spondylo construct:* Once alar rod distraction and posterior translation from overhead traction have raised L5 out of the pelvis, screws can be safely inserted into L5. With the L5 root and medial pedicle cortex under direct view, the L5 pedicle is cannulated with a blunt probe, oriented 20 degrees medially to spare the L4-L5 facet capsule dorsally and engage the vertebral body ventrally. After confirmation of appropriate trajectory with biplanar C-arm views, combination connector screws are inserted into L5. S1 screws may be directed either medially through the sacral pedicle or laterally across the ala. Bicortical alar screws are preferable after generous sacral osteotomy. A second point of distal fixation is needed to effectively control sacral rotation and to provide an adequate lever-arm for sacral flexion and mechanically sound fixation. When sacral bone is weak or the patient is obese, iliac screws can provide even stronger distal fixation. Mid-sacral alar screws, however, require less dissection and do not span the SI joints. In either case, rods are attached to the distal screws and to the S1 screws using a low or medium hook linkage. Before loading the rods, apply a cross-lock to the rods between the S1 and the distal fixation points. Then remove the alar rods one at a time and attach the L5 connectors to the rods (**Fig. 50.3**).

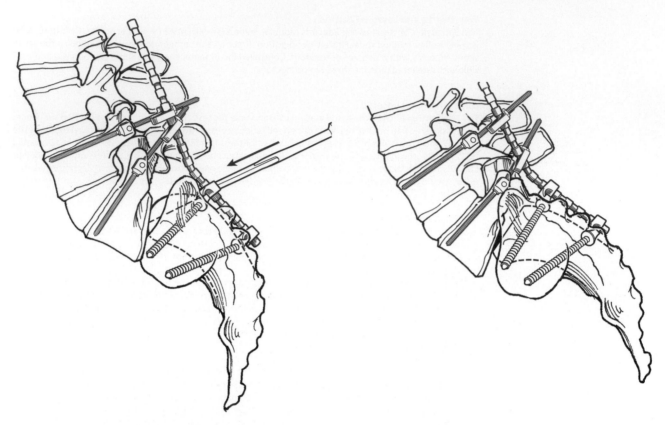

**Fig. 50.3** *Partial correction achieved with alar distraction rods and the position of the osteotome in the proximal sacrum.*

**Fig. 50.4** *The end of stage 1, with the completed sacral osteotomy, the spondylo instrumentation construct, and partial reduction.*

- *Reduction:*   The first phase of reduction is to raise L5 out of the pelvis. This is accomplished by the overhead traction and alar rods. Further correction is achieved by incrementally ratcheting and shortening the L5 connectors. First, shorten the connectors until resistance is felt, and then distract the connectors to separate the L5 body from the sacrum. Sequentially shorten (tighten) and distract (ratchet) the connectors to two-finger tightness every 10 minutes. Re-image to determine the relative amount of distraction versus translation required. Periodically check the L5 roots with a probe to ensure that they do not become overly taut or compressed between the L5 transverse process and the ala. Allow 30 to 60 minutes per grade for stress relaxation of the contracted anterior tissues to permit reduction of the deformity (**Fig. 50.4**). Reduction is continued until (1) the nerve lengthening threshold is met, (2) nerves become taut, (3) SSEP (or triggered EMG) data begin to deteriorate, or (4) function is reduced on wakeup. In the event of (3) or (4), reduction is partially released until normal function is restored.
- *Optional stage 2:*   If a subsequent stage is required to safely complete the reduction, the instrumentation is locked in place, and the wound closed. Patients are kept on bed rest for 1 week. We usually begin the second-stage reduction under local anesthesia. We have found that patients consistently experience sciatic pain from excess root stretch long before any change can be detected on EMG or SSEP. The surgeon is able to continuously monitor motor function by talking with the awake patient and observing ankle dorsiflexion. Once L5 is positioned on top of the sacrum within a few millimeters of anatomic alignment, the L5 connectors are compressed toward the sacrum to restore lordosis and further shortened until a normal alignment is achieved. Once reduction is nearly complete, the patient is given general anesthesia. The instrumentation is locked into its final position and any further needed root decompression is performed, followed by posterolateral decortication and iliac grafting (**Fig. 50.5**).
- *Postoperative bracing:*   Following surgery, our patients are routinely mobilized in a custom-made, below-the-breast thoracolumbar spinal orthosis (TLSO) with a thigh cuff. The brace serves to (1) lessen stress on the bone–implant interface, (2) counteract the flexion moment caused by contracted anterior tissues such as the rectus abdominus and iliopsoas muscles until they relax over time, and (3) prevent adjacent-segment kyphosis due to this flexion moment coupled with extensor muscle and L4-L5 facet capsular impairment from surgery.

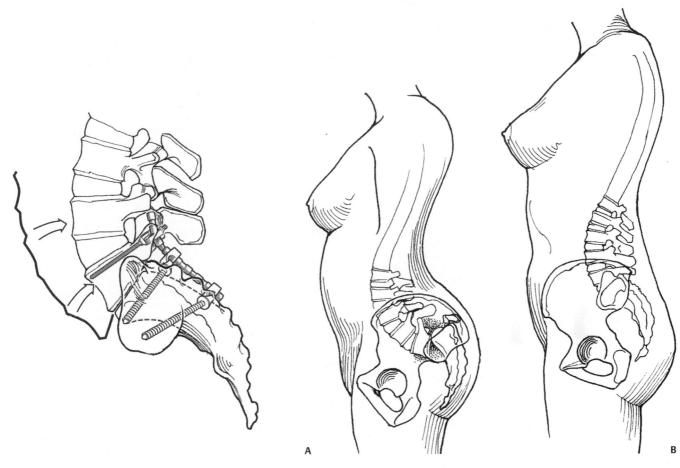

**Fig. 50.5** *Complete reduction.*

**Fig. 50.6** *Preoperative (A) and postoperative (B) illustrations demonstrating the restoration of trunk height and normal sagittal alignment.*

## PITFALLS

- The most common pitfall is the attempt to rush the reduction. Application of excess force can result in failure of implant fixation. Accelerating reduction faster than the rate of nerve root accommodation causes radiculopathy. The second most common pitfall is failure to adequately check and decompress the L5 roots at each stage of reduction. A third pitfall is to apply the concept of placing an interbody spacer between L5 and the sacrum for stabilization of low-grade spondylolisthesis to the treatment of high-grade deformities. Insertion of a spacer undermines the rapid fusion achieved with direct apposition of the decorticated inferior end plate of L5 with the osteotomized body of S1. Furthermore, to the extent that placement of an interbody device requires distraction of L5 relative to the sacrum, it increases the degree of root-stretch and likelihood of radiculopathy.

## Bailout, Rescue, Salvage Procedures

Using this method of posterior gradual instrumented reduction alone, we have successfully corrected over 100 consecutive high-grade deformities, primarily spondyloptosis, without the need for anterior surgical approaches (**Fig. 50.6**). In occasional adult cases of severe ptosis, add a third stage if stable alignment cannot be obtained due to signs of impending root stretch. If radiculopathy occurs, back off the reduction and confirm there is no root impingement, but do not abandon stable fixation. If it is not possible to obtain bilateral pedicle screw fixation at L5, extend the fixation to L4. If deep infection develops, follow the principles of sequential debridement and open wound treatment, but do not remove the instrumentation until fusion is solid. In rare spondyloptosis cases, progressive L4-L5 kyphosis develops after surgery. If it is painful or seriously impairs sagittal alignment, extend the instrumented fusion to L4. In most cases it is not necessary to fuse to L4, and we have never seen an indication to fuse to L3.

# 51

# Gaines Procedure for Spondyloptosis

*Vincent J. Devlin*

### Description

The Gaines procedure is a treatment option for spondyloptosis. This rare condition exists when the entire body of the L5 vertebra is located below the top of S1 on a standing lateral radiograph.

### Key Principles

The procedure requires a separate anterior and posterior approach to the lumbosacral junction. In the first stage, an anterior approach to the spine is performed, and the L5 vertebra, L5-S1 disk, and L4-L5 disk are removed (**Fig. 51.1**). In the second stage, the lamina and pedicles of L5 are removed to complete the L5 vertebrectomy, and the L4 vertebra is placed on top of the sacrum and held in place with pedicular fixation (**Fig. 51.2**).

### Expectations

The treatment of spondyloptosis is a major challenge. The Gaines procedure is designed to restore sagittal plane alignment and minimize the risk of complications of cauda equina syndrome and L5 nerve root deficit. In addition, the morbidity associated with long-segment instrumentation and fusion is avoided.

### Indications

The procedure is indicated only for symptomatic spondyloptosis. Lesser degrees of vertebral slippage are not indications for this procedure.

### Contraindications

Contraindications to the procedure may be related to surgeon factors, facility support issues, and patient factors. The procedure should be performed by spine surgeons with extensive experience in all types of spondylolisthesis surgery. The operating room environment should provide appropriate support services including an experienced access surgeon, an adequate number of experienced surgical assistants, appropriate spinal instrumentation, and the capacity for intraoperative spinal monitoring. The patient's

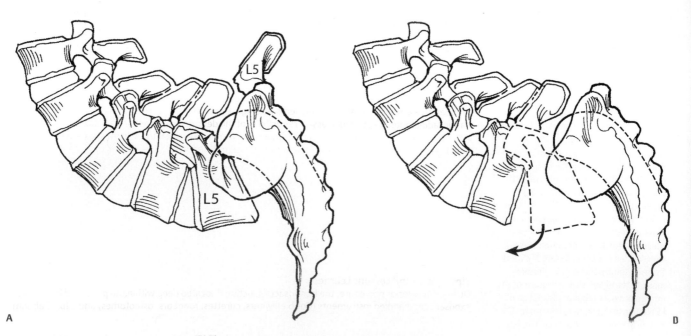

A                                                                                              B

**Fig. 51.1** **(A)** First-stage Gaines procedure. **(B)** The L5 vertebra, L5-S1 disk, and L4-L5 disk are removed.

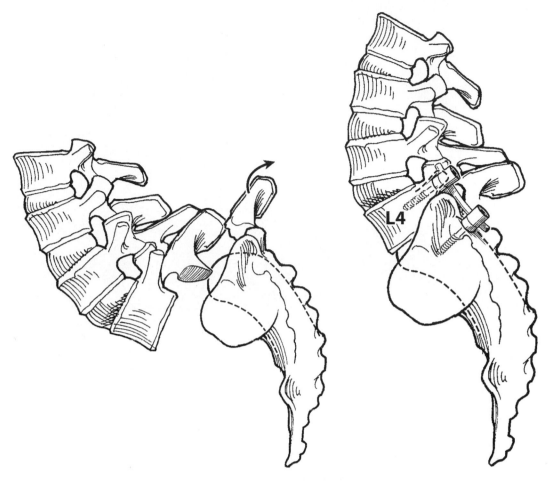

A

B

**Fig. 51.2** *Second-stage Gaines procedure. The lamina and pedicles of L5 (A) are removed to complete the L5 vertebrectomy, and the L4 vertebra (B) is placed on top of the sacrum and held in place with pedicular fixation.*

symptoms and deformity should be sufficiently severe to warrant surgery, and the patient must be informed about the risks and complications of the procedure as well as realistic expectations and goals following surgery.

### Special Considerations
Preoperative assessment includes detailed neurologic examination and appropriate imaging studies. Dynamic radiographs are utilized to assess reducibility of the deformity and to assess whether alternative procedures are a reasonable option. Neurodiagnostic imaging studies including magnetic resonance imaging (MRI) and computed tomography (CT) scans are important in planning surgical treatment. Patients with prior lumbar spine surgery, obesity, or prior abdominal surgery are more challenging surgical candidates.

### Special Instructions, Position, and Anesthesia
The first-stage procedure is performed with the patient in the supine position. The second-stage procedure may be performed on the same day or on a separate day based on multiple factors including duration of the first-stage procedure and intraoperative blood loss. If both procedures are performed on the same day, a Jackson table facilitates repositioning the patient to the prone position for the second-stage procedure.

### Tips, Pearls, and Lessons Learned
During the anterior procedure, the lumbosacral junction is located deep within the pelvis and is difficult to expose. Long-handled instruments (Cobb elevators, curettes, rongeurs, osteotomes) and a fixed abdominal retractor with long blades are essential for work in this area. During the posterior procedure, the posterior spine is located just beneath the skin, and careful and meticulous exposure is required to prevent iatrogenic neural injury.

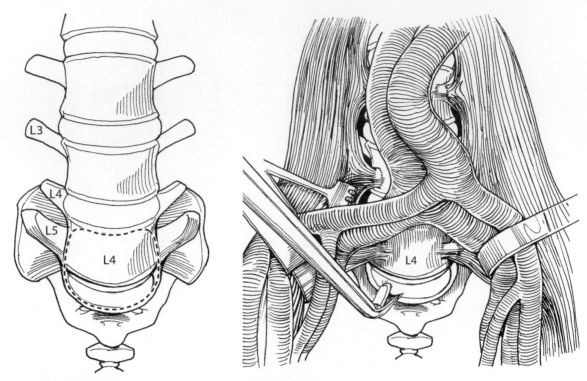

**Fig. 51.3** *(A,B) First stage. Anterior exposure for resection of the L4-L5 disk, L5 vertebral body, and L5-S1 disk.*

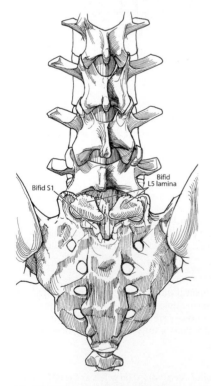

**Fig. 51.4** *Second stage. Posterior exposure from L2 to the sacrum. The L5 and S1 lamina frequently have a bifid structure.*

### Key Procedural Steps

#### Anterior Approach *(Fig. 51.3)*

The procedure may be performed through a transverse anterior abdominal incision extended across both rectus abdominus muscles or alternatively through a midline abdominal incision. Subsequent exposure of the anterior aspect of the spine and great vessels is performed through a retroperitoneal dissection. The vertebral body of L5 is located deep within the pelvis between the bifurcation of the aorta and vena cava. The external and internal iliac vessels require mobilization to permit wide exposure of the L5 vertebral body. Bilateral reflection of the medial margin of the iliopsoas muscle from L4 to S1 will permit identification of the junction of the vertebral body and pedicle as well as the anterior border of the intervertebral foramen. This provides useful landmarks for orientation during the remainder of the procedure. The first structure resected is the L4–L5 disk. It may be necessary to remove a small amount of the anterior-inferior corner of the L4 vertebral body to adequately access the L4-5 disk space. The inferior cartilaginous end plate of L4 is removed, but its cortical end plate is preserved. The second structure resected is the L5 vertebral body. Bone resection is performed using osteotomes and rongeurs to remove the vertebral body back to the base of the L5 pedicles bilaterally. The third structure removed is the L5-S1 disk. Prior removal of the L5 body permits visualization of the L5-S1 disk, which is subsequently removed with curettes.

#### Posterior Approach *(Fig. 51.4)*

The posterior spinal elements are carefully exposed from L2 to the sacrum. Initially the L5 transverse process and pedicle are located beneath the sacral ala. Distraction is applied across the L4-S1 region to bring the L5 transverse process and pedicle into the surgical field. This is most commonly achieved using bilateral temporary rods between down-going hooks placed into the sacral ala and up-going hooks placed under the upper lumbar lamina (**Fig. 51.5**). The L5 lamina, pedicles, facets, and transverse processes are carefully excised and the L5 nerve roots are identified. The cartilaginous end plate of S1 is excised but the cortical end plate is preserved. L4 pedicle screws are placed bilaterally. Medially directed bicortical S1 screws are placed. Loosening and subsequent removal of the temporary rods permits reduction of L4 onto S1 by linking the L4 and S1 pedicle screws to a rod or plate system. As the L4 and L5 nerve roots now pass through a single neural foramen, these nerve roots must be carefully explored to ensure that they are free from tension or compression following reduction. Finally, bone graft is applied to the intertransverse region between L4 and S1 (**Fig. 51.6**).

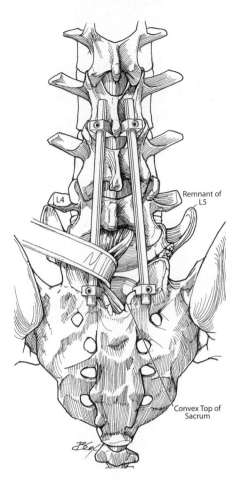

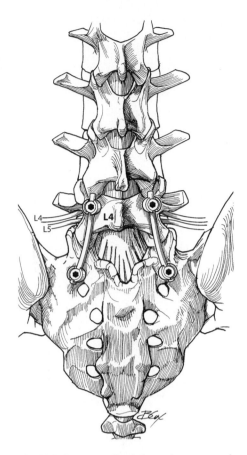

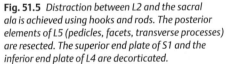

**PITFALLS**

• During initial anterior exposure of the L5 vertebra and adjacent disks, the presacral sympathetic plexus should be located in the midline. Blunt dissection should be used to mobilize this structure laterally toward each side. It is not mandatory to directly visualize the L5 nerve roots during the anterior procedure. However, the surgeon must be knowledgeable of the location of the nerve roots in relation to the L5 pedicle and intervertebral foramen to avoid iatrogenic injury. No reduction of the deformity is attempted during the anterior approach. During the posterior approach careful initial posterior spinal exposure is required to avoid dural tears due to posterior lamina dysplasia and the subcutaneous location of the posterior spinal elements. Use of an interbody cage is not necessary. Interbody devices elongate the anterior spinal column and may potentially increase the risk of neurologic deficit. The Gaines procedure is based on the concepts of spinal shortening and gentle realignment of neural structures.

**Fig. 51.5** *Distraction between L2 and the sacral ala is achieved using hooks and rods. The posterior elements of L5 (pedicles, facets, transverse processes) are resected. The superior end plate of S1 and the inferior end plate of L4 are decorticated.*

**Fig. 51.6** *Temporary distraction rods are removed and the L4–S1 interval is approximated as L4 is reduced onto the sacrum.*

### Bailout, Rescue, Salvage Procedures

If difficulties are encountered during the first-stage procedure, there is no an urgency to perform the second-stage procedure on the same day. The patient may be safely maintained at bed rest for 1 or 2 weeks prior to the second-stage procedure. During the second-stage procedure, an important goal is to achieve a stable spinal construct that will permit mobilization of the patient following surgery. If S1 screw purchase is suboptimal, supplemental distal fixation such as iliac screw fixation can be utilized to prevent failure of the S1 screws. Similarly, if L4 screw fixation is tenuous, proximal pedicle fixation can be extended to L3.

# 52

# Lumbosacral Interbody Fibular Strut Placement for High-Grade Spondylolisthesis: Anterior Speed's Procedure and Posterior Procedure

*Michael E. Janssen and Jason C. Datta*

## Description

Placement of an interbody fibular strut graft through the sacrum and L5 vertebral body for high-grade lumbosacral spondylolisthesis.

## Key Principles

Placement of the strut graft fulfills the following goals in the surgical treatment of high-grade spondylolisthesis: immediate structural support and stability, solid bony interface for fusion, and a graft placed under compression. The posterior placement of the graft requires a large decompression of the neural elements, which is advantageous in patients with neurologic complaints. Spinal fusion usually occurs within 3 to 6 months.

## Indications

High-grade lumbosacral spondylolisthesis greater than Meyerding grade III that has failed nonoperative treatment for mechanical back pain, lumbosacral neurologic dysfunction, slip progression, or revision of previous failed surgery. This procedure may be ideal for revision surgeries where the posterolateral graft bed is poor, or in the setting of a previously anterior bony strut graft procedure.

## Contraindications

- Less than 50% spondylolisthesis for the posterior procedure
- High-grade lumbosacral kyphosis >80 degrees, which may require L5 vertebral body resection

## Special Considerations

The posterior procedure is limited by the cephalad orientation of the graft tract by the patient's body. This limits the procedure to an in-situ fusion of a slip of greater than 50% or the partial reduction of a higher grade slip to 50%.

Presurgical radiographic evaluation for preoperative planning for both these procedures is essential. This includes preoperative plain films in the upright position to evaluate the posterior element dysplasia and slip angle. This defines lamina and pedicle dysplasia identifying areas at risk during decompression, and the planning of safe segmental posterior stabilization. Dysplasia of the transverse processes of L4 and L5 should be evaluated for the surface area available for posterolateral fusion. Transverse process surface area <2 cm² has been correlated with a high pseudarthrosis rate. It is strongly recommended to add the stability and superior graft bed of an interbody strut graft at the lumbosacral junction.

Magnetic resonance imaging (MRI) or computed tomography (CT) myelography should be used to evaluate the geometry and pathology of neural compression. The presence of sacral inlet stenosis should alert the surgeon to the need of a sacral dome resection. Regardless of sacral inlet stenosis, sacral dome resection may ease reduction forces required and the strain placed on the L5 nerve roots by columnar shortening. CT angiography may be a useful adjunct to define the prevertebral vascular anatomy prior to an anterior procedure in a high-grade deformity.

## Special Instructions, Position, and Anesthesia

The patient should be placed in the prone position on a radiolucent four-poster frame. Intraoperative fluoroscopy is required.

## Tips, Pearls, and Lessons Learned

The graft used, autograft versus allograft, does not appear to affect outcomes in the limited literature available. There may be a role for a vascularized fibular graft in previously radiated tissues. Reduction forces may be decreased by a wide thorough decompression, sacroplasty, and slight distraction. Resection of the iliolumbar ligament and far lateral foraminal decompression may decrease the rate of neurologic complications from the L5 root during reduction maneuvers.

A cannulated reamer from an anterior cruciate ligament reconstruction set is ideal for both the anterior and posterior procedures. An appropriate-size reamer can be chosen using the graft sizing tubes over the strut graft. The reamer sleeves in these sets serve as an excellent soft tissue protector.

The posterior placement of a fibular strut is limited to slips >50% because of limitations present with the pelvis and caudad soft tissues. Anterior graft placement can be performed in partially reduced slips, but it requires some anterior resection of the L4-L5 disk for proper positioning of the guide wire and reamer.

Both the procedures can be used without supplemental posterior segmental instrumentation, but it is felt that higher rates of successful fusion can be achieved with instrumentation. The added instrumentation is needed with dysplastic transverse processes <2 cm². This includes L4 pedicle screws, bilateral bicortical S1 fixation, and iliac screws measuring >60 mm in length and 7 mm in diameter to improve fusion rates and decrease interbody strut graft failure.

### Key Procedural Steps

The posterior placement of a strut graft requires a standard midline approach to the lumbosacral spine with exposure of the posterolateral gutters from the L4 transverse process to the sacral ala. Decompression includes partial laminectomy of the inferior portion of L4 and complete laminectomy of L5, S1, and S2 (**Fig. 52.1**). Wide foraminal decompression of the L5 nerve roots is required. Sacroplasty is needed in the setting of sacral inlet stenosis, and may be performed to ease reduction. This is best achieved with a broad curved osteotome under direct visualization. If instrumentation is to be used, it should be placed prior to reduction or graft placement. This typically requires fixation from L4 to the sacrum and in most instances the pelvis.

The starting point for the guide pin is typically midway between the S1 and S2 nerve roots and 8 mm from the lateral edge of the spinal canal. It is essential to gently retract the thecal sac and nerve roots out of harm's way with a smooth retractor or by placement of smooth Kirschner wires into the sacrum for static retraction. The guide pin is placed from lateral to medial under constant fluoroscopic monitoring (**Fig. 52.2**). The goal is to have the guide pin tip in the center of the L5 body on anteroposterior imaging, and in the superior-anterior quadrant of the L5 body on the lateral projection (**Fig. 52.3**). The reamer depth should be directly measured off the guide pin, but the length of graft should be approximately 5 mm shorter to facilitate recessing the graft 2 mm below the sacral cortex (**Fig. 52.4**). Partial reduction should be done prior to preparation and placement of the graft. The reduction can be facilitated and held by segmental instrumentation placed at the beginning of the procedure.

The anterior procedure can be performed as a stand-alone procedure for primary or revision procedures. A significant reduction of the slip can be performed by a posterior decompression, segmental instrumentation, and reduction procedure prior to anterior graft placement. If a significant reduction is achieved, then a partial L4-L5 disk removal is necessary to access the proper starting point on the L5 body. The guide pin is placed under constant fluoroscopic guidance. The remainder of the procedure is similar to the posterior procedure (**Fig. 52.5**).

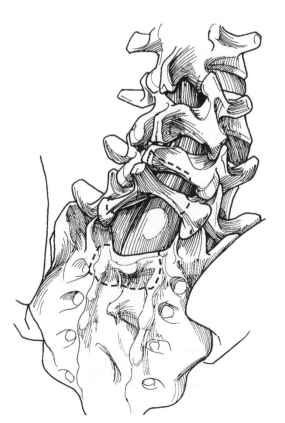

**Fig. 52.1** *Laminectomies at L4 (partial), L5, S1, and S2.*

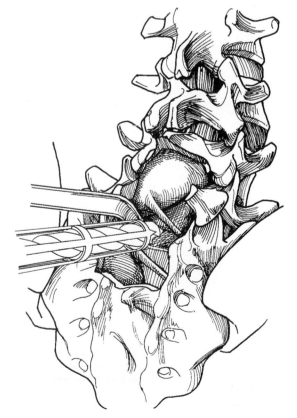

**Fig. 52.2** *Drilling the L5 vertebral body.*

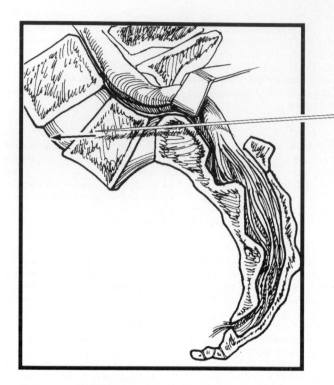

**Fig. 52.3** *Sagittal plane orientation of the guide pin.*

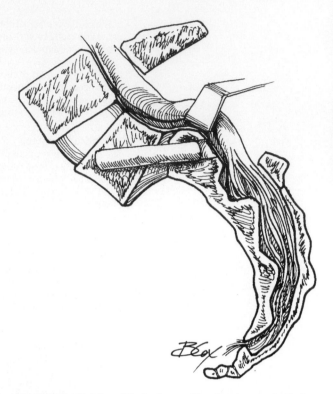

**Fig. 52.4** *Sagittal view of the lumbosacral junction showing the fibular graft in place.*

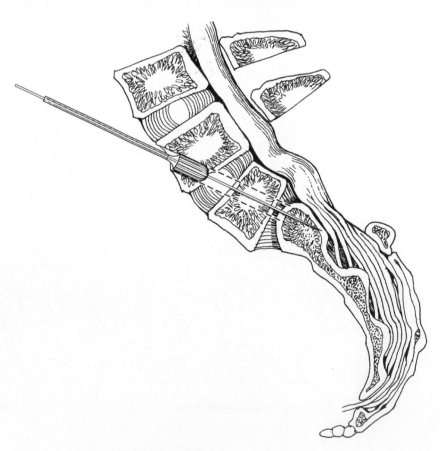

**Fig. 52.5** *Drill path through the spondylolisthesis.*

For both procedures tapering the leading end of the graft can decrease the amount of force needed for graft placement.

### Bailout, Rescue, Salvage Procedures

If the thecal sac cannot adequately be mobilized, consider a more lateral starting point. Placing the graft through the S1 pedicle is a viable bailout. Graft fracture during posterior placement can be salvaged with an anterior procedure. If a strut graft cannot be placed, a posterolateral fusion can be performed L4 to pelvis.

PITFALLS

- Aggressive retraction of neural elements, especially without proper mobilization of the dural sac
- Dural tears with the use of power equipment
- Guidewire binding within the reamer, with migration into surrounding structures

# 53

# Rib Expansion Technique for Congenital Scoliosis

*Robert M. Campbell, Jr.*

### Description

To lengthen the concave constricted hemithorax through VEPTR expansion thoracoplasty with correction of congenital scoliosis to maximize the potential for thoracic growth to benefit the underlying lungs.

### Expectations

With vertical expandable prosthetic titanium rib (VEPTR) expansion thoracoplasty, one can stabilize, or correct, rigid congenital scoliosis, without the growth inhibition effects of spine fusion, and enlarge the constricted concave hemithorax with probable benefit for the underlying lung. The thoracic spine can grow with further increase in thoracic volume. Additional benefits include leveling the shoulders, and improving both head and truncal decompensation.

### Indications

Progressive thoracic congenital scoliosis, in a patient aged 6 months up to skeletal maturity, with three or more fused ribs at the apex of the concave hemithorax, greater than 10% reduction in space available for lung, and having progressive thoracic insufficiency syndrome. Thoracic insufficiency syndrome is identified by the inability of the thorax to support normal respiration or lung growth.

### Contraindications

Inadequate soft tissue coverage for devices, poor rib bone stock or absence of proximal ribs for attachment of devices, absent diaphragmatic function, active pulmonary infection, or inability to undergo repetitive episodes under general anesthesia.

### Special Considerations

Preoperative magnetic resonance imaging (MRI) of the entire spinal cord is advised to rule out associated spinal cord pathology. An echocardiogram is performed to rule out congenital heart disease, and preoperative respiratory syncytial virus screen.

### Special Instructions, Position, and Anesthesia

Patients are placed in the lateral decubitus position with the operative side upward. Somatosensory evoked potentials and motor evoked potentials of extremities are monitored during surgery. A central line and arterial catheter are recommended.

### Tips, Pearls, and Lessons Learned

To increase the necessary soft tissue coverage, an oral appetite stimulant, Periactin, tube feeding, or gastric percutaneous endoscopic gastrostomy (PEG) feedings are useful. A body weight at the 25th percentile of normal, or greater, reduces the risk of skin slough over devices. The superior VEPTR cradle site should be placed at the superior aspect of the curve, but not into the flexible spine above it because of the risk of a proximal compensatory curve. Severe lateral contracture of the thorax can be corrected with a Harrington outrigger from a temporary rib cradle attached to chest wall in the posterior axillary line extending down to the lumbar hook site or to the pelvis with a Dunn-McCarthy hook. Acute thoracic outlet syndrome can be encountered with closure because of the altered proximal thoracic anatomy, so both pulse oximeter and upper extremity evoked potentials are monitored for loss of signal, and any changes are addressed by altering closure to let the scapula retract itself more proximal.

### Key Procedural Steps

A modified thoracotomy incision is made with the distal portion carried anteriorly in line with the tenth rib (**Fig. 53.1A**). The paraspinal muscles are reflected medially to the tips of the transverse processes, with care taken not to damage the rib periosteum (**Fig. 53.1B**). The VEPTR (Synthes Spine Co., West Chester, PA) is now ready for insertion. The superior VEPTR cradle is first placed adjacent to the tips of the transverse processes of the spine around two ribs or a fused rib mass. Next, the opening wedge thoracostomy is performed at the apex of the fused chest wall. Usually there is a fibrous cleft present anteriorly in the fused ribs in line with the planned thoracostomy. This is released with cautery, with a No. 4 Penfield retractor inserted to protect the underlying pleura, and then the thoracostomy is continued with a Kerrison rongeur, cutting a channel transversely through the rib fusion mass up to the transverse processes (**Fig. 53.2A**).

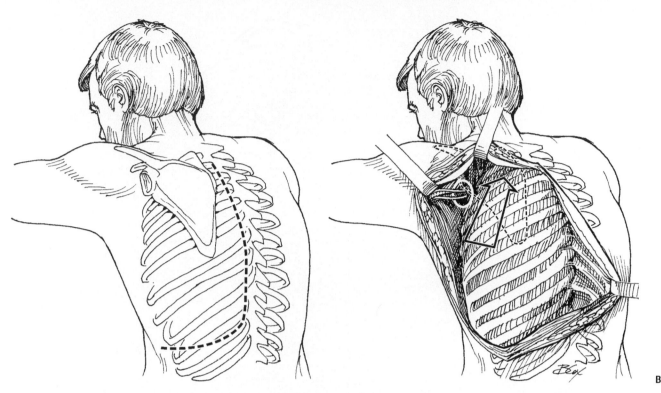

A                                                                                                                          B

**Fig. 53.1** *(A) The modified thoracotomy incision for VEPTR opening wedge thoracostomy. (B) The paraspinal muscles are reflected to the tips of the transverse processes of the spine. The "safe zone "for superior VEPTR rib cradle insertion (arrow) is posterior to the scalene muscles with the neurovascular bundle anterior.*

The osteotomized interval is gently expanded with lamina spreaders (**Fig. 53.2B**), and a Kidner sponge in a clamp is used to strip the pleura down proximal and distal. Any bone bridge remaining medial is carefully resected with a rongeur. The fused bone adjacent to the spine should be carefully pulled out laterally with a curved curette to avoid spinal cord injury. A second opening wedge thoracostomy, paralleling the first more distally, may be necessary when there is broad expanse of fused ribs of the hemithorax. The opening wedge thoracostomy is held open with a special rib retractor, and VEPTR devices are implanted to stabilize the hemithoracic correction.

In patients younger than 18 months, the spinal canal is too small for a spinal hook, so a single rib-to-rib VEPTR device is implanted on the ribs just adjacent to the spine. An inferior VEPTR cradle site is prepared on a stable, relatively horizontal rib, usually the 9th or 10th rib, and then the VEPTR is implanted and tensioned (**Fig. 53.2C**).

In patients older than 18 months, a hybrid VEPTR from ribs to spine is used for more forceful correction (**Fig. 53.3**). A longitudinal skin incision is made at the selected level of the lumbar spine, usually L2-L3, and a two-level unilateral exposure is made for insertion of a single lamina hook. Care is taken to be below any areas of junctional kyphosis. With the hemithorax deformity corrected by the rib retractors across the thoracostomy, the hybrid VEPTR size is chosen. The expandable portion of the hybrid should end at T12 and the spinal rod should be cut to extend distally only 1.5 cm past the lumbar hook. To safely form a tunnel in the muscle for the device between incisions, a Kelley clamp is threaded from the proximal incision into the lumbar incision, and used to pull a No. 20 chest tube back into the proximal wound. The VEPTR hybrid rod end is threaded into the chest tube proximally and the tube is used to guide the device into the distal wound. The hybrid VEPTR is attached to the superior cradle, and then the hook, and is then distracted. A second rib-to-rib VEPTR device is usually placed in the posterior axillary line. The medial hybrid device is once again distracted a final time.

Closure is in the usual thoracotomy fashion, but first the musculocutaneous flaps are stretched to perform closure without tension. Utilize a chest tube if there is a large pleural rent, adding two Jackson Pratt drains along with a deep pain catheter for ropivacaine infusion. Most patients remain intubated for 2 to 3 days. There is a 50% risk of a transfusion because of the dead space beneath the large flaps created. The chest tubes are removed when drainage is less than 1 cc/kg/day, and Jackson Pratt drains are removed when the drainage for each is 20 cc or less per day. No bracing is used. Patients are mobilized to ambulation as soon as tolerated. Postoperative assessment should include standing anteroposterior (AP) and lateral radiographs of the spine as well as a computed tomography (CT) scan to define position of the devices.

The devices are lengthened on schedule twice a year in outpatient surgery (**Fig. 53.4**). Device expansion access is made with 3-cm skin incisions, the distraction locks are removed, and the devices are extended slowly over several minutes, stopping when the reactive force is excessive. Expansion can be as minimal as

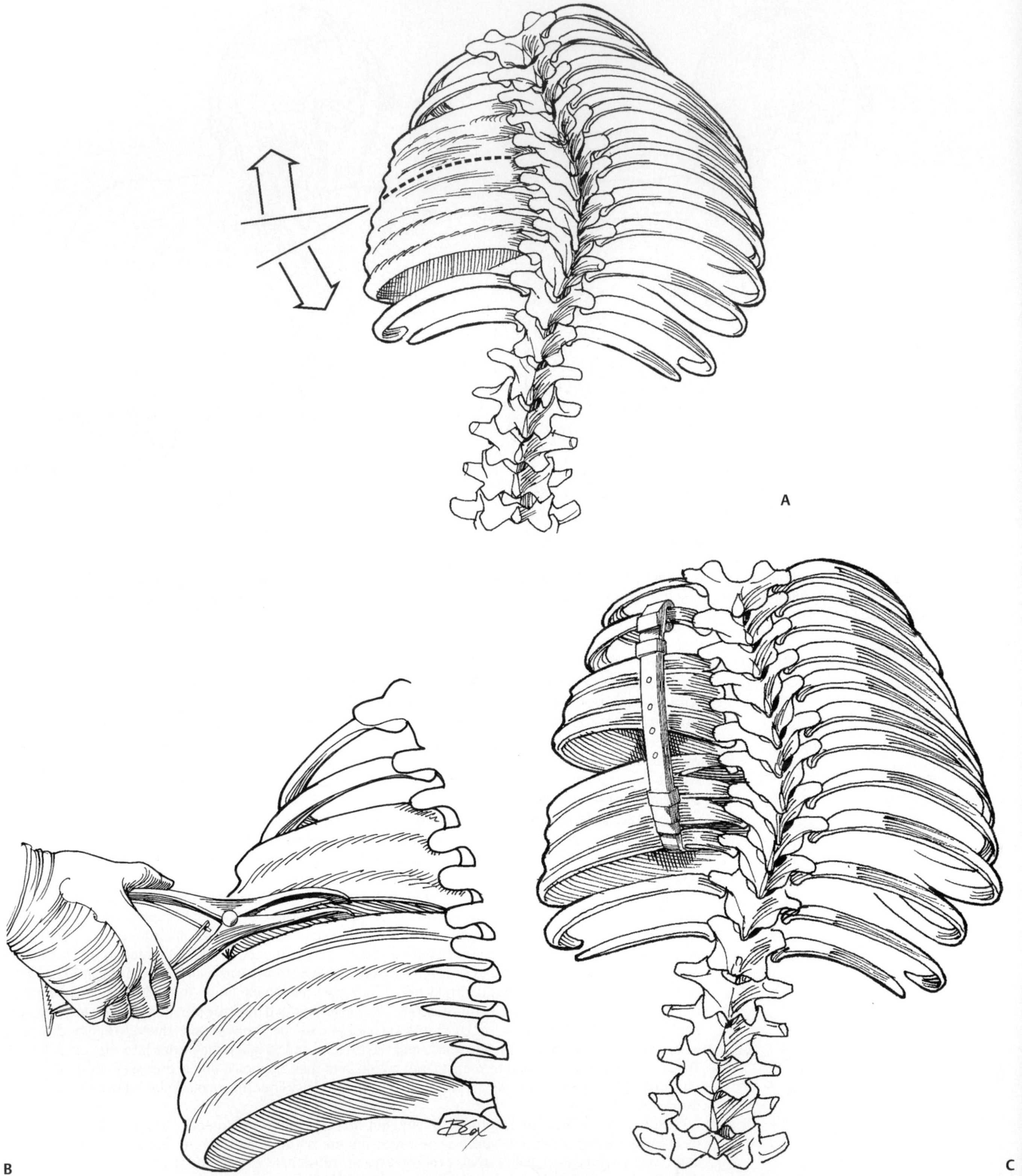

**Fig. 53.2** *(A)* *The opening wedge thoracostomy is slowly opened (arrows).* *(B)* *The constricted hemithorax is lengthened by the opening wedge thoracostomy with indirect correction of the congenital scoliosis.* *(C)* *A rib-to-rib VEPTR is implanted to stabilize the thoracic deformity correction.*

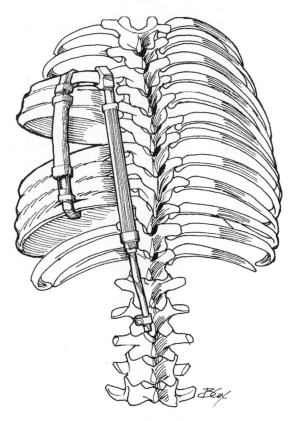

**Fig. 53.3** *A hybrid rib-to-rib VEPTR construct.*

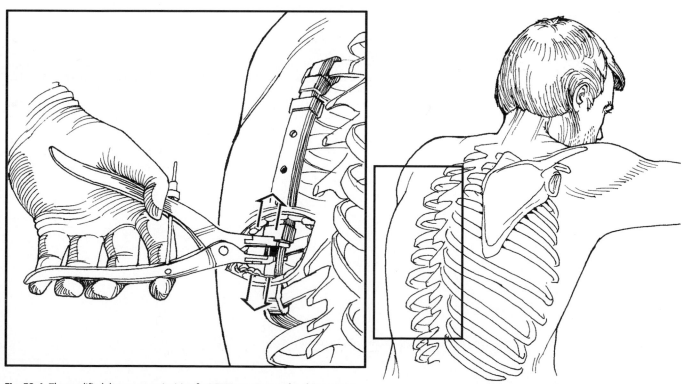

**Fig. 53.4** *The modified thoracotomy incision for VEPTR opening wedge thoracostomy.*

PITFALLS

• Inadequate correction of the thoracic deformity in the initial implant surgery cannot be addressed by expanding the devices later. Every effort should be made to completely correct the asymmetry between the concave and convex hemithorax with the initial procedure. VEPTR complications include skin slough, device infection, and asymptomatic migration devices. Skin slough is treated by debridement and primary closure. Sometimes it is necessary to use soft tissue expanders to provide skin coverage over the devices. Infections can be resolved most of the time by debridement and irrigation with loose approximation of the wound to allow granulation tissue to cover devices. Recurrent infections are best addressed by temporary removal of the central portion of the devices, with reinsertion done once the infection is resolved. Upward migration of the superior rib cradle can usually be addressed by re-anchoring it to the reformed rib of original attachment through a limited exposure. Spinal hooks that have migrated distally can be reseated at a lower level. Dunn-McCarthy hooks migrating distally into the pelvis can be removed and then re-anchored onto reformed superior iliac crest.

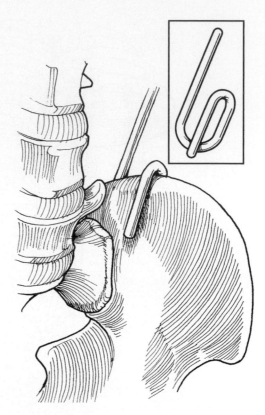

**Fig. 53.5** *Placement of a Dunn-McCarthy hook on the iliac crest.*

0.5 cm in a very tightly constricted chest and as much as 2.0 cm when the patient has had a growth spurt. Replacement of completely expanded devices can be done through limited incisions.

**Bailout, Rescue, Salvage Procedures**

When there are no proximal ribs for VEPTR attachment, this can be addressed by a first rib reconstruction through longitudinally osteotomizing the clavicle, bringing the anterior portion as a vascular pedicle underneath the brachial plexus, and joining it to an autograft rib from the contralateral side that is then attached to the spine. Within 3 months the reconstructed first rib usually has healed enough for a device attachment. When there are inadequate posterior spinal elements for hybrid VEPTR hook attachment or severe pelvic obliquity is present, then a hybrid rib-to-pelvis attachment through a Dunn-McCarthy hook can be considered (**Fig. 53.5**). A longitudinal incision is made over the posterior superior iliac spine and the abductors are reflected by cautery. A 1-cm transverse incision is made through the apophysis at the junction between the posterior third and the middle third of the iliac crest. The Dunn-McCarthy hook is then placed though the apophysis, just lateral to the sacroiliac (SI) joint, and mated by coupling to the hybrid device. The device is then distracted.

# 54

# Intervertebral Stapling for Spinal Deformity

*Linda P. D'Andrea, JahanGir Asghar, James T. Guille, and Randal R. Betz*

## Description

Vertebral stapling is a method of regulating spinal curvature development in the young patient with a coronal plane deformity. This can be accomplished using traditional or minimal access approaches.

## Expectations

Ideally, a surgeon with experience in anterior spine surgery, especially using minimally invasive techniques, should be able to perform this procedure. It may be helpful to enlist the assistance of a general or thoracic surgeon with experience in thoracoscopic and minimally invasive techniques. With the use of these techniques, scoliotic vertebrae from T2 to L4 can be stapled, while limiting the total scar length.

## Indications

Patients who have at least 1 year of growth remaining, have a scoliosis deformity that would be considered for brace treatment, or may have failed or refused bracing are ideal candidates for the stapling procedure. Lenke 1, 3, 5, and 6 scoliosis curves are ideal for treatment with vertebral stapling.

## Contraindications

Medical contraindications are the same as for any anterior spine or chest procedure and include systemic infection, active respiratory disease such as uncontrolled asthma, or conditions with increased anesthetic risk. Significantly compromised pulmonary function may be a relative contraindication.

We do not perform vertebral stapling for curves over 45 degrees, or in those whose curves do not correct to less than 20 degrees on bending films, because prior experience has yielded poor results. In children <8 years old with larger curves, it still may be desirable to perform stapling because of the ability to avoid early fusion and the potential for correction with continued growth, especially if a posterior growth device is added.

Kyphosis greater than 40 degrees is also a relative contraindication, because of the potential for the creation of hyperkyphosis with growth.

## Special Considerations

When performing thoracoscopic vertebral body stapling in small children (weighing under 50 lb), it may be difficult for the anesthesiologist to obtain or maintain single-lung ventilation. The child's airway size may not be compatible with the limited sizes of endotracheal tubes available. In these cases, the use of carbon dioxide ($CO_2$) insufflations for the thoracoscopic portion or two minithoracotomies may be used. If using $CO_2$, it is important to maintain the intrathoracic pressures at 7 to 10 mm Hg. Higher pressures can produce adverse hemodynamic effects (e.g., tachycardia, hypotension).

An important principle of insertion is to have the tines of the staples parallel and adjacent to the vertebral body end plates. In order for there to be actual correction of the scoliosis by modulation of the vertebral body growth, the patient should have at least 1 year of growth remaining.

Staple tine deployment usually occurs over 5 minutes. The staples should be placed in the inserter, with the tines straightened, and immersed in the sterile ice bath until the moment of insertion. Using flexible or rigid portal sleeves or a nasal speculum to maintain open portals allows for quick passage of the staples while protecting the skin and muscle. If tine deployment is occurring as the staple is being driven into the body, it is essential that the surgeon stop, as the tines may curl enough to penetrate the disk space. If this occurs, the staple should be removed, re-iced, and then reinserted.

## Tips, Pearls, and Lessons Learned

Although the patient is in the lateral decubitus position, often the flexible, main thoracic curve reduces. To further reduce the curve while placing the staples, lateral pressure to the apical ribs can be applied. The dull staple trial may also be used to push at the apex of the convexity, further reducing the curve prior to staple impaction. This may be important, because evaluation of data from patients who have already undergone the procedure suggests that patients who had the greatest correction at the time of surgery (curve <20 degrees on first erect radiograph) maintained that correction best.

If the staples are being placed thoracoscopically, the addition of carbon dioxide ($CO_2$) gas allows for collapse of the lung without single-lung ventilation. Specialized equipment and portals are needed for this technique. Low-pressure $CO_2$ gas also promotes hemostasis in the bleeding bone. Gas pressures should be kept low to prevent a lateral shift of the mediastinum, which may cause a drop in blood pressure. If staple or pilot holes are made but not used, then bone wax may be used to stop bone bleeding.

Previously, patients were told to wear a noncorrecting thoracolumbosacral orthosis (TLSO) for a brief time after surgery, but over the last 4 years we have found that this is usually not necessary. In a very active child with stapling of a lumbar curve, we will request that the child wear a lumbosacral corset for 6 to 8 weeks post-surgery. All patients are asked to restrict activities for 4 to 6 weeks to allow for skin and muscles incised during the surgery to heal. Only two staples of 1400 have partially moved with normal activities or vigorous participation in sports (including gymnastics) or dancing.

**Key Procedural Steps**
1. The thoracic and lumbar spine are accessible with minimally invasive techniques.
    a One-lung ventilation or $CO_2$ insufflation for thoracic visualization
    b Minimal flank incisions and nerve stimulation in lumbar surgery
    c Staple insertion aided by biplanar fluoroscopy
2. Curve reduction prior to staple insertion
    a Positioning on operating table
    b Indirect pressure on same-level ribs
    c Direct pressure with staple trial instrument
3. Placement of vertebral body staples
    a Parallel to the body's apophyses
    b Slightly anterior to rib heads
    c Use of sterile ice bath
    d Fluoroscopic verification of placement

The recommended guideline for choosing levels is to include all vertebrae that lie within the Cobb angle of the curve. The levels that may be safely stapled include T2 to L4. If the vertebrae are small, sometimes only a single two-prong staple can be placed in the upper thoracic spine.

Under general anesthesia, patients are placed in the lateral decubitus position with the convex side of the scoliosis curve in the up position. The table is not flexed, and only a small axillary roll is placed.

If video-assisted thoracoscopy is being utilized for insertion, then one-lung ventilation will be necessary, unless $CO_2$ gas insufflation is available to displace the lung for visualization of the spine and surrounding structures. After positioning the patient, biplanar fluoroscopy is used to determine the exact location for the intercostal portals before the patient is prepped and draped (**Fig. 54.1**). The incisions for staple insertion are along the posterior axillary line (**Fig. 54.2**). The incisions used for staple insertion are slightly larger than the staples themselves. Through each skin incision it is possible to make two to three internal intercostal portals. This allows several levels to be stapled through each skin incision and accommodates the size of the instruments and implants. The insertion device, which holds the single two-prong staples, is 10 mm × 14 mm wide. The staples come in many sizes, with the 12-mm four-prong, double staple being the widest, longest object (at 14 × 12 mm) that has to pass between the ribs (**Fig. 54.3**). Rigid, autoclavable plastic portals (Medtronic Sofamor Danek, Memphis, TN) have been custom made for this specific use. They allow for the maintenance of the intercostal portal space, quick removal of the staple trial, and placement of the appropriate-sized staple while protecting the muscle and pleura from repeated trauma. Small pediatric Finochietto retractors or nasal speculum distractors can also be used to enlarge the intercostal portals and may be used in place of collapsible or rigid portals.

Using fluoroscopy, the appropriate size staple trial is selected to span the distance across the disk, apophyses, and physes. The desired location in the vertebral body for the tines is as close to the end plates as possible. Once the correct size for the trial is determined, it is tapped into place where the staple is to be placed. Two single staples (two prongs) or one double staple (four prongs) is placed at each level. In very small children, the most proximal vertebra is often small, and only one single staple can be placed safely. The tines of the trial are used to create the pilot holes for the staple tines. If the tines of the trial come close to the segmental vessels, then the pleura is incised and the vessels are retracted gently while the pilot holes are created and until the staple is seated in place.

The pilot holes act as a guide for the staple tines to ensure correct placement (**Fig. 54.4**). The trial is removed and the appropriate-sized straightened staple is quickly inserted. The decision to insert a two- or four-prong staple is based on the width of the vertebral body as seen in the operating room. The four-prong staples provide the desired amount of compression with less time required for insertion and fewer instrument passes into the chest. Once the staple is in the desired position (**Fig. 54.5**), the staple inserter is removed, and if the staple is not flush against the bone, an impactor is used to drive the staple deeper. This must be done quickly before the tines are fully deployed. The dull staple trial can be used to help push at the apex of the convexity to further reduce the curve while the staple is being inserted.

The NITINOL (Nickel Titanium; Naval Ordnance Laboratory, White Oak, MD) staple's sharp, curved prong design and shape-changing abilities allow for insertion parallel to the cartilaginous vertebral apophyses to provide end-plate compression. Staple tines are sharp and are designed to pass easily through bone. The staple's prongs are straightened manually and are then cooled by immersion in a sterile ice-bath. The scrub nurse or technician can perform this ahead of time. The staples must pass quickly from the sterile ice-water bath to the vertebral bodies to prevent staple warming and tine deployment. The tines remain straight until the staple begins to return to normal body temperature. The prongs then deploy to their original curved

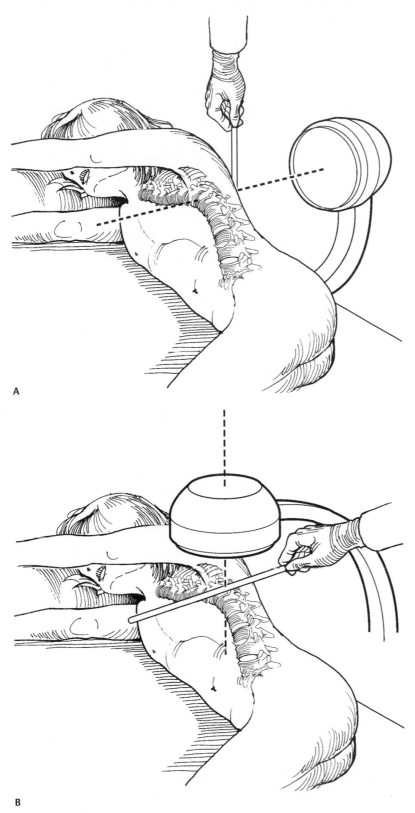

A

B

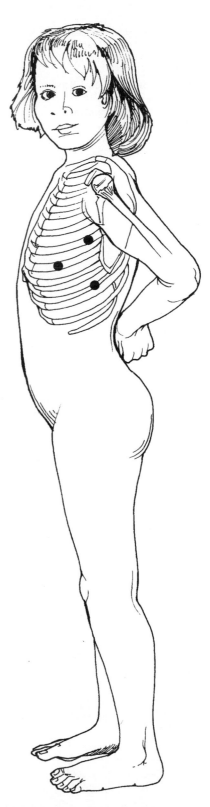

**Fig. 54.1** *(A) The patient is placed in a lateral decubitus position. Using fluoroscopic imaging, the levels of the spine to be stapled are confirmed. It is also important to ensure that access to the desired position of the spine is not inhibited by the extremities. (B) A lateral/medial fluoroscopy image is used to confirm the vertebral levels to be stapled and to center the portals in the posterior axillary line.*

**Fig. 54.2** *Generally, three incision portals in the intercostal spaces are placed, one in the anterior axillary line for the scope and two in the posterior axillary line over the levels to receive the staple instrumentation.*

**PITFALLS**

- Once a four-prong staple has been placed in a smaller vertebral body, repositioning it can be difficult, as new pilot holes will be needed.
- If segmental vessels are injured, their ligation may be necessary.
- If anatomic structures prevent the instrumentation of the entire curve, then staples should be placed where possible.
- The unstapled portion of the curve may behave differently.

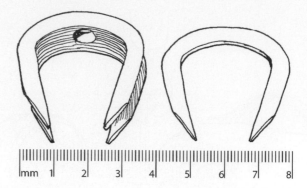

**Fig. 54.3** *Two- and four-prong staples. The NITINOL staples' sharp curved prong design and shape-changing abilities allow for insertion parallel to the cartilaginous vertebral apophyses to provide end-plate compression. The staple's prongs are straightened manually and are then cooled by immersion in a sterile ice-bath.*

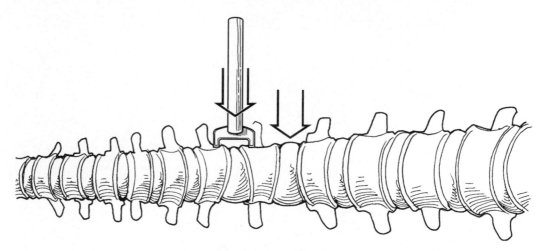

**Fig. 54.4** *The appropriate-sized staple trial is selected and used to create the pilot holes for the actual staple. The use of downward pressure with the trial allows for segmental correction of the curve.*

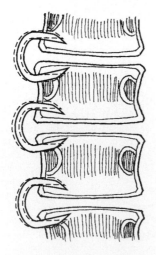

**Fig. 54.5** *After the staple is inserted, the position is confirmed with fluoroscopic image. It is important to note that the staple times have deployed and have not penetrated the end plate.*

shape. Complete tine transformation may take a minute. If the staple is completely seated within the vertebral bodies when the prongs deploy, then the staple position is secure.

Staples are placed anterior to the rib heads, and if the patient has severe hypokyphosis or thoracic lordosis, an additional staple can be placed more anterior on the vertebrae to help produce kyphosis with the patient's growth. In the lumbar spine, the staples should be placed as far posteriorly on the vertebral body as possible, at least in the posterior half of the body, to maintain a normal lordosis.

Final radiographs or fluoroscopy images are taken to ensure good position of the staples prior to closure. The incisions should be closed in the surgeon's routine manner. The use of a chest tube is left to the surgeon's discretion; not all patients have chest tubes placed. At our institution, the chest tube is removed when there is less than 2 mL of drainage per kilogram of body weight over the previous 8 to 12 hours.

**Bailout, Rescue, Salvage Procedures**

If vertebral body stapling is unsuccessful or cannot be performed thoracoscopically or open, there are other treatment alternatives. For patients who are willing to wear a TLSO for 16 to 23 hours per day, brace wear may be successful. Body casting in a molded plaster jacket may also be used. Posterior instrumentation such as a growing rod constructor or hybrid (rib to spine) is another surgical alternative.

# 55

# Posterior Rib Osteotomy for Rigid Coronal Spinal Deformities

*Bernard A. Rawlins*

## Description
A technique designed to provide additional mobility (release) to the spinal elements in a rigid deformity.

## Key Principles
The level of release should include the rib of the apical vertebrae and ribs caudal and cephalad, depending on the curve magnitude.

## Expectations
Concave rib osteotomies provide additional release to the spine beyond that provided by facetectomies, anterior diskectomies, and convex rib thoracoplasty. This becomes apparent during translation maneuvers using sublaminar wires.

## Indications
Rigid coronal curves in adult and pediatric deformities.

## Contraindications
Severe pulmonary compromise for which surgery to both pulmonary cavities would compromise the patient's perioperative recovery.

## Special Considerations
Pulmonary function testing preoperatively is usually done in large curves and provides an assessment of pulmonary reserve.

## Special Instructions, Position, and Anesthesia
Positive pressure ventilation should be requested to evaluate air leaks following the osteotomies.

## Tips, Pearls, and Lessons Learned
Rib synostosis, particularly in a congenital curve, makes dissection difficult. Comprehensive preoperative radiographic evaluation helps avoid surprises. Always obtain a postoperative chest radiograph to search for a hemothorax and pneumothorax.

## Difficulties Encountered
If a pneumothorax is suspected either intraoperatively or postoperatively, tube thoracostomy should be performed.

## Key Procedural Steps
Standard posterior exposure to the tips of the transverse processes from the caudal to the cephalic level of the spine under consideration for fusion is performed. The sequence for a routine posterior instrumented fusion is the following: place the pedicle screws, perform the facetectomies, prepare sites and place hooks, perform laminotomies for sublaminar wire placement, perform the thoracoplasty, and then consider the concave rib osteotomies.

Exposure is then carried lateral to the tips of the transverse process of the vertebrae under consideration. The dissection proceeds in a plane directly over the ribs for 2 to 3 cm. The paraspinal muscles give comparatively little resistance, given the surgeon is on the concave side of the curve. Subperiosteal dissection of the rib is performed as in a standard thoracotomy approach using the Alexander and Doyen instruments. A rib cutter is used to perform the rib osteotomy (**Fig. 55.1**). The area is filled with saline, and positive ventilation provided by the anesthesiologist is used to check for air leaks. A chest tube is placed immediately if an air

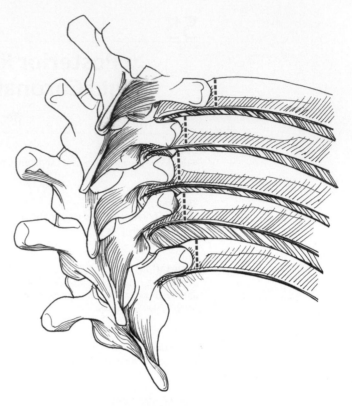

**Fig. 55.1** *Deformed spine showing rib osteotomy.*

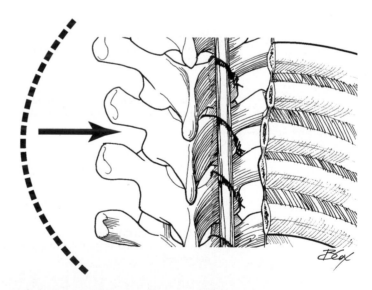

**Fig. 55.2** *Corrected deformity with instrumentation.*

**PITFALLS**

- Unrecognized pneumothorax. Anterior displacement of the lateral portion of the rib into the chest cavity.

leak is found. During the correction maneuver the rib lateral to the osteotomy should be elevated above the medial portion of the rib, transverse processes, or spinal instrumentation, as the spine is corrected in the direction of the rib osteotomy sites (**Fig. 55.2**).

**Bailout, Rescue, Salvage Procedures**

If the pleural cavity is entered during the procedure, a chest tube should be placed. Draping wide will facilitate this if tube placement is necessary.

# 56

# Thoracoplasty: Anterior, Posterior

*Carrie A. Diulus and Isador H. Lieberman*

### Description
Thoracoplasty is a technique involving rib resection to alleviate the cosmetic rib deformity associated with scoliosis.

### Expectations
Cosmetic improvement of truncal appearance.

### Indications
Rib deformity is commonly encountered with advanced curves in patients with adolescent idiopathic scoliosis or congenital scoliosis with or without a previous posterior fusion. It may be a sequela of crankshafting after a previous posterior fusion. Patients typically present with cosmetic concerns and coronal sitting imbalance. Indications include the following:

- Progressive or cosmetically unacceptable rib humps
- To balance shoulder heights
- To correct coronal sitting imbalance secondary to rib hump
- As a source of bone graft for both anterior and posterior fusion procedures

### Contraindications
- Patients without a cosmetically noticeable rib deformity
- Patients who cannot tolerate the pulmonary compromise of a thoracoplasty due to poor compliance of the chest cage, resection of numerous ribs, division of accessory respiratory muscles, or detachment of the diaphragm

### Special Considerations
To prevent reoccurrence, delay thoracoplasty until the patient is physiologically mature.

### Special Instructions, Position, and Anesthesia
There are three techniques to perform a rib resection thoracoplasty: (1) open internal transthoracic, (2) open posterior single or double incision, and (3) endoscopic internal transthoracic. Each has its merits, and the technique used depends on the clinical circumstances. Each case should be judged on its individual merits and ultimate expectations.

#### Open Anterior Transthoracic Internal
- Selective double-lumen endotracheal intubation
- Lateral position
- Drape arm free to facilitate intraoperative evaluation of scapular position (**Fig. 56.1**)
- Drape from midline posteriorly to sternum anteriorly

#### Open Posterior with Single Midline, or Midline and Posterior Axillary Line Incisions
- Prone position
- Drape field from one anterior axillary line to the opposite anterior axillary line

#### Endoscopic Transthoracic Internal
- Selective double-lumen endotracheal intubation
- Lateral position
- Drape arm free to facilitate intraoperative evaluation of the scapular position (**Fig. 56.1**)
- Drape from midline posteriorly to sternum anteriorly

### Tips, Pearls, and Lessons Learned
- Trim rib flush with transverse process at each level to avoid scapular impingement with motion
- Thoracotomy instruments should be quickly available during endoscopic procedure for emergency open exposure

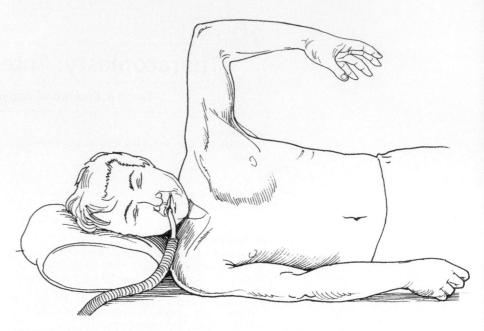

**Fig. 56.1** *Operative positioning.*

### Difficulties Encountered

- To estimate the correction required, one must evaluate and record the extent and location of scoliotic curve, the flexibility of the structural and compensatory curves, coronal and sagittal balance, shoulder heights, and the extent of scapular winging. Evaluating the curve parameters allows the surgeon to decide if the spine, the ribs, or both need to be addressed. Documenting the shoulder heights and scapular winging establishes a benchmark to advise on expectations.
- Three-dimensional computed tomography (CT) reconstruction with vector plane analysis can help estimate the locations and the extent of ribs to be resected (this technique, by creating a virtual plane parallel to the left scapula and intersecting the right-sided rib deformity, allows for an estimate of which ribs, and their lengths, are to be resected). This resected amount allows the right scapula to descend into the resection bed to balance with the left side (**Fig. 56.2**).
- Pulmonary function tests to assess feasibility of single lung ventilation if thoracotomy or endoscopic approach is considered

### Key Procedural Steps

#### Open Posterior Approach: Midline-Only Incision
- Midline incision
- From the midline incision, bluntly raise the trapezius, rhomboids, and serratus anterior as a sheet.
- Attempt to peel the paraspinal muscles from their lateral margin toward the midline over each rib.
- Strip rib by cauterizing the surface, and then use a Cobb elevator and rib stripper around the circumference of the rib.
- Take care to protect the neurovascular bundle under the inferior edge of the rib.
- Mark the resection margins.
- Osteotomize using a sagittal saw with a soft tissue protector beneath the rib.
- Oblique the osteotomy with a long power burr in the coronal plane to leave a smooth chest contour.

#### Open Posterior Approach: Two Incisions
- Parallel and paramedian incisions
- Dissection similar to single midline incision technique
- Distal rib portion exposed by raising the latissimus dorsi muscle from lateral to medial
- Ribs are osteotomized through both incisions.

#### Open Anterior Approach
- Perform thoracotomy to expose chest.
- Perform any associated procedures first, for example, anterior releases.
- Mark rib resection margins from outside-in with 18-gauge spinal needles through the chest wall.

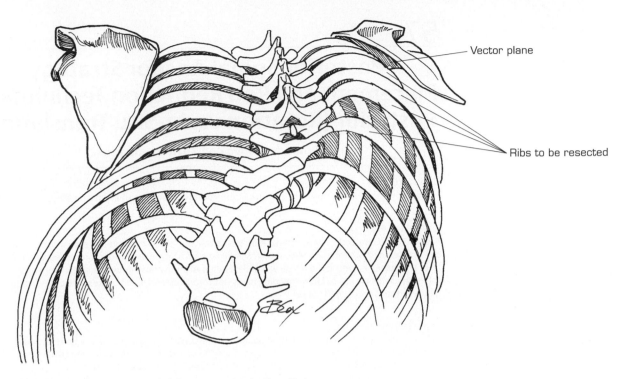

Vector plane

Ribs to be resected

**Fig. 56.2** *Axial view of cosmetic rib deformity associated with scoliosis.*

PITFALLS
- Delay thoracoplasty until the patient is physiologically mature to prevent recurrence, although adolescents tend to have improved return of pulmonary function compared with adults.

- With cautery, raise the pleura over each rib and then complete the subperiosteal rib dissection.
- Oblique the osteotomy with a long power burr while protecting the neurovascular bundle.

### Endoscopic Approach
- Create three portals in a triangular configuration with the apex just lateral to the nipple line.
- Perform any associated procedures first, for example, anterior releases.
- Mark rib resection margins from outside-in with 18-gauge spinal needles through the chest wall.
- With cautery, raise the pleura over each rib segment, and then complete the subperiosteal rib dissection with an endoscopic angled Cobb elevator.
- Grasp the rib at the distal osteotomy and complete the stripping by pulling it forward, and then create the proximal osteotomy and remove the rib through the most convenient portal.

### Bailout, Rescue, Salvage Procedures
Having a firm understanding of the open posterior, open anterior, and endoscopic transthoracic techniques provides the surgeon greater flexibility in limiting unsightly cosmetic incisions by tailoring the surgical approach to each specific patient's anatomic deformity.

# Posterior Spinal Anchor Strategy Placement and Rod Reduction Techniques: Posterior (Rotation vs. In-Situ Translation)

*Fernando E. Silva and  Lawrence G. Lenke*

### Description
Correction of scoliosis by posterior instrumentation using rotation versus in-situ translation techniques.

### Key Principles
A 90-degree counterclockwise rod-rotation maneuver permits correction of coronal and sagittal plane deformities in right thoracic scoliosis with hypokyphosis. This type of rod-rotation maneuver mostly translates the spine, in contrast to a true apical derotation maneuver using pedicle screw constructs. Translatory maneuvers via in-situ lateral bending loads can correct essentially all Lenke curve types, not just those hypokyphotic Lenke type 1 curves.

### Expectations
Both techniques can be employed using hooks or screws. We recommend screws whenever possible, however, especially with large curves. Also, screws have the added advantage of possibly obviating the need of a thoracoplasty. Both types of corrective maneuvers should lead to a balanced spine.

### Indications
All Lenke curve types.

### Contraindications
With curves other than Lenke 1A (-) and 1A (N), the technique of a 90-degree counterclockwise rod-rotation maneuver should not be employed, especially with curves that are at risk for decompensation with a full rod-rotation maneuver.

Relative contraindications for a posterior approach are Lenke type 5C curves, where an anterior approach is preferred in an attempt to prevent adjacent segment junctional kyphosis, if this curve type is approached posteriorly.

### Special Considerations
Upright lateral radiographs are required to demonstrate mild lordosis or hypokyphosis in the thoracic profile (T5–T12). Always try to assess the curve to see if selective fusion can be performed, especially when dealing with Lenke 1–3C and 6C curves. Again, in the latter, in-situ translatory loads are recommended, along with apical derotation (as needed) and selective compression/distraction to obtain final spinal balance.

### Special Instructions, Position, and Anesthesia
Prone on Jackson frame or appropriate four-poster frame, ensuring adequate lumbar lordosis. The arms are placed in the 90–90 position. Neurologic monitoring equipment, with or without the Stagnara wake-up test, is deemed appropriate.

### Tips, Pearls, and Lessons Learned
In placing pedicle hooks, be sure not to break the superior facet so that the hook does not migrate ventrally, possibly offending the neural elements.

In using free-hand placement of thoracic pedicle screws, each level should be instrumented in the same sequential manner. The technique is equivalent for lumbar and thoracic screws. It is imperative to clearly expose the base of the corresponding superior facet to serve as a guide to the imaginary location of the ventral pedicle. Do not force the Lenke probe into the pedicle. Once cancellous bone in the pedicle has been entered, the probe is easily inserted into the pedicle with a twisting and gentle pushing motion.

### Difficulties Encountered
All implants, hooks, or screws must be well positioned and constantly checked for any plowing (screws) or pull-out (screws and hooks). A derotation maneuver might prove difficult when addressing stiffer curves, and may lead to bone–implant failure, especially with hooks. In this situation, using an all-pedicle

screw construct with in-situ translation corrective loads can circumvent the difficulty. When pedicles are very small or more than one pass has been made while placing pedicle screws, a Kirschner wire (K-wire) can be used for assistance, but only when it is *absolutely certain that the bony floor of the pedicle tract is intact.*

### Key Procedural Steps

#### Rod Rotation Maneuver (Figs. 57.1 and 57.2)

Proximal fusion/instrumentation levels extend from T4 to T5, based on clinical exam and curve flexibility; distal levels usually include T12-L1, based on clinical exam and location of the stable vertebra as defined by the Lenke Classification System. Spine flexibility is again reassessed following exposure. The rod is contoured in the coronal plane, leaving an appropriate "lordotic tail" to account for the physiologic thoracolumbar sagittal profile. This concave rod is seated into the implants. A slow and careful 90-degree counterclockwise rod-rotation maneuver is performed, ensuring continued bony purchase of all implants. The rod should not be rotated past 90 degrees. The convex holding-rod is then placed. Lateral and posteroanterior (PA) radiographs are obtained. All screws are reevaluated radiographically, ensuring

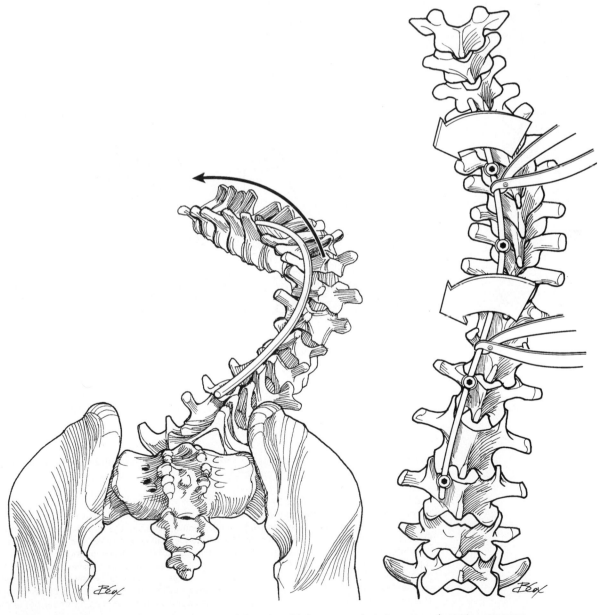

A                                                                                                    B

**Fig. 57.1** *(A) Caudo-cranial view of initial concavity rod placement. (B) Slow counterclockwise concave derotation maneuver.*

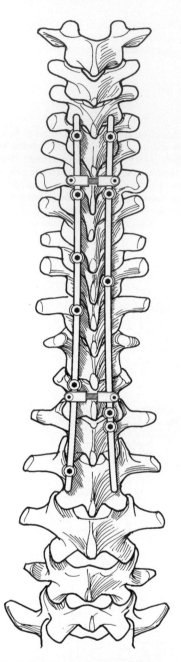

**Fig. 57.2** *Convex rod placed and tightened. Completed construct.*

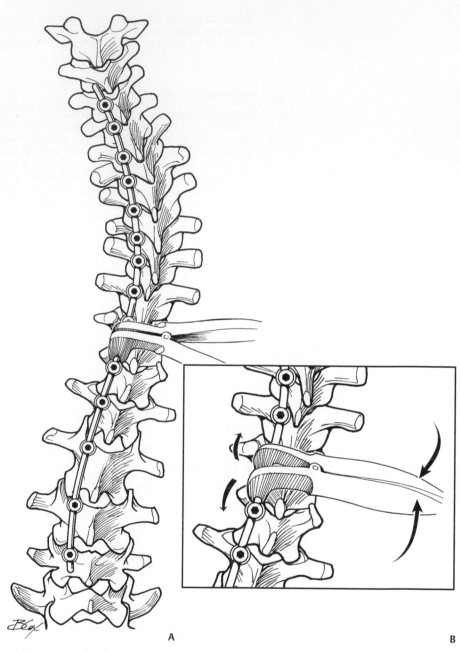

**Fig. 57.3** *(A) In-situ translation is initially applied at the apex of the concave rod. (B) Intraoperative view following multiple applications of in-situ translation.*

no changes have occurred. Appropriate-size cross-links are applied at both ends of the construct, prior to which decortication and fusion are completed.

### Rod Translation Maneuver (Figs. 57.3, 57.4, and 57.5)

Proximal fusion/instrumentation levels extend from T2 to T5, based on clinical exam, curve type, and flexibility; distal levels include T12 to L4, based on clinical exam and the location of the stable vertebra. Free-hand placement of pedicle screws is performed sequentially at each level. The rods are measured and contoured in the coronal and sagittal planes. For hypokyphotic or normokyphotic curves, the correction is performed on the concavity. Conversely, the convex side is corrected first when midthoracic hyperkyphosis is present. With the set screws loose, or locked at one end, coronal benders are used to reduce the scoliosis by placing the benders on either side of each pedicle screw, applying in-situ translatory loads. This is accomplished with several passes so as to take advantage of the viscoelastic properties of the spine.

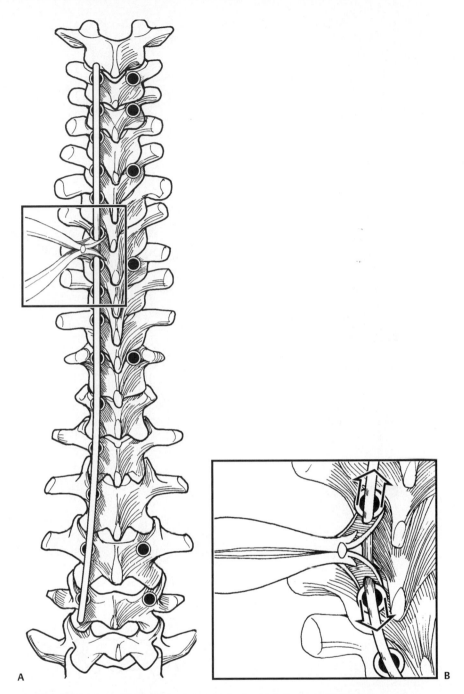

**Fig. 57.4** *(A,B) Selective distraction and compression to obtain final spinal balance.*

Direct apical derotation (midthoracic) is performed if screw placement is adequate, the thoracic spine is not overly lordotic, and when there are substantial thoracic or lumbar prominences. Careful attention must be paid at all times to the bone–screw interface, assessing any signs of screw plowing or loosening, which would indicate purchase failure, loss of correction, and possible neural element compromise. The holding-rod is then placed. Both PA and lateral radiographs are once again obtained. Proximal thoracic compression is performed as necessary. Finally, selective distal compression and distraction loads are used to horizontalize, centralize, and neutralize the lowest instrumented vertebra (LIV), leaving an appropriate tilt to the LIV. All screws are again evaluated on intraoperative radiographs to ensure that no changes have occurred and to assess overall spinal balance. Set plugs are sheared, posterior elements decorticated, bone graft is placed, and cross-links of appropriate size are secured to the rods.

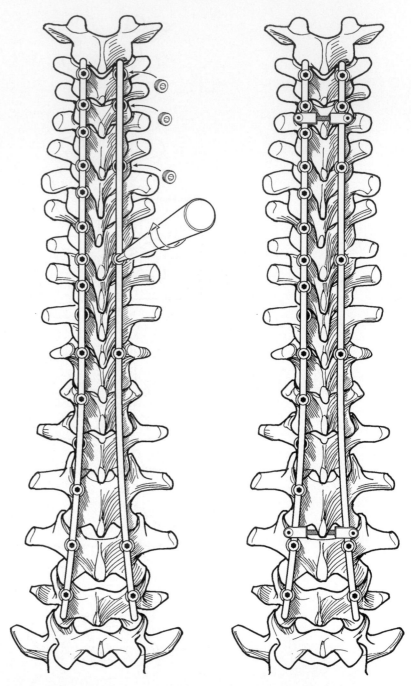

**Fig. 57.5** *(A,B) Final tightening of holding convex rod and completed construct.*

**Bailout, Rescue, Salvage Procedures**
- If the hooks pull out, pedicle screws can be placed.
- Any changes in motor evoked potentials (MEPs) or somatosensory evoked potentials (SSEPs) require checking the leads, making sure the irrigation being used is of appropriate temperature, increasing the blood pressure, checking all implant sites, and loosening the instrumentation. If need be, the instrumentation is removed, and the patient is returned to the operating room at a later time to complete the correction.

# 58

## Anterior Spinal Anchor Strategy Placement and Rod Reduction Techniques

### *Keith H. Bridwell*

### Description
Surgical technique for two-screw/two-rod construct for thoracic, thoracolumbar, or lumbar scoliosis.

### Key Principles
To correct the coronal plane deformity and to normalize the sagittal plane. Most importantly for thoracolumbar and lumbar curves, this means preserving or enhancing lumbar lordosis.

### Expectations
The expectation with a two-screw/two-rod construct is that the correction will be enhanced by either rod rotation or direct vertebral derotation through the screws. Lordosis will be maintained by eliminating the amount of compression and by utilizing anterior structural support in the anterior disk space. Finally, the construct will be stable enough with a two-screw/two-rod system that patients can return to activities at an early date. The advantages of anterior over posterior surgery include a shorter construct with more segmental correction.

### Indications
In most cases, the patient should have a coronal Cobb measurement of at least 45 degrees and usually not to exceed 70 degrees (curves over 70 degrees usually cannot be adequately corrected enough to allow for an anterior-only construct). Otherwise, the patient should be at least physiologically young and nonosteoporotic (**Fig. 58.1**).

### Contraindications
- Most curves over 70 degrees
- Curves that do not at least correct to 40 degrees or better on flexibility maneuvers
- An osteoporotic patient
- A patient with a severe sagittal plane malalignment

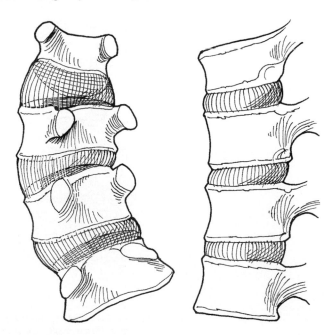

A                                                                                          B

**Fig. 58.1**  *The scoliotic spine in coronal **(A)** and sagittal **(B)** planes. Note: there is a component of kyphosis from T12 to L3.*

### Special Considerations

The screws need to be bicortical in all circumstances.

### Special Instructions, Position, and Anesthesia

Standard general anesthesia is used with the patient in a lateral decubitus position. The convex side is up, the concave side down. We do not recommend anterior constructs for thoracic curves anymore because of the impact on pulmonary functions. We have found with thoracolumbar and lumbar curves and lower thoracotomies that thoracoabdominal approaches do not have a negative impact on pulmonary functions. If the spine is exposed below T9, it is not necessary to deflate a lung.

### Tips, Pearls, and Lessons Learned

It is very important to complete the diskectomy all the way over to the concave anterior corner. Use disk spreaders to open the disk space to facilitate exposing the corner. It is also useful to perform fluoroscopy after the disks have been removed to be sure the diskectomy has been completed all the way over to the other side.

### Difficulties Encountered

For fairly large curves, it may be somewhat difficult to reach the top and bottom. There may be a tendency with the anterior screw, both proximally and distally, to inadvertently put it into the adjacent disk space. Also, it is helpful to take a rib at least one level, if not two levels, higher than the intended proximal vertebra. If the anterior fusion extends up to T11, it is best to take the ninth rib rather than the tenth rib.

### Key Procedural Steps

The procedure for a lumbar curve is described here through a thoracoabdominal approach. Typically, this is a left lumbar curve. The patient is placed in the lateral decubitus position, right side down, left side up. A curvilinear incision is made paralleling the tenth rib. The latissimus dorsi and external oblique muscles are incised down to the tenth rib. This rib is then subperiosteally stripped, exposed, and resected. The chest is then entered through the bed of the tenth rib. The retroperitoneum is then entered through the cartilage of the tenth rib. Peritoneum is swept off the undersurface of the deep abdominal muscles, which are then taken down parallel to the skin incision. The peritoneum is then swept off the undersurface of the diaphragm, which is taken down with a 1.5-cm peripheral radial cuff. Next, the segmental vessels are ligated at mid-body level from T12 to L3. Exposure of the vertebral bodies is then accomplished from the base of the pedicle around to the other side. Care is taken not to injure any segmental vessels on the opposite side.

Next, diskectomies are performed. It is very helpful to use disk distractors to be able to facilitate getting to the concave anterior corner. The next step is to place an appropriate-size cage in the anterior concave portion of the apical three disk spaces. Fluoroscopy is then performed to confirm that the cages are over far enough. The staples are then placed at T12, L1, L2, and L3. It is important that each staple be equidistant

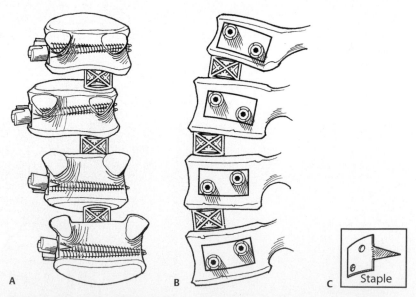

**Fig. 58.2** *The scoliotic spine in coronal (A) and sagittal (B) planes after complete disk excision, placement of the cages anteriorly, and placement of the staples and bicortical screws (C). Note that placing the cages in the anterior concave portion of the disk space has a tendency to facilitate correction of the scoliosis and also lordosization of the spine.*

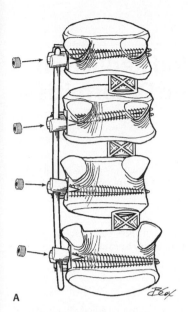

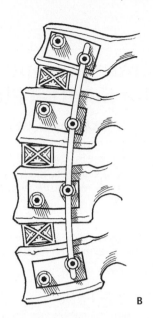

A

B

**Fig. 58.3** *Correction of the deformity. (A) The first step is to place screwdrivers into the anterior screws and accomplish derotation by pushing from the convex dorsal side*

*of the spine to the concave ventral side of the spine. (B) Once this derotation is accomplished, then the rod is engaged into the posterior screws.*

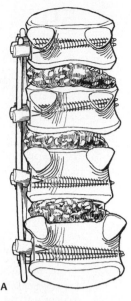

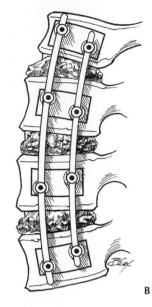

A

B

**Fig. 58.4** *(A) Coronal plane. (B) Sagittal plane. Depicting morselized rib bone graft in the disk space(s). Bone graft placed into the disk space at the apical three levels. Finally, placement of the anterior rod is accom-*

*plished. Some compression force may be applied through the posterior screws. Usually no force is placed through the anterior screws. The anterior rod is simply a holding fixation rod.*

---

### PITFALLS

- It is important that all screws be bicortical. It is absolutely critical that the screw tips be directed away from the canal and the foramen. At times it is possible to reach around the front with a gloved finger to feel the tip of the screw. If this is not possible, another option is to put the screw in and then take it out and palpate with a sounder to feel whether or not the screw is bicortical. It is also critical to not reduce segmental lordosis.

from the pedicles. It is important not to inadvertently place the staples around the front. If this is inadvertently accomplished, there will be a tendency to direct the screws into the spinal canal. In placing the screws through the staples, the surgeon needs to visualize the posterior longitudinal ligament (PLL) and be absolutely sure the screws are being directed anteriorly well away from the PLL. The surgeon will be leaning his hand back further on the more apical segments than the end segments. The staples and screws will appear to sit more posteriorly at the apical segments than the end segments, but in fact, they are all equidistant from the base of the pedicle. After placing the staples and screws, it is helpful to verify under fluoroscopy that the screws are all placed correctly and that they are bicortical. Having the cages in the anterior disk spaces facilitates opening up the disk space enough to visualize the PLL (**Fig. 58.2**).

The next step is to accomplish direct derotation through the anterior vertebral body screws. Then contour and engage the posterior rod. Before placing the rod, place the rest of the morselized bone graft in each disk space. After placing the posterior rod, apply a moderate amount of compression force posteriorly. The goal is to shorten the posterior disk space, but lengthen the anterior disk space (**Fig. 58.3**). The anterior rod is purely a stabilizing rod. Most commonly the diameter of the screws is 6.0 mm and the length is usually 35, 40, or 45 mm. The rods are usually 4.5 mm (**Fig. 58.4**).

### Bailout, Rescue, Salvage Procedures

If screw purchase is deemed not adequate or if the screws pull out during correction, the appropriate salvage is a posterior instrumented fusion preferably with pedicle screw implants. This is not likely to occur if the procedure is performed on a patient under the age of 30. It is usually possible and feasible to instrument to L4. It is often not feasible to instrument anteriorly below L4, because the vena cava and bifurcation is often in the way at L5.

# 59

# Fixation Strategies and Rod Reduction Strategies for Sagittal Plane Deformities

*Kirkham B. Wood*

### Description

To safely and effectively stabilize the hyperkyphotic thoracic or thoracolumbar spine with bilateral rigid posterior segmental instrumentation while reducing the sagittal curvature into a more physiologic range.

### Key Principles

By first securing the longitudinal members (rods) proximally into multiple hook or pedicle screw anchors, careful judicious cantilever bending is used to deliver the rods into increasingly caudad sites of fixation and the hyperkyphosis is reduced.

### Expectations

Modern instrumentation systems with their multiple sites of fixation and increased rigidity over those from previous eras allow not only improved construct rigidity and a higher rate of fusion, but also an ability to safely and consistently correct hyperkyphosis toward a more physiologic sagittal contour and to maintain that correction over time.

### Indications

Thoracic or thoracolumbar hyperkyphosis.

### Contraindications

- Preexisting fusion of the anterior column
- Tumor or infection
- Some congenital kyphosis

### Special Considerations

Hooks (pedicle, transverse process, or laminar) have been historically the principal means of fixation. Although the transverse processes of the upper thoracic spine are potential sites of hook fixation, those of T10–T12 are frequently insufficient for adequate purchase, dictating the use of the laminae or pedicle screws for fixation. Pedicle screws, however, are increasingly recommended as anchors because of their increased pullout strength. Screws may also be used in all levels; however, the risk of a pedicle breach or neurologic injury should always be considered.

### Special Instructions, Position, and Anesthesia

The patient is positioned prone on either a four-poster frame or transverse rolls under the chest and pelvis. The operating table may be flexed slightly initially in severe cases, so that returning to the horizontal position aids in the reduction maneuver.

### Tips, Pearls, and Lessons Learned

Individuals with long-standing spinal deformity are often more osteopenic than control populations; thus, undue force should not be used to avoid fracture of the laminae or transverse processes if hooks are used. Pedicle screw fixation is strongly recommended in these situations.

Because of the risk of proximal or distal fixation cutout during the reduction maneuver, especially in the elderly, wires can be passed around and through the end spinous processes or around the laminae, further securing the instrumentation. Additionally, a supra- or infralaminar hook at the ends of the constructs helps protect against pullout of the end pedicle screws.

Posterior fusion alone typically works well, but in kyphosis surgery the incidence of pseudarthrosis is greatly affected by the degree of deformity. Hence, curves over 70 or 75 degrees usually require concomitant anterior fusion. In the event of insufficient posterior elements for hook fixation in the middle to upper thoracic region, pedicle screws should be used.

Because of altered anatomy, intraoperative lateral radiographs or even C-arm imaging is strongly recommended to aid in the successful placement of pedicle screws.

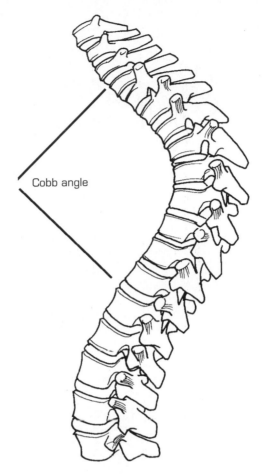

Cobb angle

**Fig. 59.1** *The levels of instrumentation should include all kyphotic vertebrae as measured by the Cobb method, including the first lumbar lordotic segment.*

Currently, many pedicle screw systems have extended threaded connectors that can allow, first, the capture of the rods to the screws, and then the gentle and gradual final reduction of the rods to the base of the screw.

Care must be taken when performing this technique for shorter segment fixation situations such as thoracolumbar fractures. Often, after reducing the malalignment from the posterior approach, a significant "gap" may exist anteriorly from the deficient anterior column. A secondary anterior procedure to restore the column's integrity may well be necessary.

**Difficulties Encountered**

The major complication following the reduction of thoracic kyphosis is the development of a junctional kyphosis beyond the levels of instrumentation. Reasons for this include failing to include all kyphotic vertebrae proximally as well as distally including the first lumbar lordotic segment. Overcorrection of the kyphosis (>60%) is also associated with increased risk of proximal deformity. Careful preoperative hyperextension radiographs over a bolster will help define the spine's rigidity and suggest expected degrees of correction. Age, osteopenia, and previous spine surgery should also be taken into consideration during the reduction maneuver as far as correction expectations are concerned.

**Key Procedural Steps**

In cases of thoracic kyphosis (e.g., Scheuermann's), the levels of posterior fusion and instrumentation should include the entire kyphosis as measured by the Cobb method to include the uppermost level of kyphosis down and including the first lordotic disk (often T12-L1) (**Fig. 59.1**). The basic instrumentation construct consists of a minimum of two claws, preferably three hooks or four to six pedicle screws on both sides above the apex of the kyphosis, and six to eight hooks or pedicle screws distally. Two ¼-inch rods

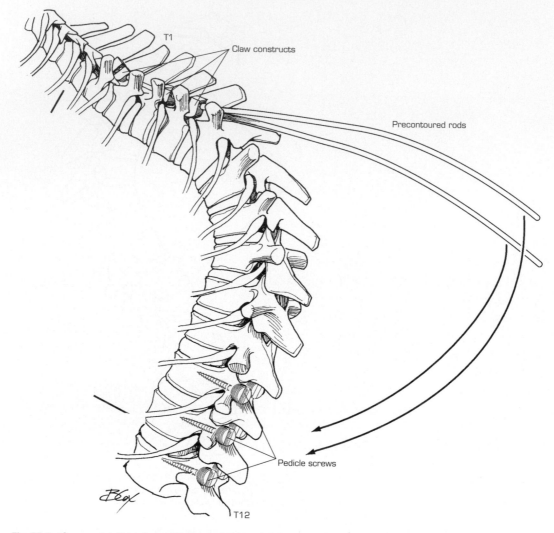

**Fig. 59.2** *After securing the rods proximally into the clawed anchors, the underbent rod is gently introduced and fixed into more caudal segments, correcting the hyperkyphosis.*

are bent to represent the desired kyphosis and then introduced first into the most proximal anchors and secured. Then, by careful cantilever bending, the rods are sequentially introduced into the more caudal hooks or screws (**Fig. 59.2**). Finally, segmental compression toward the apex of the kyphosis is applied.

In cases of thoracolumbar kyphosis (e.g., fracture) depending on the osseous quality, pedicle screws with or without supporting laminar hooks can be placed one or two levels above and below the pathology. With advancing osteopenia, more levels should be included both proximally and distally.

**Bailout, Rescue, Salvage Procedures**
The use of postoperative external immobilization helps protect instrumentation at risk of either bone or instrument failure.

# 60

# Vertebral Column Resection

*Timothy R. Kuklo and Alexander R. Vaccaro*

### Description
Severe rigid spinal deformity is a difficult problem for the spinal surgeon (**Fig. 60.1**). The traditional approach to severe rigid spinal deformities has included a stabilizing posterior spinal fusion with instrumentation, or an anterior release and fusion followed by a posterior spinal fusion with segmental instrumentation. Both of these approaches have resulted in variable, but mostly limited, correction, as a true translation of the spinal column is limited by these approaches. Vertebral column resection (VCR) is the only means of achieving significant vertebral column translation in these difficult deformities. It has traditionally been most commonly utilized for congenital scoliosis.

### Key Principles
Vertebral column resection implies complete resection of the posterior elements, pedicles, and the entire vertebral body. It can be achieved through either an anterior-posterior approach (on a single day or staged), or through a posterior only approach. Generally, VCR does not result in direct bone-on-bone contact, as is common with Smith-Petersen and pedicle subtraction osteotomies; therefore, reconstruction of the anterior and posterior columns is required. As well, the procedure is considered a vertebral column *shortening* procedure. Compromised pulmonary function, which is frequently encountered, may be a contraindication to an anterior approach, and thus may tip the surgeon toward a posterior-only VCR. The posterior-only procedure, however, is more technically demanding. Mastery of an anterior-posterior VCR is necessary prior to attempting a posterior-only VCR. The larger the resection, the greater the associated blood loss, risk of neurologic deficit, and other significant complications.

### Indications
Vertebral column resection is indicated for any severe fixed deformity, such as:

- Solid anterior and posterior spinal column after previous fusion or congenital scoliosis (fixed multiplanar deformity)
- Solid posterior spinal column in kyphosis or kyphoscoliosis (especially for thoracic deformity)
- Severe kyphotic deformity (with or without neurologic compromise)
- Severe coronal and sagittal imbalance
- Spondyloptosis
- Spinal tumors

The most dominant aspect of the clinical presentation is often sagittal plane decompensation; however, patients generally complain of difficulty with standing or sitting secondary to pelvic obliquity with imbalance, apparent leg length discrepancy, and cosmetic concerns. After evaluation of the deformity, consideration should be given to the surgical approach, technique (i.e., multiple Smith-Petersen osteotomies, pedicle subtraction osteotomy, or vertebral column resection), levels of resection, and levels of instrumentation.

### Contraindications
A VCR is not recommended for medically compromised patients who cannot undergo an extended period of anesthesia or potentially significant blood loss, as the procedure can entail extended operative time or excessive blood loss. Like other procedures, spinal instrumentation is generally contraindicated with active infection.

### Special Considerations
A thorough understanding of the complexity of the multiplanar deformity is mandatory. Ideally, this should be evaluated with a complete radiographic scoliosis series (standing anteroposterior [AP], lateral, side-bending, and hyperextension lateral over a bolster) if possible. This series assists the surgeon in assessing the potential flexibility of the deformity, as well as overall sagittal and coronal decompensation. If standing radiographs are unobtainable, then sitting AP and lateral radiographs should be obtained. Further radiographic evaluation should also include a thin-section computed tomography (CT) scan with sagittal, coronal, and three-dimensional (3D) reconstructions. The CT images greatly assist in defining and understanding the bony anatomy and in assisting with preoperative planning. The CT also assesses pedicle size and location, and postoperative screw placement.

Magnetic resonance imaging (MRI) is helpful in assessing associated spinal canal abnormalities, especially in congenital scoliosis, as well as in detecting potential areas of central or foraminal stenosis.

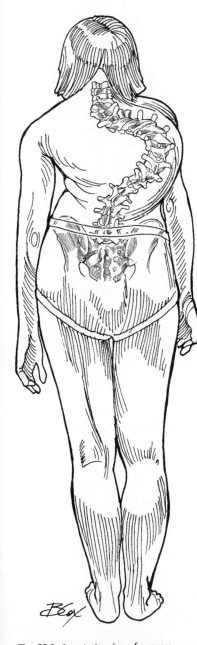

**Fig. 60.1** *A posterior view of a severe coronal plane deformity.*

The segmental blood supply can also be quite tenuous, especially in revision or congenital scoliosis surgery. For this reason, it is generally advisable not to ligate these arteries if at all possible. As an alternative, the artery should be clipped and only ligated if there are no motor evoked potential monitoring changes after waiting for several minutes.

### Special Instructions, Position, and Anesthesia

For an anterior-posterior vertebral column resection, the patient is placed in the lateral decubitus position on a bean bag with an axillary roll, usually the right lateral decubitus (left-side approach) on a radiolucent table. Following this, the patient is flipped to the prone position on an open Jackson frame. For a posterior-only VCR, the patient is placed directly in the prone position on a well-padded radiolucent table. The arms are placed with the shoulders abducted 90 degrees and the elbows are flexed 90 degrees. General anesthesia is used, and the neck is placed in a neutral to slightly flexed position.

### Tips, Pearls, and Lessons Learned

Generally, only one or two vertebrae are necessarily resected along with the associated disks (three disks for two-level resection), especially for sharply angulated deformities. This is determined by both the magnitude of the deformity, as well as the acuteness of the angulation. For long sweeping rigid curves, more than one vertebra may need to be resected. In either case, the goal is to achieve a balanced correction without stretching or compressing the spinal cord.

With potentially large expected blood loss, all efforts should be made to control bleeding from the onset of the procedure. This includes meticulous dissection and control of soft tissue bleeders, with liberal use of powdered thrombin-soaked Gelfoam (Pharmicia & Upjohn Company, Kalamazoo, MI), or similar available commercial products such as FloSeal (Baxter Healthcare Corporation, Fremont, CA). For tumor resections, consideration should be given to preoperative arterial embolization; however, this may also increase the risk of spinal cord compromise or loss of function secondary to the embolization. As well, it is recommended to keep the blood pressure at the resting mean arterial pressure during correction, and to closely watch for an acute drop in pressure during correction. Spinal cord monitoring, specifically somatosensory and motor evoked potentials, should also be closely watched during correction. After correction, a wake-up test should be considered. Inherent to this is a close working relationship with the anesthesia team.

### Difficulties Encountered

The most important difficulty encountered is compromised neurologic function during or following VCR. Consequently, meticulous attention to complete visualization, and slow steady correction, as outlined above, are mandatory. As well, VCR is an inherently destabilizing procedure; therefore, rigid internal

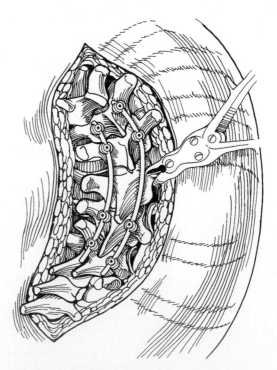

**Fig. 60.2** *Once the spinal anchors (screws) are placed posteriorly, the posterior vertebral resection is commenced.*

fixation with at least two or three levels of fixation is required both proximal and distal to the level of resection. Attention should also be given to the condition of the bone, as osteoporotic or compromised bone quality may necessitate additional levels of fixation. As well, pseudarthrosis or loss of fixation are significant concerns. Persistent imbalance or loss of lumbar lordosis may also be encountered during the correctional procedure.

Small pedicles, which make pedicle screw fixation difficult, may be particularly difficult to identify, and alternative fixation strategies should be considered at these levels if it is thought to be a critical level of fixation.

## Key Procedural Steps

### Anterior-Posterior (Circumferential) Vertebral Column Resection

The anterior procedure is done through either a thoracotomy or thoracoabdominal approach on the convex side of the deformity. An anterior osteotomy is performed if there is a solid fusion. Ideally, an osteoperiosteal flap is elevated, but this is often too difficult. Often the area to be resected is removed to the level of the adjacent disk, which is also removed along with the articular cartilage of the adjacent end plate back to a bleeding subchondral bone. All of the bone back to the posterior longitudinal ligament (PLL) is removed piecemeal. It is optional to remove the PLL, as infolding of the PLL into the spinal canal could result in spinal cord compression during a correctional maneuver. The entire vertebral body, and convex pedicle are removed. A lamina spreader is helpful to maintain or improve visualization of the area to be resected; however, overdistraction should not be applied. After complete resection, an autologous tricortical iliac crest, femoral allograft, titanium mesh with allograft or autograft, or an expandable cage is placed. Whatever the chosen interbody spacer, a vertebral column shortening will be the ultimate final corrected spinal alignment. Instrumentation is often applied following grafting. The patient is then flipped to the prone position for a posterior element resection and segmental instrumentation, or returned at a later date for this procedure (**Fig. 60.2**).

### Posterior-Only Vertebral Column Resection

After complete dissection through a midline incision, segmental bilateral pedicle screw instrumentation is performed. The posterior VCR is done through the same midline approach, with an extracavitary approach to the anterior column. This includes complete resection of the involved transverse processes, and associated ribs; the more lateral the rib resection, the better the visualization of the anterior column (**Fig. 60.3**). This is necessary to limit spinal cord retraction, which should be avoided. The thoracic nerves are also resected

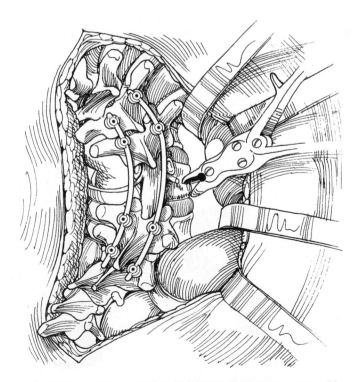

**Fig. 60.3** An extracavitary approach allows for simultaneous resection of the anterior and posterior spinal elements. Temporary rods are placed to maintain alignment until the vertebral resection is completed.

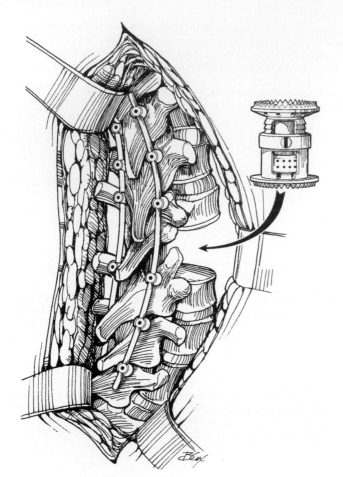

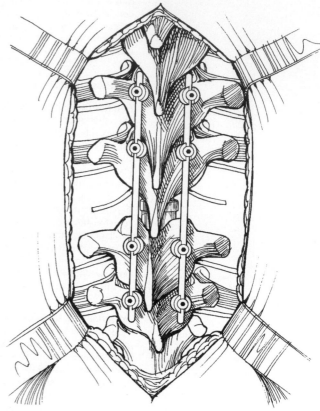

**Fig. 60.4** *Following the vertebral resection, a cage or spacer is then placed in the anterior column defect as the spine is shortened using the cage as a fulcrum.*

**Fig. 60.5** *Following anterior and posterior vertebral element resection, the spinal deformity is slowly corrected.*

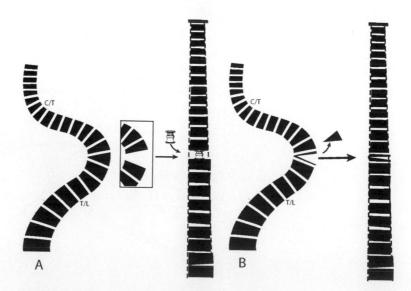

**Fig. 60.6** *A vertebral resection can involve the entire vertebral body* **(A)** *or involve a wedge resection with incomplete removal of the vertebral body* **(B).**

at the level of involvement to improve anterior visualization. After complete resection, autologous tricortical iliac crest, femoral or humeral allograft, titanium mesh cages, or expandable cages are utilized to stabilize the anterior column as well as to serve as a fulcrum for deformity correction. Posteriorly segmental pedicle screw instrumentation is used for both correction and stabilization of the spine deformity (**Figs. 60.4, 60.5,** and **60.6**). The use of multiple cross-links should be considered to improve the torsional stability of the construct, which is severely compromised after vertebrectomy.

### Bailout, Rescue, Salvage Procedures

For inadequate fixation, pedicle screw augmentation techniques such as cement injection can be utilized; however, these also are not without risk, including extravasation through a fractured cortex, thermal damage, difficult removal in the event of infection or misplacement, and the potential for neurologic compromise.

Additional levels of fixation and cross-links should be utilized in the osteoporotic compromised spine, and if extension to the sacrum is necessary, iliac screw fixation should be used. Postoperative bracing may be helpful to limit forward bending and additional pullout forces on posterior instrumentation.

Intraoperative somatosensory and motor evoked potentials should be utilized throughout the procedure to detect potential spinal cord injury. Steroids should be considered in the case of spinal cord injury.

# 61

# Posterior Cervicothoracic Osteotomy

*Paul Licina and Geoffrey N. Askin*

## Description

This extension osteotomy is performed posteriorly at the cervicothoracic junction to correct cervical kyphosis. Although originally described as being performed under local anesthesia with the patient in the seated position, the preferred technique entails general anesthesia, prone positioning, and spinal cord monitoring.

## Expectations

The procedure should improve sagittal balance and restore forward gaze.

## Indications

Severe cervical kyphosis associated with the following:

- Sagittal imbalance
- Loss of forward gaze
- Difficulty eating (jaw opening and swallowing)

Kyphosis severe enough to require corrective osteotomy is usually associated with ankylosing spondylitis or rheumatoid arthritis. Less commonly, kyphosis can result from trauma or cervical laminectomy.

## Contraindications

Severe kyphosis localized to the thoracic spine may be more effectively corrected with thoracic osteotomies. Severe osteoporosis is a relative contraindication.

## Special Considerations

### Level of Osteotomy

The accepted osteotomy level is at C7-T1. This level is sufficiently cephalad for correction of the cervical deformity, while being sufficiently caudad to avoid the vertebral artery in the foramen transversarium. It is also at a level of the spinal canal that is relatively wide.

### Positioning and Anesthesia

Head Control
It is best to use a halo ring attached to the bed. It facilitates precise and secure positioning as well as subsequent head manipulation.

Torso Support
A four-poster frame is usually employed. It may need to be elevated off the bed to accommodate the cervicothoracic kyphosis, and it allows the head to be attached to the bed via the halo ring.

Visualization
The required degree of correction is difficult to estimate. The use of transparent plastic drapes allows the surgeon to see the relative position of the head and torso to facilitate visual confirmation of adequate reduction.

### Intubation

The flexed position and stiffness of the neck usually poses intubation problems. Preoperative anesthesia assessment includes reviewing lung and cardiac function, and developing an intubation plan. An awake intubation is usually undertaken, using a nasotracheal tube or fiberoptic laryngoscope.

### Neurologic Assessment

Spinal cord injury during reduction of the osteotomy, and even during positioning, is a significant risk. For this reason, spinal cord monitoring, ideally both motor and somatosensory, is required.

## Tips, Pearls, and Lessons Learned

### Preoperative Planning

The following needs to be obtained:

- A lateral photograph to measure the chin–brow angle and to estimate the required degree of correction
- A standing lateral radiograph to assess the desired level and size of osteotomy

- A magnetic resonance imaging (MRI) scan to assess the space for the cord and the vertebral artery anatomy at the proposed site of osteotomy
- A computed tomography (CT) scan to confirm the bony anatomy in the region of the osteotomy

A useful way to gauge the degree of correction required on the lateral x-ray is to trace the spine on tracing paper, cut the paper at the osteotomy level, and then rotate the pieces until sagittal balance has been achieved. The angle between the cut edges then gives the required osteotomy angle (Webb technique).

It may also be helpful to obtain a biomodel (a custom polymer model of the spine based on the CT scan data). The osteotomy and fixation can be planned preoperatively, and the model can be sterilized and used intraoperatively to facilitate three-dimensional visualization.

### Control of Osteotomy Reduction

Correction of the osteotomy is often rapid, and precise control may not be possible. Resultant translation can cause spinal cord injury. A way of minimizing this risk is to use a modular cervicothoracic fixation system with cervical lateral mass and thoracic pedicle clamps that allow the rod to slide through them. Once the osteotomy is completed, a temporary malleable rod (a useful trick is to use an intubation stylette) is inserted and the cervical clamp screws are tightened to secure the rod cephalad to the osteotomy. As the osteotomy is corrected, traction is applied to the caudad end of the rod, allowing it to bend and slide through the thoracic clamps in a controlled fashion, thereby minimizing the risk of translation (Mehdian technique).

### Key Procedural Steps

#### Preparation

The patient is intubated, positioned, and monitored as described above. A long midline approach is made, exposing C3 to T4. Imaging is used to confirm the level.

#### Instrumentation

An instrumentation system that can span the cervicothoracic junction is employed. Lateral mass screws are prepared in C3 or C4 to C6, and pedicle screws are prepared in T2 to T4 or T5 (**Fig. 61.1**).

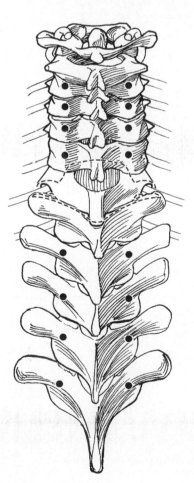

**Fig. 61.1** *Lateral mass and pedicle screw holes with planned resection.*

### Osteotomy

Using a high-speed burr, the inferior lamina of C6, the whole lamina of C7, and the superior lamina of T1 are removed. The C8 roots are thoroughly decompressed by removing adjacent parts of the C7 and T1 pedicles, and the osteotomy is extended laterally at this level through the C7-T1 facet joints (**Fig. 61.2**). The dura is often adherent to the lamina necessitating caution to avoid inadvertent durotomy.

### Reduction

If the malleable rod technique is to be used, the rod is inserted and the cervical clamps are tightened to the rod (**Fig. 61.3**). If not, rods are precontoured to the anticipated degree of correction and fixed to the cervical spine above the osteotomy. One surgeon unscrubs and performs the reduction. The halo ring is detached from the bed, and the surgeon grasps the ring and gently and slowly extends the head, while the other surgeon observes the osteotomy and especially the dura (and guides the malleable rod if this technique is employed). As the reduction approaches completion, the degree of correction is assessed through the transparent drapes. A gap should remain between the C6 and T1 laminae to allow room for the buckled dura (**Fig. 61.4**).

### Fixation and Fusion

The correction is then fixed with the instrumentation. If the malleable rod technique is used, the thoracic clamps are secured to the malleable rod, the other side is fixed with a contoured titanium rod, and finally the malleable rod is replaced (**Fig. 61.5**). Decortication is performed, and osteotomy bone together with bone from the iliac crest is laid down. The wound is closed (**Fig. 61.6**).

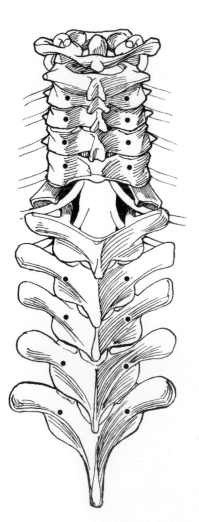

**Fig. 61.2** *Resection of posterior elements and decompression of C8 roots.*

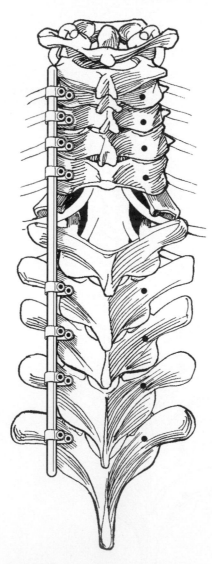

**Fig. 61.3** *Unilateral insertion of clamps and malleable rod on the left side.*

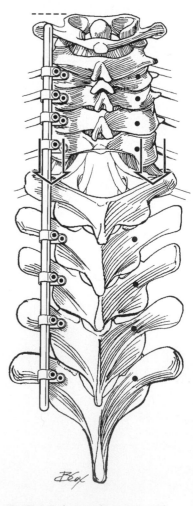

**Fig. 61.4** *Reduction of osteotomy with bending and sliding of malleable rod.*

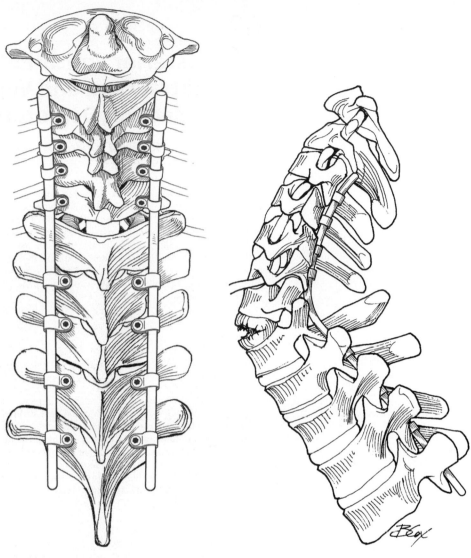

**Fig. 61.5** *Insertion of clamps and definitive rod on the right side.*

**Fig. 61.6** *Lateral appearance of completed osteotomy with definitive rods.*

PITFALLS

• Difficulties may be encountered with intubation and patient positioning. The most significant potential problem is spinal cord or nerve root injury, due to translation during reduction, kinking, and compression of the cord or roots, or from instrumentation misplacement. Internal fixation may be inadequate, leading to loss of correction. Finally, undercorrection or (especially) over-correction of the deformity may pose functional problems postoperatively.

### Postoperative Immobilization

Depending on the adequacy of fixation and bone stock, either an occipito-cervico-thoracic orthosis or a halo-thoracic brace is used for 3 months.

### Bailout, Rescue, Salvage Procedures

If monitoring indicates impaired spinal cord function, the correction should be reversed. If function does not return, the implants should be removed. If correction is lost postoperatively, a supplemental anterior approach may be required. If an inappropriate degree of correction severely compromises function, remedial corrective surgery may be required.

# 62

# Posterior Smith-Petersen, Pedicle Subtraction, and Vertebral Column Resection Osteotomy Techniques

*Stephen L. Ondra and Brian A. O'Shaughnessy*

## Description

Although modern spinal implants enable the surgeon to exert powerful force on the spine in the correction of deformity, the limiting factor remains the bone–metal interface. As a result, there is a limit to the force that can be applied to the spine. Osteotomies are the primary tool in the surgical armamentarium by which the surgeon can introduce mobility into the spinal column, thereby decreasing the forces required to obtain a correction. Osteotomies also alter the anatomy of the spinal column, and when combined with spinal implants and interbody devices, enable the surgeon to manipulate the axis of rotation to more effectively obtain the desired correction. The three most commonly implemented osteotomies in deformity surgery are the Smith-Petersen osteotomy, pedicle subtraction osteotomy, and vertebral column resection osteotomy.

## Expectations

The choice of osteotomy is dependent on the goals of the procedure, the correction requirements, the native bone quality of the patient, and the anatomic variations that may be present. Each of the osteotomy techniques has specific advantages as well as inherent limitations. They can be used individually or in combination to achieve the desired correction. In theory, the Smith-Petersen osteotomy offers up to 10 degrees of correction per level; however, 3 to 7 degrees per level is more commonly achieved. It can be performed at any level in the thoracolumbar spine and is best accomplished at a level where there is a disk that is not ankylosed. The taller the disk, the more effective the osteotomy, as this technique requires posterior osteotomy closure and simultaneous anterior opening. The pedicle subtraction osteotomy, a more powerful technique that hinges on the anterior column and involves middle and posterior column shortening, can reliably achieve between 30 and 40 degrees of correction at a single level. A vertebral column resection procedure, an extension of the pedicle subtraction technique, typically yields a bit more correction than a standard pedicle subtraction osteotomy due to the distance and height of the anterior pivot, which places the correction arc point anterior to the vertebral body.

## Indications and Contraindications

The indications for each of these osteotomy techniques include fixed segmental kyphosis or globally positive sagittal imbalance. The Smith-Petersen osteotomy requires a mobile anterior column, which is not always the case. A pedicle subtraction osteotomy, by contrast, does not possess the same limitation because the bony resection is carried through into the anterior column. Although a pedicle subtraction osteotomy is commonly performed for fixed sagittal correction, it can also be used for coronal correction or combined sagittal–coronal correction. The pedicle subtraction osteotomy can also be utilized in nonfixed deformity if other techniques will not give the needed correction.

A vertebral column resection procedure, the most powerful osteotomy technique, is particularly valuable in the setting of sharp, angular deformities.

## Special Considerations

The choice of osteotomy is based on the bone quality, patient needs, local anatomy, pathology, and the amount of correction needed. The desired correction is often either estimated or calculated by doing cumbersome radiographic cutouts. We have developed a method that allows rapid, easy, and precise mathematical calculation of the degrees of correction needed in any plane. This has translated into the operating room by allowing the degrees of correction to the osteotomy to be translated into millimeters of bony resection throughout the osteotomy. Our method, which takes advantage of simple trigonometry, has had a high level of correlation between the calculated degrees, the bony resection based on these parameters, and the clinical result.

The distance from the planned osteotomy to C7 is measured. The distance from C7 to the S1 plumb line on a standing 36-inch film is then measured. This establishes a right triangle and a simple trigonometric calculation is performed: $(Opposite/Adjacent)^{-1} = Angle$. In this case it is (C7 – S1 Plumb Line Distance/Osteotomy to C7 Distance)$^{-1}$ = Angle Needed for Correction.

Once the degrees needed for correction are known, the surgeon can make the decision as to what single osteotomy or combination of osteotomies is needed to accomplish the planned correction based on the expected correction with each type of osteotomy and the unique patient characteristics that may enhance or limit an osteotomy correction. For instance, if the surgeon knows that 45 degrees of correction are needed, it is unlikely to be achieved by three or four Smith-Petersen osteotomies. More likely, a single pedicle subtraction coupled with one or two Smith-Petersen osteotomies would be adequate. This type of calculation and information enables the surgeon to develop a comprehensive surgical plan that realistically achieves the goals of correction.

### Tips, Pearls, and Lessons Learned

The patient is positioned prone on a radiolucent frame with four to six posts allowing the abdomen to be free of pressure. The patient is typically "built up" on a chest pad so as to render the lumbar spine as lordotic as possible. Particularly when there is a mobile anterior column, patients often sustain a reasonable degree of correction simply by proper positioning.

In general, it should be noted that stainless steel rods are preferred in all the osteotomy correction techniques as microfractures in titanium is more common with large bends and can lead to rod failure at an increased rate.

In performing the Smith-Petersen osteotomy, we often initially prepare the screw or other implant sites, but we do not actually place the implant until just prior to the osteotomy closure. A Gelfoam product can be used to minimize bleeding until the implant is placed. This approach has the advantage of allowing screw hole placement and preparation while all anatomic landmarks are present. It also allows for much of the work to be done while minimizing the time that the osteotomy is present, as this may be a source of blood loss. Not placing the screw until the osteotomy is done prevents the screw head from getting in the way and decreasing the efficiency of the bone removal at the superior facet.

### Key Procedural Steps

#### Smith-Petersen Osteotomy

The most important aspect of this osteotomy is removal of the superior facet. The osteotomy is begun by using an osteotome to resect the inferior facet the desired number of millimeters. A drill is then utilized to create a chevron-like resection of the inferior and superior facet complex and the inferior edge of the superior lamina of the osteotomy level. The ligamentum flavum is then resected to expose the dura (**Fig. 62.1A,B**). Gelfoam is used to decrease bleeding. Once all osteotomies are completed, the pedicle screws or other implants are placed. Closure is achieved by compression, postural effects, table manipulation, or some combination of these (**Fig. 62.1C**).

At times, to maximize the correction at a level and improve fusion, an interbody device is placed in the anterior one third of the disk space. This increases the height of the disk and provides an anterior pivot. The axis of rotation moves forward to the pivot, increasing the correction angle of closure. It also has the advantage of providing graft in the anterior column for fusion. This can be done using a unilateral or bilateral transforaminal lumbar interbody fusion (TLIF) technique as the facets are already resected by the osteotomy. It is important not to place an implant that does not taper or that covers a large part of the end plate, as this has the potential to block the closure of the posterior disk space and, as a result, the osteotomy.

#### Pedicle Subtraction Osteotomy

After placing pedicle screws above and below the osteotomy level, the precision-cut pedicle subtraction osteotomy begins with placement of a pedicle preparatory hole. With no implant in place, a prepped and tapped pedicle is very useful to maintain orientation while the bony removal is taking place. The bony removal of the posterior elements then begins. The removal should be centered at the pedicle that is to be removed. The amount of bone to be removed should be calculated to match the amount of closure needed. It should involve the superior and inferior facet of the osteotomy level and the inferior facet of the cephalad level and the superior facet of the level below. In the case of a prior posterior fusion mass, a fusion mass removal is performed. This is done with osteotomes, rongeurs, and curettes to save all bone for later fusion. The osteotomy can be fine-tuned with a high-speed drill. It is helpful to undercut the posterior bone edge in a "keystone" fashion. This decreases any dural impingement. Others will cut a small hole in the bone overlying the dura.

The pedicle is then fully removed with a rongeur and a drill. Care should be used to fully remove the pedicle base. Small spicules of bone can result in radiculopathy once the osteotomy is closed. In revision cases, it is also important to remove all scar tissue from the dura to avoid soft tissue crowding once closure has been done. Once the pedicle has been removed, dissection of the vertebral wall is done bilaterally. Penfield dissectors and elevators are used, with the dissection being performed from the level of the disk that immediately lies above the resected pedicle caudally as much as the resection needs to go. The body should be dissected all the way to the anterior vertebral body to get adequate exposure and resection.

The segmental artery is swept caudally subperiosteally. This can typically be done without difficulty over two thirds of the vertebral body. If the vessel begins to bleed, bipolar cautery at a higher setting can be used. If this does not work, pack the area. Bleeding typically resolves with osteotomy closure. We have not had to stop and move to a flank incision for control of the aorta, but this would be a reasonable maneuver should all else fail.

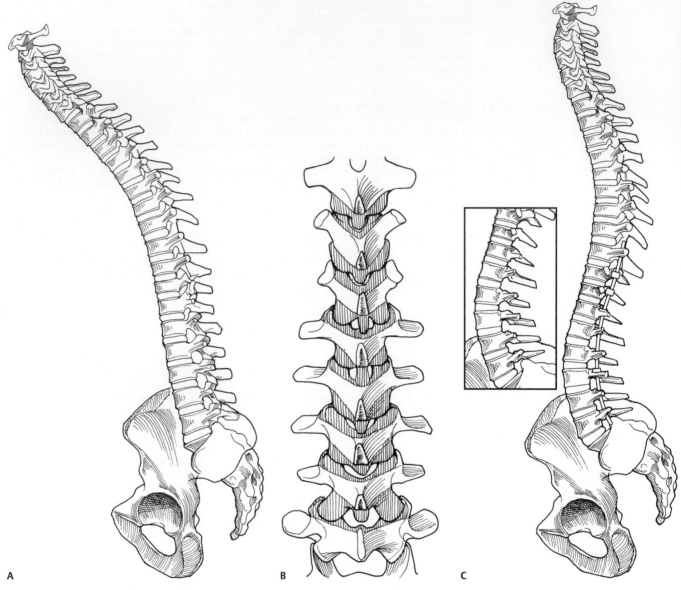

**A**

**B**

**C**

**Fig. 62.1** *(A) A sagittal view of an obvious flat bone deformity of the lumbar spine. (B) An illustration of the Smith-Petersen osteotomy. Note resection of the superior facet, inferior facet, and ligamentum flavum. (C) Following multilevel Smith-Petersen osteotomies, closure of the defects is performed through compression, postural manipulation, or table manipulation.*

The bone is removed with rongeurs and a drill, in a precise wedge based on the calculated degrees of closure. The apex of the wedge is at the anterior vertebral body wall. This wall should be preserved as a pivot point. The base of the osteotomy is at the floor of the spinal canal. This is more easily done today with specialized vertebral body retractors to assist in exposure. The cancellous bone is then removed with curettes and rongeurs in a wedge-shaped fashion matching the cuts on the lateral walls. Again, all bone is saved for later grafting. Drills can be used for final shaping. The final bone resection is the posterior vertebral body wall, or the floor of the spinal canal. The lateral edge can be removed with rongeurs. The final removal is an impaction technique into the vertebral body cavity created by the resection. This can be done with curettes or with specialized impactors, which again makes the procedure a bit smoother (**Fig. 62.2**).

It is important to place a temporary holding rod to maintain vertebral body orientation and prevent early collapse of the body when the posterior wall is removed. This is occasionally necessary earlier in the procedure. With all bone resected and the canal and root exit zones inspected for any tissue that could impinge on neurologic structures, the osteotomy is closed. Typically, very little compressive pressure is needed on the screws above and below the osteotomy. The osteotomy is closed by gentle pressure by hand on the spine on each side of the osteotomy. If a standard operating table is used, the patient's body can also be flexed. The closure is further completed by hyperlordosing the rod in the area of the osteotomy and adding cantilever force. Final closure is performed by gentle rod compression. If more force is needed and there are posterior elements, a compression hook combination can be put in the bone above and below the osteotomy. A third rod can be used to get added compression. Once the final rod is in place, the third rod and its hooks

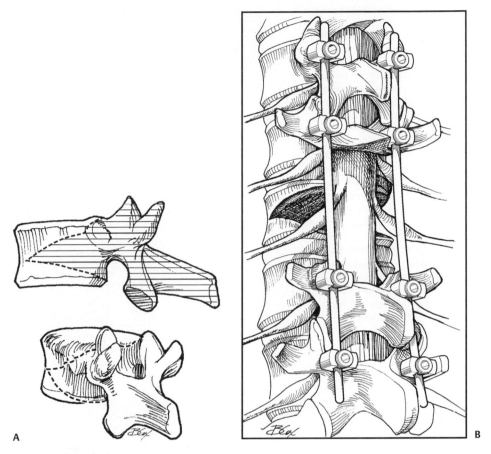

A                                                                              B

**Fig. 62.2** *(A) The highlighted area on the vertebral body indicates the anticipated bone that will be removed for a pedicle subtraction osteotomy. (B) An intraoperative illustration showing the neural elements after a pedicle subtraction osteotomy. Note that the spinal column is stabilized by bilateral temporary rod fixation.*

are generally removed. Anteroposterior and lateral 14- × 36-inch scoliosis radiographs are used to confirm osteotomy closure and ensure there is no translation. The posterior elements should be completely or nearly completely closed and not translated (**Fig. 62.3**). The lateral wall closure and the root exit zones are inspected. The roots above and below the pedicle are now both contained in a superforamen.

The advantage of precision cut technique is the precise closure of the bone, giving the exact calculated resection. Ideal bone contact leads to improved rates of fusion and less stress on the construct before fusion. All bone cuts should be symmetric unless coronal correction is then needed. If this is the case, the side to which coronal deviation is needed is cut larger than the other side by the amount needed to obtain coronal correction.

### Vertebral Column Resection Osteotomy and X Osteotomy

This technique is an extension of the pedicle subtraction precision cut technique. It can be performed effectively from T3 to L1 (inclusive). All implants are placed via a midline incision, with the exception of the osteotomy levels. Again, the osteotomy level pedicles are prepped. The erector spinae muscle is then dissected on its lateral border and mobilized. Access and dissection of the ribs that articulate with the disks above and below the osteotomy level is then performed. Up to 10 cm of the ribs are removed unilaterally and saved for graft. Somewhere between 2 and 3 cm of the ribs can be removed from the opposite side to enhance closure of the osteotomy and help with vertebral resection. A lateral extracavitary dissection is then performed to the anterior vertebral body. It is often necessary to coagulate one and at times both segmentals at the level of resection. With the rib heads removed, attention is turned to the vertebral resection.

The vertebral resection begins with a posterior removal of the lamina (or fusion mass) and the pedicles. The vertebral body is then fully resected to include the disks above and below the body. The end plates of the bodies above and below the resection are feathered with curettes and drills. The posterior vertebral body wall is then carefully removed with impactors.

In vertebral column resection, an anterior cage is placed as a pivot point and gradual posterior closure is performed while pivoting on the cage. In an X osteotomy, the anterior longitudinal ligament is cut. The pivot point is either the preserved posterior vertebral body wall or a posterior vertebral body pivot cage that is placed after resection. If the posterior vertebral body wall is used as a pivot, care must be taken that it pivots and does not buckle back into the canal. For this reason, many prefer a structural implanted pivot cage.

PITFALLS

- The most important aspect of the Smith-Petersen osteotomy is removal of the superior facet. If it is not completely removed, it will limit closure and cause foraminal stenosis and potentially radiculopathy by migrating into the foramen during compression and closure. The remainder of the posterior resection is to remove enough of the inferior articular facet and inferior lamina edge of the cephalad vertebra and ligamentum flavum to attain the desired number of millimeters at the osteotomy level.
- When placing an interbody graft as an anterior pivot point in a Smith-Petersen osteotomy, it is important to place a tapered implant that is situated as anteriorly as possible. If the interbody spacer is not tapered or covers a large part of the end plate, it has the potential to block the closure of the posterior disk space and, as a result, the osteotomy.

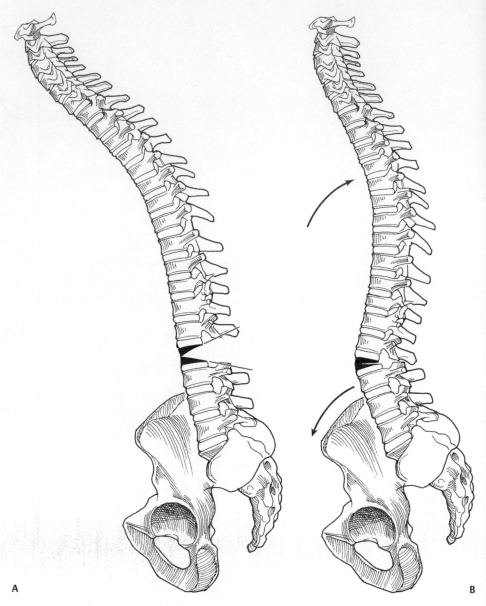

A                                                                                                B

**Fig. 62.3** *Preoperative **(A)** and postoperative **(B)** lateral scoliosis illustrations before and after a pedicle subtraction osteotomy in a patient who was fused in kyphosis. Note the marked improvement in sagittal contour in the postoperative film.*

This X osteotomy technique is an anterior opening and posterior closing osteotomy done from a posterior approach. The axis of rotation moves to the pivot that is near to or at the spinal canal. As a result, this has the advantage of minimal canal length change, either in compression or extension. This allows the largest amount of closure of any osteotomy. It has the disadvantage of instability through translation during closure.

**Bailout, Rescue, Salvage Procedures**

Occasionally, a patient in whom multiple Smith-Petersen osteotomies were planned, the osteotomies will not close down, implying that there is an ankylosed disk space anteriorly. If the desired correction cannot be achieved as planned, two adjacent Smith-Petersen osteotomies can be converted into a single pedicle subtraction osteotomy. Such a maneuver reliably allows one to salvage a situation in which a Smith-Petersen osteotomy plan does not close and yield the correction previously anticipated.

# 63

# Laparoscopic Surgical Technique

*Harvinder S. Sandhu*

## Description

Availability of surgical instruments and advances in minimally invasive surgical techniques have enabled surgeons to use laparoscopic methods to access the anterior lumbar spine. The first reported laparoscopic approach for lumbar diskectomy was performed by T.G. Obenchain in 1991. The first two cases of anterior L5-S1 fusion via a laparoscopic approach were performed in September 1993 by J. Zuckerman et al. A variety of interbody implants, such as titanium cages, carbon cages, and allograft, have been utilized to provide stability across the intravertebral segment. These devices permit restoration of lordosis and disk space height and provide immediate intervertebral fixation via the flexion-distraction concept. The techniques are potentially demanding and involve a significant learning phase.

## Indications

Laparoscopic anterior fusion is indicated for reconstituting the foraminal volume (indirect decompression), increasing lordosis, obtaining fusion of the symptomatic degenerative spinal motion segment, and obtaining fusion following posterior pseudarthrosis.

## Contraindications

Because adhesions might prevent safe and adequate exposure, patients with previous abdominal surgery are generally not ideal candidates for laparoscopic exposure of the spinal column.

## Key Procedural Steps

The technique involves accessing the anterior disk space, allowing disk removal, and distraction across the intravertebral space. The space is then prepared for placement of the fixation implant. Frequent fluoroscopic assessment is done throughout the procedure.

The technique involves the following steps:
1. Preoperative planning
2. Operating room setup
3. Positioning of the patient
4. Access
5. Intraoperative localization and templating

## Preoperative Planning

Preoperative planning is performed to facilitate accurate implant placement. Computed tomography (CT) or magnetic resonance imaging (MRI) scans are mandatory to evaluate the location of the vessels (superior vena cava, aorta, and the common iliac arteries and veins) and their respective bifurcations, and to plan the optimal and safest approach.

The preoperative preparation requires that patients be treated with a routine mechanical large bowel prep to empty the sigmoid colon.

## Operating Room Setup and Patient Positioning and Equipment

General anesthesia is utilized, and a Foley catheter and a nasogastric tube are inserted. The patient is placed in the supine position on a radiolucent operating table. Narrow folded blankets or inflatable supports are placed underneath the pelvis to elevate the spine, to increase lordosis, and to obtain better visualization with the C-arm fluoroscope. Furthermore, careful placement of both forearms at the sides and below the level of the spine, or across the chest, or suspended using finger traps is performed to clear the forearms from the C-arm lateral view (**Fig. 63.1**). The standard laparoscopic equipment is utilized, including a 0- and 30-degree 10-mm endoscope, camera, light source, $CO_2$ insufflator, and two monitors to provide visualization for two surgeons on either side of the table. The patient is then placed in a steep Trendelenburg position using straps to prevent the patient from sliding. This position allows the bowel to fall cephalad, providing an unobstructed view of the lumbosacral spine. The patient may be placed in the supine closed leg position with the surgeons at the sides of the patient or may be placed in a split leg position with the primary surgeon positioned between the legs. The split leg position may be preferable if the spine surgeon wishes to gain a midline caudad to cephalad orientation of the lumbar spine.

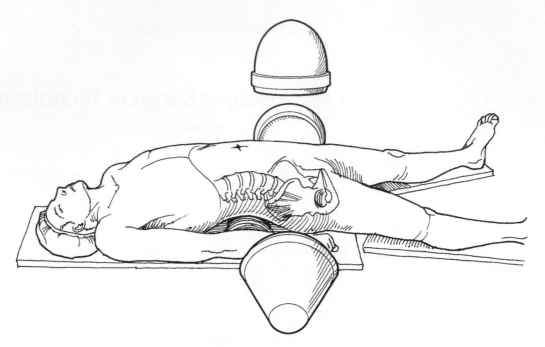

**Fig. 63.1** *Patient in the supine position on a radiolucent operating table.*

### Access and Surgical Technique

Before an incision is made, confirmation of the involved level with an external marker in both the antero-posterior (AP) and lateral planes with the C-arm is accomplished. This allows the correct and proper placement of the *access*, *retracting*, and *working* portals. After the proper visualization is obtained, the patient is prepped and draped in the usual sterile fashion.

Typically, four portals for a one-level fusion and five or six portals for a two-level fusion are required (**Fig. 63.2**). A periumbilical incision below the umbilicus is made, and finger dissection may be used to the level of the fascia (**Fig. 63.3**). The fascia is incised and grasped with a Kocher clamp. A U-suture of 1-0

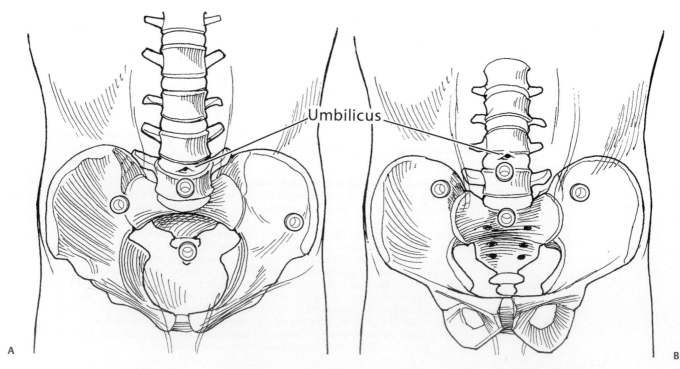

Umbilicus

A                                                                                                              B

**Fig. 63.2** *(A,B)* Four portal placement.

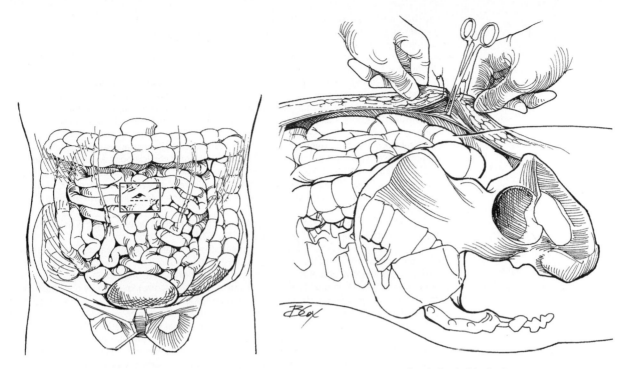

**Fig. 63.3** **(A)** *A periumbilical incision below the umbilicus is made.* **(B)** *Finger dissection is used to the level of the fascia.*

Vicryl is placed on either side of the fascia. This helps to prevent leakage of $CO_2$ via the trocar stem. All trocar sites should be airtight, and occasional use of a laparoscopic balloon-type trocar may be needed. The peritoneum is grasped and opened, and a trocar is placed in a controlled fashion. The balloon is insufflated and $CO_2$ is allowed to insufflate the abdomen to approximately 15 mm Hg (**Fig. 63.4**). The laparoscope is then placed. Under direct visualization of the abdominal wall, additional trocars are placed. Commonly, one is placed in the right lower quadrant and another in the midline above the pubis. The

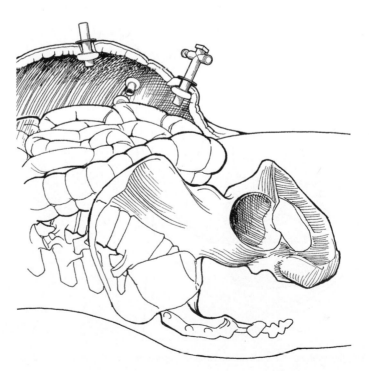

**Fig. 63.4** *The balloon is insufflated and $CO_2$ is allowed to insufflate the abdomen to approximately 15 mm Hg.*

patient can now be placed in maximum Trendelenburg position. The colon is retracted to the left and the mesentery over the aorta and common iliac vein and artery and the inferior vena cava is incised with the ultrasonic Harmonic scalpel (Ethicon, Somerville, NJ). This area is then dissected free, and numerous small vessels that are usually identified going to the left iliac vein can be cut and coagulated with the Harmonic scalpel.

The middle sacral vessels are identified and also cut and coagulated with the Harmonic scalpel and clipped with a right-angle clip applier. Dissection proceeds to expose the anterior interbody space between L5 and S1 from one side to another, mobilizing both the left and the right common iliac vein and artery and the distal portion of the inferior vena cava depending on the level of the bifurcation. If iliac crest bone grafting is desired, the $CO_2$ is allowed to escape from the abdomen at this point. Extending the right lower quadrant trocar site and bringing it over the anterior iliac crest allows harvesting of autologous bone. Cancellous bone graft is removed with a curette through a small cortical bony window. An epidural catheter can be placed in the subperiosteal position and instilled with 0.5% Marcaine solution. The periosteum is then closed and the catheter is bought out though a separate stab wound and secured with Tegaderm. At this point, the fascial and skin defects are closed and the trocar reintroduced into the medial aspect of the incision site.

The abdomen is then reinsufflated. Retraction of the iliac veins on either side is now possible, and the L5-S1 disk space is well exposed and accessible (**Fig. 63.5**).

For the *L4-L5 level*, MRI or CT scan review is mandatory to localize the bifurcation level and to determine if it is high enough to perform the procedure within the bifurcation. If not, the approach may need to be from the left side with retraction of the left common iliac vein within the bifurcation and ligation of one to five iliolumbar veins to allow mobilization. The camera trocar is usually placed *above* the umbilicus and additional trocars are placed based on fluoroscopic visualization of bony landmarks. The posterior peritoneum is incised more proximally, about 3 cm. The colon is retracted laterally, and with careful blunt dissection using a Kitner surgical sponge, the aorta is exposed anteriorly at the bifurcation. The L4-L5 disk is usually located at this point. Left lateral dissection is performed over the left common iliac vein and artery, retracting these vessels to the right. To accomplish this maneuver in a safe fashion, the ascending segmental iliolumbar vein(s) must be identified and transected (there may be more than one). After these vessels are doubly ligated or clipped, the artery and the vein can be retracted to the right to expose a significant amount of the disk. Sometimes this is not necessary in patients with a high bifurcation, and one can proceed in the same fashion mentioned above for the L5-S1 disk access.

Once access to the involved disk level is obtained, the midline suprapubic working trocar (10/12 mm) is placed. A wire is first placed percutaneously and the proper position is verified in two planes with the C-arm fluoroscope. Ideally, the trajectory of the wire should be parallel to the disk space under treatment. Once the trajectory is verified, a 10/12-mm trocar is placed.

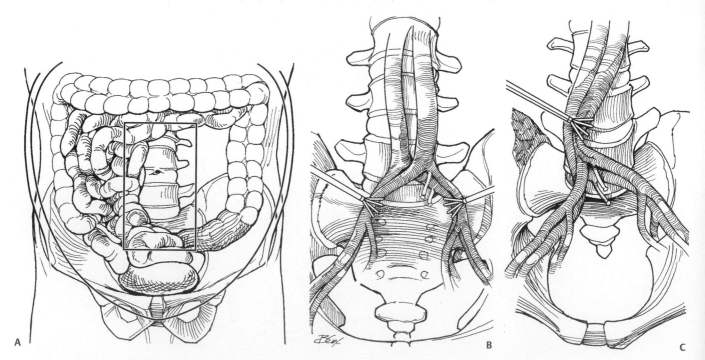

A    B    C

**Fig. 63.5** *(A–C) Retraction of the iliac veins on either side is now possible and the L5-S1 disk space is well exposed and accessible.*

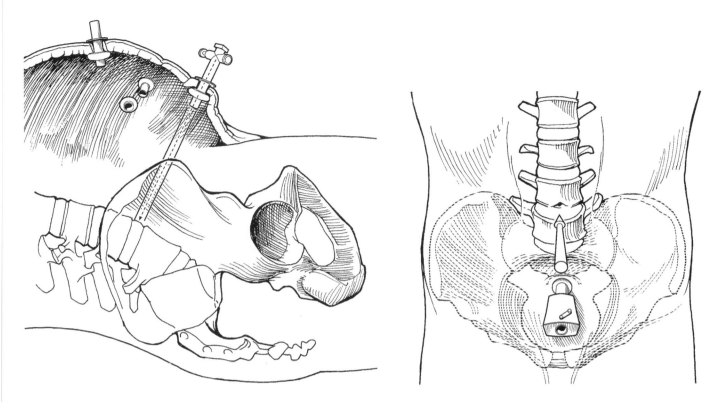

**Fig. 63.6**  *Locating the center of the disk space.*

**Fig. 63.7**  *A wire is placed through the working trocar.*

### Intraoperative Localization and Templating

The initial step is to locate the center of the disk space (**Fig. 63.6**). A wire is placed through the working trocar and the disk space is marked, and confirmed with both AP and lateral fluoroscope views (**Fig. 63.7**). The surgical procedure is then completed utilizing the technical protocol associated with the fixation implants.

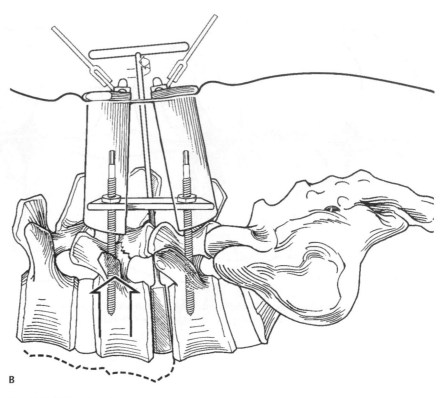

**B**

**Fig. 64.5** *(B) Continued*

**PITFALLS**

- The major pitfall of this technique is the learning curve associated with the confines of operating through the tubular retractor. Once this is mastered, the procedures and pitfalls are essentially the same as the conventional techniques. The majority of these problems can be avoided by appropriately progressing from simple diskectomies and decompressions to more advanced techniques. Further, the use of an expandable retractor may shorten this learning curve. Due to muscle preservation, following larger procedures, patients may have significant muscle spasms that necessitate routine use of antispasmodic medications for 24 to 48 hours postoperative.

is made for pedicle screw placement. For a TLIF, the skin incision is 4 to 5 cm paramedian. The fascia is split in line with the incision. Blunt finger dissection facilitates identification of the intermuscular plane. At the dorsal level of the facet, a Cobb elevator can be used to release the facet muscular attachments from lateral to medial. This maneuver facilitates access to the dorsal laminar interval (allows medial and contralateral decompression as necessary) and medial retraction of the multifidus from the dorsal surface of the facet. The tubular retractor is then docked directly onto the facet and a TLIF may be performed. When desired, a facet fusion can be easily accomplished by docking an 18-mm retractor directly onto the facet, decorticating the joint with a burr or curette and packing it with bone or an alternate fusion material. The use of an expandable tubular retractor provides a greater degree of exposure and is necessary to perform pedicle screw instrumentation using conventional screw systems.

With the retractor in the intermuscular interval (**Fig. 64.5**), the trajectory for pedicle screw insertion is ideal. The facet-traverse process junction can be directly visualized and the pedicles cannulated using anatomic landmarks, followed by placement of a rod or plate directly down the retractor. Specialized compressor and distractors may be required.

### Bailout, Rescue, Salvage Procedures
Inability to obtain adequate visualization or the appropriate trajectory to adequately complete the procedure may necessitate conversion to a standard open exposure. Prior to converting, ensure that the incision has been appropriately placed. If not, then repeat the initial steps with the appropriately localized incision. Otherwise, conversion to an open procedure is simple: extend the paramedian incision and utilize a standard retractor within the intramuscular or intermuscular plane. Alternatively, subfascially mobilize to the midline from the extended paramedian incision or make a separate midline incision and perform a conventional exposure with a standard retractor.

# 65

# Minimally Invasive Posterior Surgical Approaches to the Lumbar Spine Through Tubular Retractors

*James D. Schwender, Kevin T. Foley, and Langston T. Holly*

## Description

Minimally invasive techniques have revolutionized the management of pathologic conditions in various surgical disciplines. The objective is to reduce the approach-related morbidity and at the same time allow the surgery to be performed in an effective and safe manner. The systems currently available consist of a series of concentric dilators and thin-walled tubular retractors of variable length. The tube circumferentially defines a surgical corridor through the erector spinae muscles.

## Expectations

This technique is appropriate for the surgical treatment of lumbar disk herniation, spinal stenosis, or in cases that require stabilization. The current retractor systems are designed to allow exposure of one and two lumbar levels. In the case of stenosis, ipsilateral and contralateral decompression of central, subarticular, and foraminal stenosis is possible through a single paramedian incision.

Published outcomes for decompression surgery compare favorably to the traditional midline open technique. Same-day surgery has become the rule. Concerning one- and two-level fusions, in experienced hands, the blood loss and hospitalization are typically reduced by 50%. Outcomes again compare favorably to traditional techniques. Operative times and complication rates for both decompression and fusions are similar compared with open techniques.

## Indications

The indications are the same as the surgeon would use for tradition open procedures at one or two levels in the lumbar spine for either decompression or fusion.

## Contraindications

Relative contraindications currently include the following:

- More than two-level pathology
- Requirement to correct kyphosis. It is possible to correct 3 to 5 degrees of kyphosis with the transforaminal lumbar interbody fusion (TLIF) procedure; if more is required, an anterior approach continues to provide better lordosis.
- Obesity (body mass index >40). Working within a tubular retractor greater than 8 cm significantly reduces the degrees of freedom of the instruments, particularly if performing interbody fusions.
- Previous surgery. This approach appears to be easier because less scar tissue is encountered. Skin-related complications are rare, even if a previous midline incision scar exists.

## Special Considerations

Knowledge of three-dimensional spinal anatomy is fundamental in the mastery of less invasive techniques. Not infrequently, the surgeon relies on live or virtual fluoroscopic images displayed on a monitor or three-dimensional images from an image guidance system for anatomic orientation. This can be challenging for surgeons who have not had significant experience using two-dimensional images to determine their three-dimensional surgical position.

## Tips, Pearls, and Lessons Learned

Patient positioning and good intraoperative imaging are essential. It is also important to choose the correct size retractor for the given procedure. For decompression, a smaller diameter retractor is required to allow placement medial to the facet joint. This minimizes the amount of soft tissue creep into the wound. The same holds true for fusions. In this case, a larger diameter retractor is docked over the facet joint to be fused again to prevent muscle creep. This allows for identification of the anatomy for decompression and fusion. Once the retractor is in the correct position, resist the temptation of moving the retractor often, which leads to creep of the muscle into the wound.

The treatment of an incidental durotomy should proceed in a similar fashion as if this complication was encountered in an open procedure. A primary suture repair is preferable if it is possible. If a watertight repair cannot be achieved, TisseelTM (Baxter, Deerfield, IL), DuraGenTM (Integra Life Sciences Corp., Plainsboro, NJ), or other dural repair products are useful. In our experience, the minimal dead-space created by the less invasive procedures seems to limit the formation of a symptomatic pseudomeningocele.

Epidural bleeding needs to be proactively controlled. There are several ways to reduce the likelihood of problematic bleeding. First, positioning of the patient on the Jackson frame with or without the Wilson attachment reduces intraabdominal pressure. When in the epidural space, find the bleeders before they find you and use bipolar electrocautery. Liberally use a thrombotic paste product such as Gelfoam paste and cottonoids. When performing the facetectomy for a TLIF, preserve the capsule during bone resection and only remove it once the facetectomy is complete. This allows for easier identification of the epidural veins for cauterization. Finally, the larger more difficult-to-control epidurals are typically medial in the vicinity of the posterior longitudinal ligament and far laterally in the foramen. Avoid exposure of these anatomic areas unless necessary.

**Key Procedural Steps**
1. Patient selection
2. Intraoperative positioning of the patient in the prone position
3. Identification on orthogonal imaging of correct level of surgery
4. Placement of skin incision(s)
5. Correct diameter and depth of tubular retractor
6. Minimize movement of the retractor once in position to prevent tissue creep
7. Address pathology to avoid failure of execution

The working retractor size for decompression varies between 12 and 18 mm and for fusions between 22 or 26 mm. The patient is positioned prone on a Jackson or Wilson frame to allow a C-arm fluoroscope to be used in a biplanar fashion. It is important to confirm that both views are technically possible and the anatomy of the spine is well visualized prior to prepping and draping. The position of the skin incision is determined based on the pathology to be addressed and is localized using the orthogonal fluoroscopic images. Typically, the incision is 2 to 3 cm off midline for disk herniations and stenosis that require assessment through the interlaminar space and 4 to 5 cm for foraminal herniations, TLIF, or posterolateral fusion (**Fig. 65.1**).

For decompression, a unilateral incision based 1:1 on the tubular retractor size is made and carried down through the subcutaneous tissues and then through the lumbodorsal fascia. This position is confirmed by palpation of the bony landmarks and by fluoroscopy. Serial dilators are then placed until the diameter of the working retractor is obtained. A light source to allow for tubular illumination is positioned, and visualization is obtained with either loupe magnification or a microscope. In most cases, there is little soft tissue to remove from within the retractor prior to visualization of the bony anatomy. Anatomic landmarks are again defined with fluoroscopy and confirmed with direct visualization. Bayonetted instruments have been designed to work within the tubular retractors without the surgeon's hand obscuring visualization. These are used to perform the soft tissue and bone resection required for the appropriate decompression.

For fusion, the incisions are 2 to 3 cm in length and typically 4 to 5 cm off midline. The positioning of the patient and identification of bony landmarks using orthogonal fluoroscopy cannot be overstated. A Kirschner wire (K-wire) is used to identify the facet joint at the correct level. Sequential dilators are used, and the distal end of a 22- or 26-mm diameter tube of appropriate length is positioned over the facet joint complex

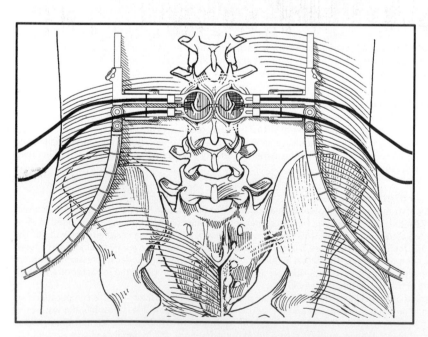

**Fig. 65.1** *Bilateral paramedian placement of Quadrant retractor system (Medtronic Sofamor Danek, Memphis, TN).*

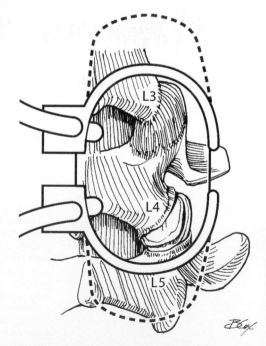

**Fig. 65.2** *Posterior exposure at the L4-L5 level. Facet joint capsule removed at L4-L5 and preserved at L3-L4. Subperiosteal exposure of the pars interarticularis and lamina.*

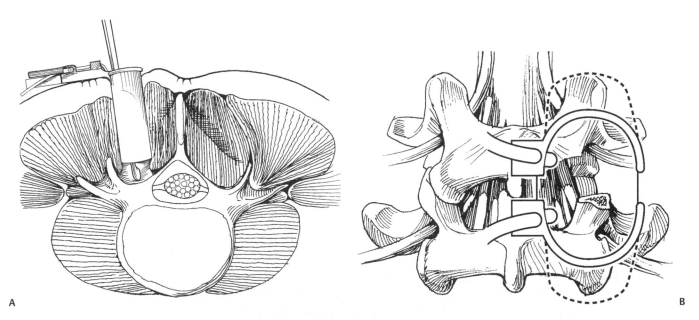

**Fig. 65.3** *(A,B) Complete facetectomy for transforaminal lumbar interbody fusion (TLIF) with decompression of the foramen and subarticular space. Note epidural fat (A) exiting the nerve root and the view of the TLIF working portal without the requirement of retraction.*

(**Fig. 65.2**). For the TLIF procedure, a total facetectomy is performed using a bayoneted osteotome, Kerrison rongeur, or a high-speed drill. This bone is denuded of all articular cartilage and soft tissue, and saved for later use as interbody graft material.

The complete facetectomy allows for ipsilateral decompression of central, subarticular, and foraminal stenosis (**Fig. 65.3**). Contralateral decompression through the ipsilateral incision is possible through rotation of the retractor toward midline to the junction of the lamina and spinous process. The lamina is resected to the base of the spinous process, at which point the ligamentum flavum is resected bilaterally.

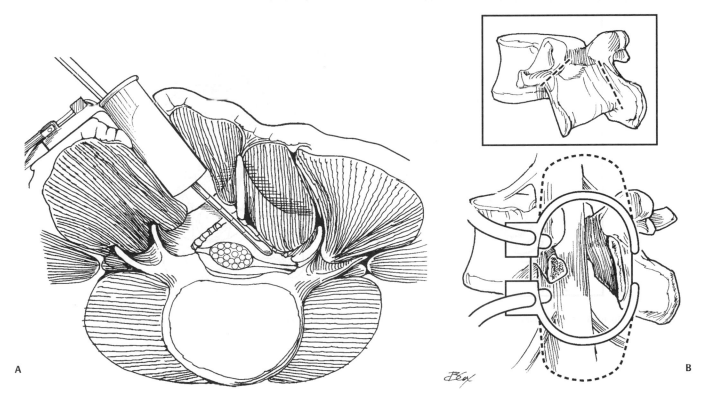

**Fig. 65.4** *(A,B) Contralateral over-the-top decompression accomplished by medial angulation of the retractor and lamina resection.*

# 66

# Percutaneous Cement Augmentation Techniques (Vertebroplasty, Kyphoplasty)

*Choll W. Kim and Steven R. Garfin*

## Description

Percutaneous vertebral augmentation (vertebroplasty, kyphoplasty) is used to treat painful vertebral compression fractures due to osteoporosis or lytic tumors via injection of bone cement into the vertebral body.

## Key Principles

Immediate stabilization of vertebral body fractures to decrease pain or prevent further collapse of the vertebral body. Fracture reduction can be obtained in some circumstances using postural techniques or with the use of an inflatable bone tamp (kyphoplasty).

## Expectations

Patients with painful vertebral compression fractures may have severe pain for prolonged periods of time. This treatment provides a minimally invasive method of stabilizing the micromotion of the fracture and thereby decreasing pain. Pain relief occurs within 1 or 2 days in most cases. Pain relief has been correlated with fracture reduction. However, fracture reduction via kyphoplasty is best accomplished when fractures are treated within 2 to 3 months.

## Indications

Percutaneous vertebral augmentation is indicated for the treatment of painful, low-energy thoracic and lumbar vertebral body fractures due to osteoporosis and certain lytic lesions, such as multiple myeloma.

## Contraindications

Percutaneous vertebral augmentation should not be used in the setting of infection and certain mass-occupying lesions, including solid tumors and arteriovenous malformations. This technique is intended to stabilize the micromotion associated with low-energy fractures. It is not recommended in high-energy injuries with concomitant ligamentous or posterior element injuries. Care should be taken in vertebral body fractures with posterior wall involvement (discussed later).

## Special Considerations

The proper identification of the painful vertebrae can be challenging. In addition to radiographs, advanced imaging studies must be obtained. Magnetic resonance imaging (MRI) is the most useful method of evaluation. Technetium bone scan is useful in patients with a contraindication to MRI, such as brain aneurysm clips or cardiac pacemakers. Clinical localization of the fracture using percussion of the spinous processes can be helpful in distinguishing distant sites (e.g., T6 versus L4), but not nearby sites.

The posterior wall is often involved, but is not always an absolute contraindication to vertebral augmentation. In low-energy injuries with an intact posterior longitudinal ligament, the cement is often prevented from entering the canal. A secondary indicator of posterior wall compromise is the presence of an epidural hematoma. This suggests that the fracture communicates directly with the epidural space and thus may be a conduit for cement leakage. Percutaneous vertebral augmentation should be pursued only with great caution.

Vertebral compression fractures may be caused by pathologic conditions such as tumor or infection. Unless the diagnosis of osteoporosis is well established, a biopsy is recommended. In patients who have a dual-energy x-ray absorptiometry (DEXA) study consistent with osteoporosis, no history of malignancy, and a previously known osteoporotic vertebral compression fracture, a biopsy is not necessary.

## Special Instructions, Position, and Anesthesia

Gentle lordotic positioning allows some postural reduction in certain fractures. The procedure can be performed with local anesthetic in many patients. The patient should be able to lie prone for at least 1 hour without significant pain or respiratory difficulties. Attention to injecting the periosteum of the entry point decreases pain during trocar insertion. Some pain may be encountered during balloon inflation or during injection. This is best treated with reassurance and gentle intravenous sedation.

If general anesthesia is utilized, the patient must be handled gently. Rib fractures may occur as a result of undue pressure in the course of patient positioning and during impacting maneuvers to insert the trocar into the vertebral body.

During multilevel injections, the cement load is greater. Toxic monomeric constituents have the potential to cause cardiorespiratory collapse. The anesthesiologist must be alerted at the time of each injection procedure. Vasoactive substances to treat sudden hypotension must be readily available.

### Tips, Pearls, and Lessons Learned

The use of biplanar fluoroscopy greatly aids cannula insertion and cement injection. Biplanar fluoroscopy is readily obtained by using two separate C-arms (**Fig. 66.1**). The lateral image is brought over the top and the arc, leaning away toward the head. The anteroposterior (AP) image is brought in diagonally with the image intensifier directly over the target site. It is most convenient to obtain the true AP image first because the diagonal entry makes this process challenging. The lateral image is then adjusted around the AP image. Meticulous attention should be exercised to obtain true AP and lateral images of the target vertebrae.

Treatment of multiple levels can be performed using a single batch of cement. The cement is stored in a sterile ice-water bath to slow the polymerization process. With vertebroplasty, all the cannulas are inserted first, and then each site is injected sequentially. With kyphoplasty, the guide wires are inserted into all the target vertebral bodies (as described later). The first site is then drilled, the balloon tamp deployed, and the cement injected. The next level is then drilled, treated with the balloon tamp, and subsequently injected. A third site can be treated thereafter in the same sequence. This stepwise sequence allows use of a single pair of balloon tamps for the treatment multiple levels. The limitation of the number of levels is dictated by the cement load. The risk of cement toxicity increases with the number of levels treated. As a general rule, no more than three levels are treated at one operation.

Special consideration related to cement fill is needed for kyphoplasty. In addition to filling the void created by the balloon tamp, additional cement is needed to allow integration of the cement into the surrounding trabecular bone. This serves to "lock in" the cement. Inadequate filling may lead to further collapse of the surrounding bone due to excessive motion at the bone–cement interface. In general, the volume of cement injected should be greater than the volume of the inflated balloon.

The method of cement injection is geared toward proper cement fill and prevention of extravasation. It is important to inject the cement in small aliquots with fluoroscopic images taken at each step. Leakage can continue even after the injection is halted due to back pressure or blood flow. By limiting the injection volume, the severity of cement leakage can be mitigated.

Maintenance of reduction via kyphoplasty may be difficult in certain fractures, particularly in vertebrae plana. Once the balloon is deflated, the fracture may collapse again. The reduction can be maintained by the "eggshell" technique. A small amount of cement (0.5 to 1 cc) is injected into the cavity. The balloon tamp is reinserted and gently reelevated. The small cement bolus is then spread around the balloon to create a thin eggshell of cement. When the balloon is removed, the eggshell mantle holds the reduction until the remainder of the cement is injected. This technique can also be utilized to control cement leakage (described later).

### Difficulties Encountered

Intraoperative fluoroscopic imaging of the midthoracic spine can be challenging in the severely osteoporotic patient. The image can be improved by halting respiration and bringing the x-ray tube closer to the patient. This magnifies the image and decreases beam scatter.

Cement polymerization can occur rapidly, making injection difficult. Avoid handling the cement or placing the cement under bright lights as polymerization rate increases with higher temperatures. Chilling cement prior to use is helpful. Slower setting cements are available (e.g., KyphX cement, Kyphon, Sunnyside, CA).

### Key Procedural Steps

With the patient prepped and draped in the prone position (under either general or local anesthesia), two C-arms are brought into the field (**Fig. 66.1**). True AP and lateral images of the involved vertebral body are obtained. In the AP plane, the pedicles should be symmetric in shape. The lateral edge of the vertebral body should be equidistant from both pedicles. Some fractures have an asymmetric configuration, making alignment of the pedicles and the lateral vertebral body wall somewhat challenging. In this case, the spinous process can be centered between the pedicles. Caution should be exercised when using the spinous process to obtain a true AP image because there is significant anatomic variation in the shape of the spinous process.

The entry point to the pedicle is marked using high-quality biplanar images. Use of local anesthesia, even in patients under general anesthesia, is recommended for perioperative and postoperative pain control. The periosteum must be anesthetized if the patient is awake. A trocar needle is inserted into the vertebral body either with a transpedicular or extrapedicular approach (**Fig. 66.2**). The transpedicular approach is best suited for large pedicles such as those in the lumbar spine and lower thoracic spine. The extrapedicular approach is best suited for the midthoracic spine. The entry point for the extrapedicular approach lies between the lateral edge of the pedicle and the costovertebral joint. The rib head helps direct the needle into the vertebral body. The extrapedicular approach allows a more medial trajectory, thereby accessing the central portion of the vertebral body. With this technique, adequate cement distribution into the vertebral body may be accomplished through a unilateral injection site.

During vertebroplasty, the cement injection needle is inserted through the same trocar. The tip of the needle is placed anteriorly and medially. Optimal needle placement is in the anterior one third of the vertebral body. During kyphoplasty, this trocar (usually a Jamshidi needle) is used to insert a guidewire into the vertebral body. The Kyphon cannula is inserted over the guidewire and into the vertebral body. Vigilance

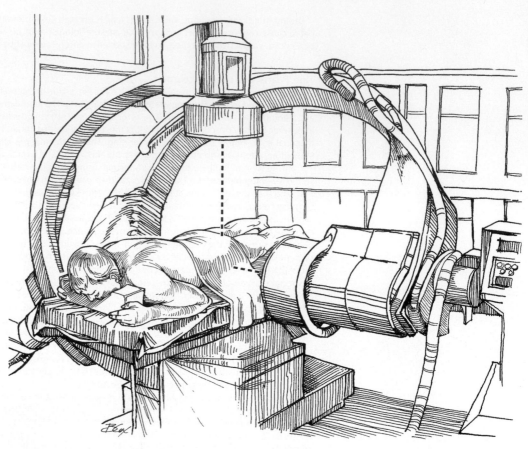

**Fig. 66.1** *Biplanar fluoroscopy is best accomplished with two simultaneous C-arms. The patient is placed prone on a well-padded, radiolucent table (e.g., Jackson flat table). The C-arm for the lateral image is brought in first (C-arm 1). By placing the arc over the top of the patient, the arc can be leaned over and away from the incoming C-arm used for the anteroposterior (AP) image. The C-arm for the AP image is brought in diagonally from the same side (C-arm 2). The surgeon stands on the opposite side of the C-arms. Entry of C-arm 2 in a diagonal fashion can make adjustments challenging. Thus, it is best to move the lateral C-arm 1 up slightly to provide adequate working room to obtain a true AP image of the target site. Once the AP image is captured, C-arm 2 is adjusted to obtain a true lateral image of the target site.*

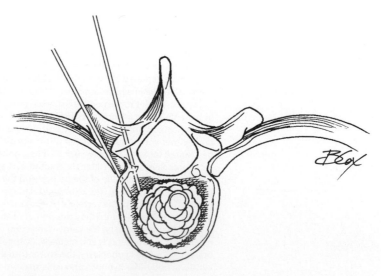

**Fig. 66.2** *Superior view of vertebroplasty, using pedicular and parapedicular approaches.*

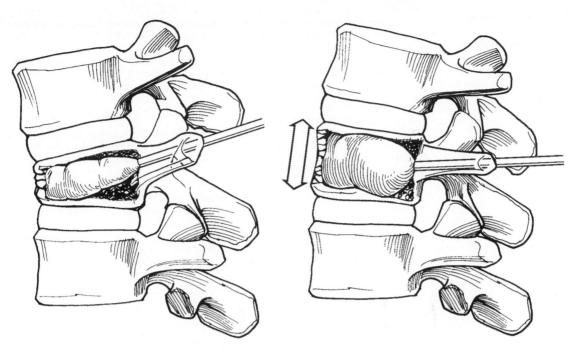

A                                                                                              B

**Fig. 66.3** **(A)** *Lateral diagram showing inflatable balloon tamp is inserted into the vertebral body via a transpedicular approach.* **(B)** *Inflation of the balloon tamp elevates the vertebral end plates to achieve fracture reduction.*

is recommended to avoid advancing the guidewire inadvertently. The cannula is inserted approximately 2 to 3 mm past the posterior vertebral body wall. The guidewire is removed and a drill is used to create a path for the inflatable balloon tamp. If a biopsy is planned, a biopsy trocar is used to sample the vertebral bone prior to drilling the vertebral body. Once both balloons are in the vertebral body, they are inflated simultaneously under biplanar fluoroscopy (**Fig. 66.3**). The use of the balloon tamp produces a void in which cement can be deposited under low pressure (**Fig. 66.4**). In some cases, reduction of the vertebral body can be accomplished. The reduction maneuver is best accomplished when the balloon pushes up

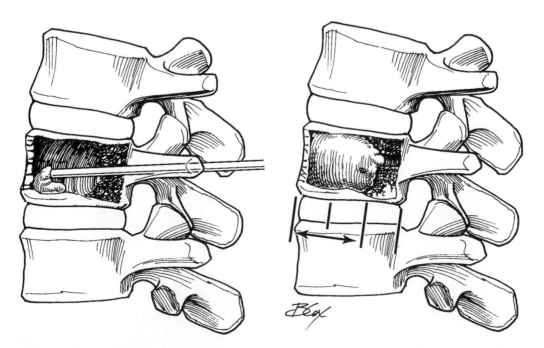

A                                                                                              B

**Fig. 66.4** **(A)** *Lateral diagram showing injection of cement into cavity created by the balloon tamp.* **(B)** *Cement is filled until small appendages can be seen infiltrating the trabecular bone around the cavity. Cement volume should be* greater than the volume of the balloon. The cement is kept in the anterior two thirds of the vertebral body to minimize the risk of cement leaks through posterior wall defects or venous channels.

**PITFALLS**

- Poor fluoroscopic visualization due to severe osteoporosis
- Cement embolization
- Cement extravasation into neuroforamina or spinal canal
- Medial wall breach
- Pedicle fracture
- Inadequate cement fill

against the end plate and shows a flattened appearance on fluoroscopic image. The inflation of the balloon should be stopped before causing a cortical breach, which is revealed by the appearance of a small outward bleb in the balloon.

Small volumes of cement (about 0.2 to 0.5 cc) are injected in a stepwise fashion with fluoroscopic visualization. The cement should be injected into the anterior two thirds of the vertebral body. By avoiding the posterior one third, the risk of cement leakage into the spinal canal is minimized.

**Bailout, Rescue, Salvage Procedures**

When cement leakage is observed, injection should be halted immediately. The cannula is repositioned to another location and another attempt at injection may be pursued after adequate time has passed to allow the first injection to polymerize. Gelfoam or bone wax can be used to further plug the breach. A new cannula is inserted to resume the injection.

If kyphoplasty is performed, the balloon tamp can be used to create an eggshell mantle (described above) that will contain the cement. The balloon is then removed and cement injected within the mantle. If there is persistent leakage, injection from that side is aborted and the procedure is performed from the contralateral side only.

In most cases, cement leakage is clinically inconsequential. If a significant leak is suspected, a wake-up test is performed prior to departing the operating room. If there are clinical signs and symptoms of neurologic compromise, emergent decompression should be considered.

# 67

# Minimally Disruptive Lateral Approach to the Lumbar Spine: Extreme-Lateral Lumbar Interbody Fusion

*Luiz Pimenta*

## Description

The extreme-lateral lumbar interbody fusion (XLIF) procedure is a minimally disruptive direct-lateral, retroperitoneal, trans-psoas approach to the lumbar spine. It incorporates blunt finger dissection of the retroperitoneal space, stimulated electromyogram (EMG) guidance of blunt dilators through the psoas muscle, and advancement of a split-blade retractor system for illuminated direct visualization of the lateral portion of the spine. The approach is described here for interbody fusion, but has also been used as a revision strategy for failed anteriorly placed total disk replacement and as a primary procedure for laterally placed total disk replacement.

## Key Principles

The direction of the approach avoids the muscle, bone, and ligament disruption of a posterior approach and the vascular and visceral mobilization and potential concomitant risks of an anterior approach. The minimal dissection and tissue damage result in quick operative times, minimal blood loss, minimal morbidity, and quick patient recovery. The lateral exposure allows for more complete disk space preparation and optimal placement of a large interbody device, which, when coupled with preservation of both anterior and posterior longitudinal ligaments, provides for an exceptionally stable construct.

## Expectations

Working in a lateral position through the retroperitoneal anatomy may feel foreign to those accustomed to the more traditional anterior or posterior approaches. However, because the exposure procedure itself is relatively simple, and the intervertebral disk work is conventional, the learning curve is not steep. XLIF can be performed without the assistance of an approach surgeon in about an hour, with barely detectable blood loss. Disk height, foraminal volume, and spinal alignment can be superbly achieved using a large implant, positioned optimally in the anterior half of the disk space and sitting along the biomechanically sound ring apophysis. Patients tend to have few postoperative complaints, aside from a transient hip flexor pain or weakness (depending on how delicately the psoas muscle is dissected), and can generally ambulate within hours of surgery and be discharged from the hospital the next day.

## Indications

The indications for XLIF fusion surgery are those for any L1–L5 interbody fusion, and include, but are not limited to, degenerative disk disease with instability, recurrent disk herniation, low-grade degenerative spondylolisthesis (less than grade 3), degenerative scoliosis, adjacent level syndrome, postlaminectomy instability, and posterior pseudarthrosis. The XLIF surgery, as a stand-alone procedure, relies on indirect decompression of the neural elements from restoration of disk height and spinal alignment, but the need for direct decompression does not necessarily contraindicate XLIF. Performing a conjunctive posterior microdecompression adds minimally to the surgical time and retains the minimally disruptive benefits of the procedure.

## Contraindications

Contraindications include those for interbody fusion surgery in general, such as infection, unless an autograft is placed, or there are significant comorbidities. Interestingly, although osteoporosis may contraindicate other fusion procedures, low bone quality is better tolerated by the XLIF procedure due to the size and position of the interbody implant. The direct lateral approach is specifically contraindicated at L5-S1 due to the location of the iliac crest, and in patients with bilateral retroperitoneal scarring, such as from prior surgery. Although degenerative scoliosis is a growing application for the XLIF approach because of the potential for alignment correction and low morbidity for a typically elderly population, lumbar deformities with greater than 30 degrees of rotation can confuse the approach and present risk. Similarly, high-grade degenerative spondylolisthesis (higher than grade 2) may require more demanding techniques for slip reduction.

## Special Considerations

Large patients tend to be more difficult than thin patients from most approaches. However, in XLIF the patient is in a lateral decubitus position, which allows the abdomen to fall anteriorly away from the spine, shortening the distance from skin to spine (which is more dependent on the width of the hips than the girth of the waist), and opens the retroperitoneal space to provide a large safe approach trajectory. In all patients, it is important to consider the nerves of the lumbar plexus within the psoas muscle, which typically lie in the posterior third of the muscle. Given variation in anatomy and surgical approach, care is warranted and EMG-assisted nerve avoidance is recommended.

### Special Instructions, Position, and Anesthesia

Patient positioning is key to an unencumbered successful XLIF procedure. The patient should be positioned on a radiolucent breakable surgical table in a true lateral decubitus position. A true lateral position should be confirmed with fluoroscopy prior to taping and draping and reconfirmed periodically. It is easiest if the patient or surgical table is positioned to provide a true lateral, such that the fluoroscope C-arm will be used at a 0- or 90-degree angle for lateral or cross-table anteroposterior (AP) images only, rather than adjusting the angle of the C-arm to fit the angle of the patient. This helps to ensure that access exposure and instrument manipulation occur in the true lateral direction, maximizing implant placement and minimizing risk to anterior or posterior structures. The patient should be securely taped to the table in this true lateral position, with the iliac crest at the break in the table, and the tape securely leveraging motion of the iliac crest inferiorly away from the waist. Breaking the table then at the crest provides for added working space between the rib cage and the ileum and facilitates exposure, especially at L4-L5. The patient's hips should be flexed to relieve tension on the psoas muscle.

For EMG nerve monitoring during the trans-psoas approach and during interbody distraction and implant insertion, anesthesia should not include muscle relaxants or paralytic agents subsequent to initial short-acting agents given for intubation, or they should be reversed prior to the start of the approach. Four out of four twitches from a train-of-four test is required.

### Tips, Pearls, and Lessons Learned

A good fluoroscopic image is extremely helpful. Adjust the cephalocaudal angle of the C-arm to provide a clear lateral view of the end plates. There is a tendency to cheat the initial exposure anteriorly to avoid the nerves posteriorly. However, because the XLIF retractor is designed to prevent pressure on the posterior elements, the aperture is preferentially expanded anteriorly. Therefore, the ideal initial target spot is the direct center of the lateral aspect of the disk, which will result in retractor exposure of the anterior half of the disk space. Multilevel procedures can be performed using the same skin incision but separate fascial incisions and psoas muscle dilations. In degenerative scoliosis cases, coronal alignment can be achieved from either side, but access is easier from the convex side because of osteophyte formation on the concave side. The contralateral annulus must be disrupted to achieve parallel distraction, optimal biomechanical position of the implant, and optimal coronal alignment.

### Difficulties Encountered

Symmetrical cephalocaudal expansion of the retractor can be deflected by the iliac crest at L4-L5 or by the ribs at L1-L2 or L2-L3. Access difficulty at L4-L5 can be overcome with proper positioning and aggressive bending of the patient. At L2-L3, the 12th rib may need to be retracted or partially resected. At L1-L2, an intercostal approach may be necessary between the 11th and 12th ribs. If nerve monitoring warns of a too posterior position within the psoas, slight translation of the dilators away from the indicated direction of the nerve(s) should still provide adequate exposure. A stimulating ball-tipped probe can be used to identify tissue structures within the exposure if necessary. Proper targeting of the disk space should prevent a too anterior exposure, but care should be taken to limit retractor excursion or disk work to posterior to the anterior longitudinal ligament. Lateral fluoroscopic images should be obtained to ensure AP position.

### Key Procedural Steps

1. *Exposure:* With the patient in a true lateral decubitus position, target the disk of interest using lateral fluoroscopy and mark the skin over the direct-lateral center of the disk space. Make a second incision posterolateral to this direct-lateral marking, just large enough for finger access (**Fig. 67.1**). Alternate finger and reverse-scissor dissection through the posterolateral muscle and fascia in a 45-degree trajectory until resistance gives and the retroperitoneal space is entered (**Fig. 67.2**). Sweep the finger within the retroperitoneal space to ensure a clear working channel and use it to guide dilators through the lateral incision to the surface of the psoas muscle (**Fig. 67.3**). Attach stimulated EMG nerve avoidance to the blunt dilators to gently and safely split the fibers of the psoas (**Fig. 67.4**). Advance the split-blade expandable retractor over the dilators, rigidly lock it to the surgical table, and expand it over the anterior half of the lateral aspect of the disk space (**Fig. 67.5B**).
2. *Annulotomy and disk space preparation:* Make an annulotomy wide enough in the AP dimension to accommodate a large XLIF implant. Perform disk removal and end-plate preparation as in conventional techniques using conventional instruments such as pituitary rongeurs, curettes, shavers, and scrapers. Disk removal can be facilitated by using a Cobb elevator along both end plates to release the disk and to disrupt the contralateral annulus.
3. *Insertion of XLIF implant:* Use a trial to both size the disk space and help gain parallel distraction. Impact the implant across the disk space under AP fluoroscopy, ensuring the central implant marker is

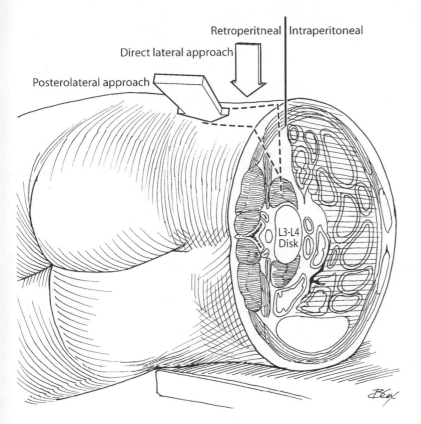

**Fig. 67.1** *Direct lateral and posterolateral skin incision sites.*

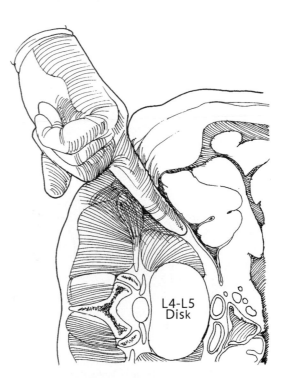

**Fig. 67.2** *Finger dissection through the posterolateral musculature to the retroperitoneal space.*

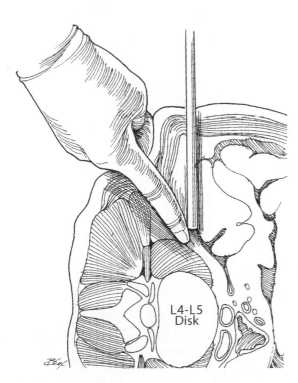

**Fig. 67.3** *Finger guidance of the initial dilator safely to the surface of the psoas muscle.*

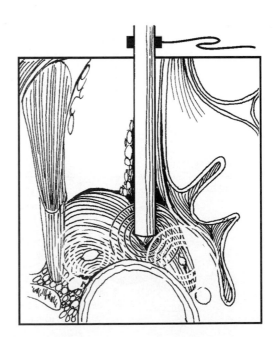

**Fig. 67.4** *Stimulated electromyogram (EMG) on the initial dilator for safe approach through the psoas muscle to the spine.*

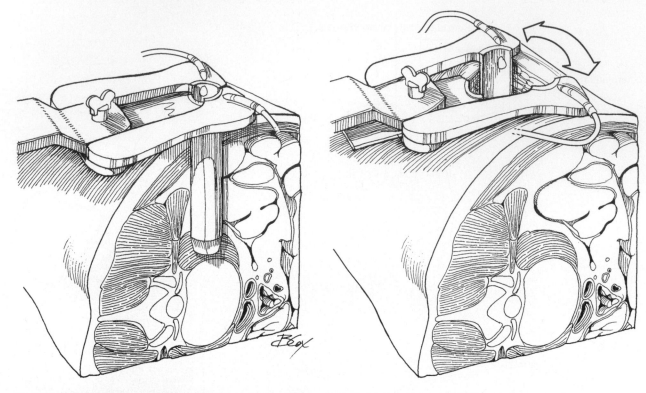

**Fig. 67.5 (A,B)** *Split-blade retractor advanced and expanded over the anterior half of the lateral aspect of the disk space. Incorporated light cables provide for direct illuminated visualization.*

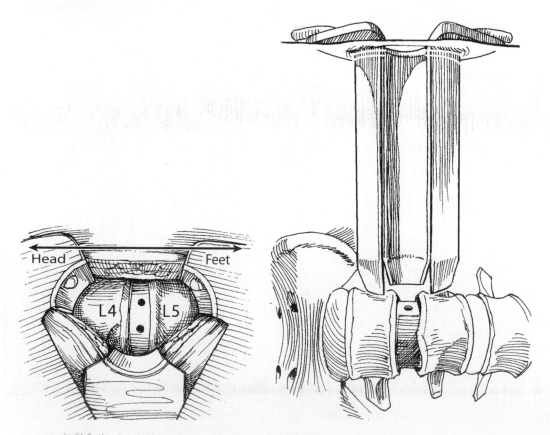

**Fig. 67.6 (A,B)** *Optimal implant placement, with strong end plate support.*

PITFALLS

- Failing to properly position the patient makes for a tedious procedure. A few extra minutes in the beginning will save a lot of time in the end. Disk removal and end-plate preparation should be complete to facilitate fusion and should extend clear across the disk space through the contralateral annulus. Failure to release the contralateral annulus could result in difficulty in implant positioning, which can lead to coronal imbalance if the implant is inserted asymmetrically, or in subsidence if a short implant is chosen. End-plate compromise should be avoided using careful end-plate–sparing preparation techniques. Oversizing of the implant in height could cause rupture of the anterior longitudinal ligament, displacement of the implant anteriorly, or difficulty in distracting adjacent levels in multilevel procedures.

positioned centrally within the disk space and that the length of the implant spans both sides of the ring apophysis for strong end-plate support (**Fig. 67.6**).

4. *Close:*   Close and gently remove the retractor. Close the fascia and skin using standard technique.

**Bailout, Rescue, Salvage Procedures**

Because the expandable retractor allows for customizable exposure, the incision can be widened as needed if confined by the minimally disruptive exposure. If construct integrity is questionable (e.g., due to end-plate compromise or anterior longitudinal ligament [ALL] disruption), supplemental instrumentation can be used for stabilization.

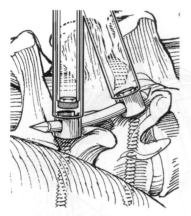

**Fig. 68.4** *Medtronic Sofamor Danek Sextant system rod insertion.*

made proximally, and the rod is advanced through the musculature into the top-loading portions of the screws (**Fig. 68.4**). The locking nuts are then advanced to the rod, tightened, and countertorqued. The rod is released from the CD Horizon Sextant II system guide, and the system extensions are removed from the wound. The entire process is then repeated on the opposite side.

### *Minimal Access Surgical Technology Quadrant™ Retractor System*

In this system, the Jamshidi needle and wire is centered over the facet joint between the pedicles. Sequential dilators are passed over the wire, and the MAST Quadrant retractors are placed around the dilators in the closed position. The dilators are removed and the MAST Quadrant retractors are expanded in a proximal and distal direction (**Fig. 68.5**). Next, medial-lateral retractors are connected to the MAST Quadrant frame. The pedicle entry sites can then be exposed under direct vision and prepared in the usual fashion. The transverse processes can be exposed and decorticated and fusion graft material can be placed prior to placing the pedicle screws. Once the screws are in the pedicle, a rod can be dropped directly on top of the screws through the MAST Quadrant retractor without the need for a radial alignment guide or proximal incision (**Fig. 68.6**). The locking nuts are then placed under direct vision.

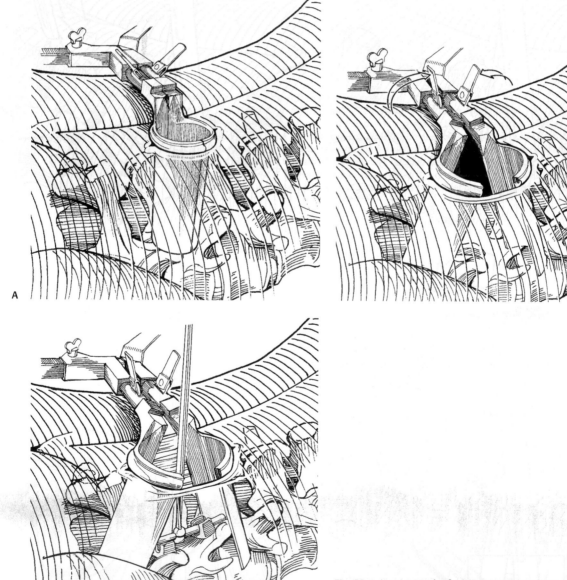

**Fig. 68.5 (A–C)** *Example of mini-open retractor system. Shown here Medtronic Sofamor Danek's Quadrant system.*

## PITFALLS

*Misplaced Screw: Medial Malposition*

- This is the most dangerous screw malposition because it can cause nerve injury. This may be apparent on the fluoroscopic view but usually the surgeon is alerted to this situation by the nerve monitoring. If the nerve depolarizes at a current of <15 mA, there is a possibility of a pedicle wall breach. If the nerve depolarizes at a current of <10 mA, there is significant pedicle wall distortion and nerve root irritation. At this time, the screw should be removed; however, the pedicle can still be salvaged if so desired. Another Jamshidi needle or pedicle awl can be placed in the starting hole and directed in a more vertical orientation to redirect the screw. Also, a more lateral starting hole can be made. However, nerve monitoring may be abnormal even with good positioning because of decreased electrical resistance to the failed bone. If the malpositioned screw is the middle of three screws, it can be removed and the construct spanned by a rod between the proximal and distal screws. This is more acceptable if there is an interbody graft. If there are only two screws in the construct, then a unilateral construct may be necessary. If a patient wakes up with hip or leg pain that was not present preoperatively or can possibly be secondary to nerve root irritation, then the most accurate test is a computed tomography (CT)/myelogram with reformatted images. If the CT is not definitive and the patient has strong radicular symptoms or weakness, then the pedicle can be explored with a minimally invasive or open decompression. If the pedicle is breached, then the screw must be removed.

*Misplaced Screw: Lateral Malposition*

- Lateral malposition can occur and must be corrected to maintain screw pullout strength. This situation becomes apparent because the screw insertion torque feels less than normal. In addition, any wire passed through the screw will pass around the vertebra and anterior to the spine. Remove the screw, use the same starting hole, and redirect the pedicle preparation tool in a more medial direction. Then place another screw as usual.

*Rod Will Not Pass*

- The rod may not pass the soft tissue. In that case, make a larger skin and fascia incision for the rod to pass. If the rod will not pass through the screw head, you must check a few things. If a nut dropped prematurely from the screw holder, it will not allow the rod to pass. Push a guidewire through the screwdriver into the screw and into the bone. Then, remove the screw and reassemble the screw/nut/holder assembly. Next, reinsert the screw over the wire into the pedicle and start again. This may also happen if the screw disassembles from the screw holder and the solution is the same. In a multilevel construct, you can rotate the screw extensions slightly and gently tap the rod holder to advance the rod. If this does not work, remove the middle screw and span the construct between the proximal and distal screws. Alternatively, you can extend the skin and fascia incisions, bluntly dissect the muscle tissue to the screw heads, and drop the rod directly into the screw heads.

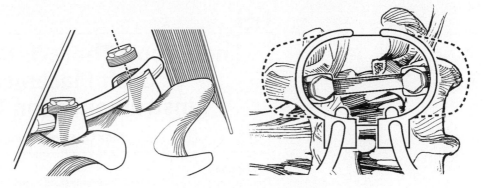

**Fig. 68.6** *(A,B) Medtronic Sofamor Danek's Quadrant system rod insertion.*

There are other percutaneous screw systems not explained in detail here. Each system differs in the details of exposure, pedicle insertion, and especially how the rods are placed. Regardless of these differences, the primary understanding must be in preparing the pedicle in a safe and accurate manner.

### Bailout, Rescue, Salvage Procedures

Many of these techniques have already been described; however, be patient and think through the problem. If for any reason, you must reinsert a tubular or percutaneous retractor, always pass a guidewire through the instrument you have in the wound. That way, you will always keep your exposure without having to redo your positioning or the fluoroscopy. Remember, you can always convert the case to an open procedure by extending the skin and fascia incisions and use blunt dissection through the muscle planes to the spine. Rescue and salvage procedures rely on knowledge of spine and instrumentation biomechanics to create the best construct possible.

### Conclusion

Percutaneous pedicle screws systems offer the advantages of the open pedicle screw systems without the disadvantages of exposure-related muscle damage. When following the key principles of percutaneous lumbar pedicle screw fixation, the surgeon may safely and accurately implant percutaneous pedicle screws for the current indications. The systems are being modified and improved to expand their indications in static stabilization and future applications in dynamic stabilization. Compared with traditional open techniques, the minimally invasive techniques have shown marked reductions in surgical time, blood loss, and postoperative pain.

# 69

# Endoscopic Thoracic Decompression, Graft Placement, and Instrumentation Techniques

*Max C. Lee and Daniel H. Kim*

## Description

Thoracic decompressions include diskectomies and corpectomies with intervertebral grafting with anterior instrumentation, as well as thoracoscopic decompression and stabilization in the setting of trauma to the thoracolumbar junction (TLJ).

## Expectations

The goals of operative treatment include (1) adequate decompression of the spinal canal to provide the maximum chance of neurologic recovery; (2) correction of the spinal deformity and restoration of anatomic alignment to prevent delayed spinal deformity and neurologic deficits; and (3) immediate rigid fixation for early mobilization and rehabilitation with fixation of the least number of motion segments. The approach and instrumentation selected should be able to achieve all these goals with minimal trauma to the patient.

## Indications

Early on in our experience, we often reserved the thoracoscopic approaches for thoracic fractures involving the T4 to T10 vertebrae. With increasing experience, we extended the indications to thoracolumbar injuries. As many of these patients have multiple injuries, all major injuries are stabilized before the spinal procedure is done.

## Contraindications

Thoracoscopic procedures are contraindicated in patients with previous cardiopulmonary disease with restricted cardiopulmonary function, acute posttraumatic lung failure, severe pleural adhesions, and severe medical instability. Routine bowel preparation is required to reduce intraabdominal pressure and facilitate the retraction of the diaphragm. A detailed informed consent is obtained after explaining the various risks involved in the procedure, such as visceral injury, vascular injury, blood loss, instrumentation failure, failed fusion, and possible conversion to open procedure.

## Special Considerations

The thoracoscopic transdiaphragmatic approach (TTA) presents several unique challenges to spine surgeons that necessitate a clear understanding of the diaphragmatic, thoracic, and retroperitoneal anatomy. The entire TLJ can be exposed thoracoscopically with minimal diaphragmatic detachment. This is made possible by an anatomic peculiarity of the pleural cavity and the diaphragmatic insertion, the lowest point of which, the costodiaphragmatic recess, is projected onto the spine perpendicularly just above the base plate of the second lumbar vertebrae.

## Tips, Pearls, and Lessons Learned

To avoid inadvertent injury to the lungs, the diaphragm, and the organs beneath the diaphragm, the most cranial portal is inserted first by a mini-thoracotomy approach. Through a 1.5-cm skin incision placed above the intercostal space, the muscle layers of thoracic wall are cut through in a zigzag fashion following the direction of the fibers. The 30-degree scope is introduced through the portal, and the other trocars are inserted under direct thoracoscopic vision. The endoscopic image is rotated to obtain an orientation of the spine parallel to the lower edge of the video monitor screen. The cephalocaudal axis of the camera is oriented to the view of the primary operative surgeon to allow for normal translation of his or her hand movements to the monitor (**Fig. 69.1**).

## Key Procedural Steps

With the patient in a supine position, double-lumen endotracheal intubation is performed. A Foley catheter, central venous line, and arterial line for continuous blood pressure monitoring are inserted.

The patient is placed in a stable lateral decubitus position. The top-lying arm is placed flat on an arm support and raised to 90 degrees of elevation to avoid a collision during placement and manipulation of the endoscope. Sterile draping extends from the middle of the sternum anteriorly to the spinous processes posteriorly as well as from the axilla down to approximately 8 cm caudal to the iliac crest. Monitors are placed at both lower ends of the operating table on opposite sides to enable free vision for the surgeon and

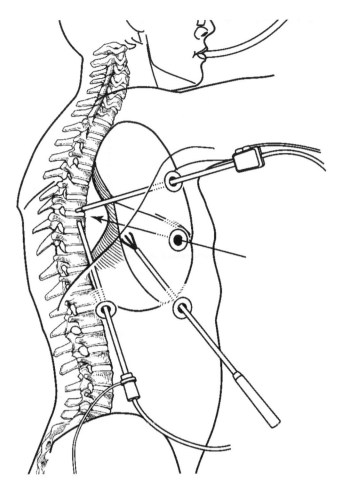

**Fig. 69.1** *Orientation using a three- or four-portal approach.*

the assistant. The surgeon and the assistant holding the camera stand behind the patient. The C-arm monitor and the second assistant are placed on the opposite side.

Under direct fluoroscopic guidance, the target fracture vertebra is projected onto the skin level. The borders of the fractured vertebra are marked on the skin. The working channel (10 mm) is centered over the target vertebrae. The optical channel (10 mm) is placed two or three intercostal spaces cranial to the target vertebra. The approach for suction/irrigation (5 mm) and retractor (10 mm) is placed approximately 5 to 10 cm anterior to the working and optical channel.

The fractured area is now exposed with the help of a fan retractor inserted through the anterior port. The fan retractor performs the dual function of holding down the diaphragm and exposing the insertion of the diaphragm on the spine. Exposure of the spine below L1 usually requires detachment of the diaphragm. Then the extent of the planned corpectomy is defined with an osteotome. The disk spaces are opened to define the borders. Trauma can obscure normal anatomic landmarks. After resection of the intervertebral disks, the fragmented parts of the vertebra are removed carefully with rongeurs. Resection close to the spinal canal is facilitated with the use of high-speed burrs. If decompression of the spinal canal is necessary, the lower border of the pedicle should first be identified with a blunt hook. The base of the pedicle is then resected in a cranial direction with a Kerrison rongeur and the thecal sac can be identified. Finally, the posterior fragments, which occupy the spinal canal, are removed.

The preparation of the graft bed is completed by aggressive preparation of the adjacent end plates and complete removal of all soft tissue. The length and depth of the bone graft/spacer required are measured with a caliper. For vertebral fractures, autologous iliac crest is used in most patients. Distractible titanium cages may also be used. The graft or cage is mounted on the graft holder and inserted through the working portal incision. Longer bone grafts (>2 cm) are inserted along their long axis through the opening and then mounted onto the graft holder inside the thoracic cavity. It is best to place the graft/cage under distraction. With the distractible titanium cages, additional reduction can be achieved by further increasing the height of the cage within the graft site.

Insert a self-tapping screw under fluoroscopic control in the vertebra superior to the fractured one, as well as in the fractured vertebra. Next, insert the first screw of the MACS-TL system (Aesculap, Tuttlingen, Germany) into the caudal vertebral body. Afterward, place the polyaxial, posterior screw over a Kirschner

PITFALLS
- Chronic donor-site pain, neurologic injury, vascular injury, cosmetic deformity, abdominal injury or herniation of abdominal contents, ASIS avulsion fracture, iliac wing fracture, disruption of SI joint, and superficial or deep infection.

for interbody fusion. In the lumbar spine cancellous bone can be harvested from the iliac crest using the "trapdoor" technique for packing interbody fusion cages.

If the abdominal compartment is entered during iliac crest harvest, a general surgery consult is recommended for exploration and closure of the peritoneal defect. If the lateral femoral cutaneous nerve is injured, repair should be attempted with 5-0 monofilament suture.

### Posterior

Unicortical-cancellous strips or cancellous graft is most often harvested for posterior procedures. The "trapdoor" technique can be utilized for cancellous bone graft harvest utilizing straight and curved curettes. The sacroiliac (SI) joint is best avoided by standing on the opposite side of the table from where the graft is being taken. Avoid violating the inner table of the pelvis with either technique. Avoid overaggressive retraction into the sciatic notch due to potential injury to the gluteal vessels or sciatic nerve.

If the gluteal vessels are injured, do not attempt to blindly clamp them due to the proximity of neurologic and urologic structures. If vigorous bleeding occurs as a result of gluteal vessel injury, isolate the bleeding vessel and apply a vessel staple or ligature. If bleeding cannot be controlled due to retraction of the vessel into the true pelvis, the superior aspect of the sciatic notch can be resected to visualize the gluteal vessels. If this is unsuccessful, pack and close the wound and seek interventional angiography for embolization of the vessel.

### Key Procedural Steps

#### Anterior

A 6- to 8-cm skin incision should be made at least 2.5 cm lateral to the ASIS inferior to the iliac crest to avoid compression by the belt line. Bluntly dissect through the subcutaneous fascia. Incise the deep fascia off the lateral edge of the iliac crest. Elevate the periosteum and deep fascia off of the iliac crest in line with the skin incision. When harvesting cancellous bone, use the "trapdoor" technique and replace the roof of crest before closing. If harvesting a structural bi- or tricortical graft, mark the depth of the saw cut on the blade. Thrombin-soaked Gelfoam can be applied for hemostasis. Sharp edges should be rounded off with a burr or rasp to decrease postoperative pain. Close the periosteum, deep fascia, and skin in layers. A drain may be placed in the deep or superficial layer of closure.

#### Posterior

A limited vertical incision should be made within 8 cm of the PSIS. Bluntly dissect through the subcutaneous fascia. Sharply dissect the iliolumbar fascia off the periosteum. Dissection should not extend medially to the SI joint or inferiorly to the sciatic notch. When harvesting cancellous bone use the "trapdoor" technique and replace the roof of crest before closing. If corticocancellous strips are necessary, straight or curved osteotomes may be used. Thrombin-soaked Gelfoam can be applied for hemostasis. Sharp edges should be rounded off with a burr or rasp to decrease postoperative pain. Close the periosteum, deep fascia, and skin in layers. A drain may be placed in the deep or superficial layer of closure.

### Bailout, Rescue, Salvage Procedures

If the volume of the graft is inadequate, combine with an allograft source or the contralateral iliac crest.

# 71

# Autologous Fibula and Rib Harvesting

*Joshua D. Auerbach and Kingsley R. Chin*

### Description
To harvest autologous fibula or rib bone graft for spinal reconstructive procedures while minimizing donor-site morbidity.

### Key Principles
Although autologous fibula and rib strut grafts are not routinely used for spinal reconstructive surgeries, they remain excellent options for those procedures that require long strut grafts. Autologous graft harvesting from the fibula or rib carries minimal added infection risk, achieves favorable rates of fusion, provides a source of vascularized cortical bone, and can be safely performed with minimal donor-site morbidity. Autologous fibular strut grafts have superior compressive strength compared with iliac crest and rib grafts.

### Expectations
Safe harvest of autologous fibula or rib grafting for use in spinal reconstructive procedures.

### Indications
Multilevel cervical corpectomies, posterior cervical reconstruction, posterior occipitocervical fusion, anterior thoracic spinal fusion and reconstruction for tuberculosis spondylitis, infection, neoplasm, and progressive kyphosis.

### Contraindications
- Fibula: ankle pain, instability, lower extremity weakness, sensory or motor deficit, or lower extremity vascular compromise
- Rib: previous fracture and deformity

### Special Considerations
In situations at high risk for delayed union or nonunion, such as multilevel fusions, thoracic/thoracolumbar kyphosis, or in tumor patients receiving perioperative radiation, vascularized fibular or rib grafts may be indicated to provide a solid initial biomechanical construct and facilitate a quicker time to fusion. If a vascularized fibular graft is considered, it is recommended to obtain preoperative arteriography to evaluate for anomalous vascularity or previous vascular injury of the fibular pedicle graft.

The fibula is a straight cortical bone that can provide a graft up to 26 cm in length. The vascular pedicle, which may be from 1 to 5 cm in length, is composed of the peroneal artery (1.5 to 2.5 mm in diameter) and its accompanying two vena comitantes (2 to 3 mm in diameter).

The rib is a curved, flexible bone that can provide a graft up to 30 cm in length. The shape of the graft can be modified by the choice of the rib and section of rib excised (from the flatter posterior portion to the curved anterior portion) to optimize contact between the graft and recipient bed. Its vascular pedicle, which may be from 3 to 5 cm in length, consists of the posterior intercostal artery (1.5 to 2 mm in diameter) and single intercostal vein (1.2 to 2.5 mm in diameter).

### Special Instructions, Position, and Anesthesia

#### *Fibula*
The fibular graft site can be approached using either a posterior or lateral approach. The lateral approach is preferred, as it is simpler and quicker and can be done simultaneously with the majority of the indicated primary procedures. With the patient supine, a sandbag or roll is placed underneath the ipsilateral buttock for optimal visualization of the lateral leg. A tourniquet is applied to the thigh to maintain a bloodless field. General anesthetic is typically used, with or without supplementation with local long-acting anesthetic.

#### *Rib*
The patient can be placed in either the prone position if a posterior spinal procedure is anticipated, or in the lateral decubitus position with the graft side up, which allows for visualization of the rib along its entire course. In the lateral decubitus position, the ipsilateral arm is elevated anteriorly and cephalad away from the ribs and the table flexed at the midthoracic region to increase the intercostal space. The table is tilted anteriorly to allow the ipsilateral lung to fall anteriorly. A double-lumen tube is used to allow single lung ventilation. General anesthesia is typically used, with or without supplementation with local long-acting anesthetic.

### Tips, Pearls, and Lessons Learned

- For posterior occipitocervical fusions in children, the rib is uniquely shaped to permit maximal graft-recipient bed contact. In children the rib is also an abundant source of graft material and rapidly regenerates, compared with iliac crest bone graft.
- Identify the intercostal neurovascular bundle running on the caudad surface of the rib before performing rib stripping to avoid intercostal neurovascular injury.

### Difficulties Encountered

Obese patients may increase the difficulty of localizing the anatomy, especially the middle ribs. Have a low threshold to use fluoroscopy or plain radiographs to identify the correct rib. Excessive bleeding may occur after releasing the tourniquet, requiring reinflation and a vascular consult.

### Key Procedural Steps

#### Fibular Harvest

To avoid damage to the peroneal nerve, proximal fibular osteotomy should be performed at the junction of the middle and distal thirds of the fibula, whereas ankle instability can be safely avoided by staying 10 cm above the ankle joint for the distal fibular osteotomy. A straight lateral approach to the midportion of the fibula is used. Dissection is initially performed between the posterior and lateral compartments of the leg. Incise the superficial fascia overlying the peroneus longus and soleus muscles (**Fig. 71.1**), and continue to dissect in a plane posterior to the peroneus longus and anterior to the soleus muscle. The peroneal vessels lie just deep to the soleus and are almost in contact with the fibula. After identification and protection of the vessels, incise the fibular origin of the soleus muscle and retract posteriorly (**Fig. 71.2**). Identify and protect the superficial peroneal nerve in the proximal aspect of the incision. Attention is then turned to the distal aspect of the fibula, where the interval between the peroneal muscles and the more posteriorly

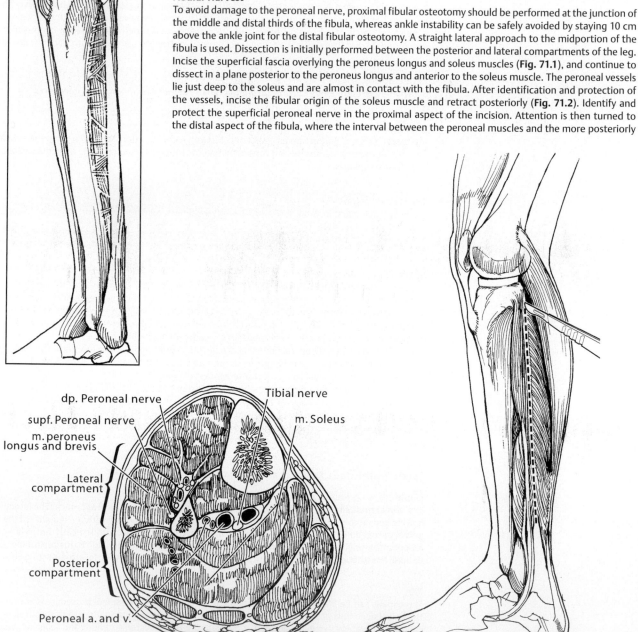

**Fig. 71.1** *(A–C) Identification of the fascial interval between the soleus and the peroneus longus muscles.*

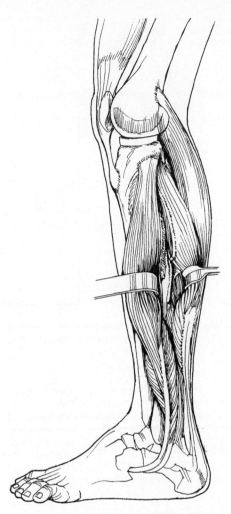

**Fig. 71.2** *Following identification and protection of the underlying peroneal vessels, the fibular origin of the soleus muscle is carefully incised.*

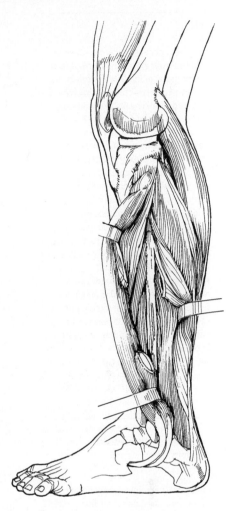

**Fig. 71.3** *Retraction of the anterior tibial artery and deep peroneal nerve anteriorly.*

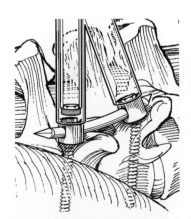

**Fig. 71.4** *Following peroneal vessel ligation distally, the fibula is elevated from the wound proceeding distally to proximally.*

located flexor hallucis longus is identified. The peroneal vessels travel within the substance of the flexor hallucis longus muscle and are therefore protected with careful retraction. For anterior exposure, retract the peroneal muscles anteriorly and dissect them off the fibula in an extraperiosteal plane. Continue extraperiosteal dissection distally, being sure to protect the anterior tibial artery and deep peroneal nerve anteriorly (**Fig. 71.3**). If no vascularized graft is warranted, however, dissection can be performed in a subperiosteal plane to maximize protection of the neurovascular structures. A Gigli saw is used to osteotomize the fibula with careful retraction of the peroneal vessels posteriorly, and the superficial and deep peroneal nerves and anterior tibial artery anteriorly.

After identification, ligate and divide the peroneal vessels distally to gain maximal access to the fibula, but it is preferable to leave these vessels intact. The fibula is carefully elevated from the wound, proceeding distally to proximally while the intact pedicle is maintained proximally if a vascularized graft is to be performed. The peroneal vessels are then clipped at their origin at the posterior tibial vessels (**Fig. 71.4**). Finally, the tourniquet is released, meticulous hemostasis is obtained, the wound is closed over suction drainage (do not close the fascial compartments for risk of compartment syndrome). The patient is made weight bearing as tolerated on the donor extremity following a brief period of splint immobilization for comfort. Passive stretching exercises at the ankle may help prevent postoperative contractures.

### Rib Harvest

Most importantly, identify the correct rib. An oblique incision is made over the rib. The specific rib, as well as the specific portions to be used, is determined by the desired shape and length of graft necessary for arthrodesis. Dissect through the superficial fascia and the latissimus dorsi and erector spinae muscles to expose the rib. The periosteum overlying the rib is circumferentially dissected off and the

**PITFALLS**

*Fibula*

- Failure to adequately identify baseline ankle or lower extremity neurovascular compromise, or inability to protect the neurovascular structures during harvest may lead to ankle pain, instability, leg weakness (predominantly the leg evertors), nerve injury, muscle contractures, postoperative hematoma, pulmonary embolism, lower extremity vascular compromise in patients with aberrant vascular anatomy, and delayed wound healing due to compromised lateral skin vascular supply (peroneal artery and vein). Be sure to stay at least 10 cm proximal to the ankle joint to minimize risk for syndesmotic injury and subsequent instability.
- Failure to recognize aberrant vascular anatomy when performing autologous fibular harvest may result in significant vascular compromise. In one case, a patient had only two dominant vessels in the lower extremity, and the peroneal vessel turned out to be the predominant vessel. A reverse saphenous vein graft was successfully performed to maintain perfusion into the foot. Therefore, consider preoperative arteriography especially in cases where there is vascular compromise in the contralateral lower extremity.

*Rib*

- Intercostal neuralgia, pneumothorax, dysesthetic chest pain, and intercostal neurovascular injury. In 80% of cases the artery of Adamkiewicz arises from the left side off an inferior intercostal artery and enters the intervertebral foramina near the costotransverse joints, accompanying one of the ventral roots of T9 to T12. To limit the risk of injury to this artery or collaterals and resultant paraplegia, avoid ligature of a vessel close to the foramen and be careful when disarticulating a costotransverse or costovertebral joint. Consider preoperative angiography prior to left-sided approaches between T8 and T12, although the artery can enter the canal from T5 to L5.

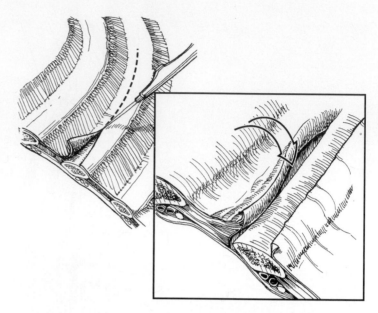

**Fig. 71.5** *Entering the pleura above the rib to avoid damage to the neurovascular bundle that runs along the posteroinferior rib border.*

rib is elevated (**Fig. 71.5**). The pleura and intercostal muscles are sectioned in the intercostal space just above the rib to avoid damaging the neurovascular structures lying directly beneath. A rib-stripper is used to completely subperiosteally remove the pleural surface from the rib. Disarticulation at the costovertebral joint is then performed, and dissection is performed to the costochondral region using a rib-cutter. The rib may be harvested lateral to the costovertebral joint to avoid injury to the artery of Adamkiewicz. Care is taken to remove enough bone for strut graft and for morselized graft. The pleura is then inspected visually, and by hyperinflating the lungs and inspecting for air leaks. If no leaks are present, the chest is then closed in layers and a chest tube is considered.

### Bailout, Rescue, Salvage Procedures

If the volume or shape of autologous strut graft is inadequate, anterior iliac crest bone graft can be used instead. Allograft bone can be substituted at any time for inadequate or insufficient autologous strut bone graft. If using rib autograft, a second rib can be used to augment the first graft. If pleural injury is noted at the time of rib harvest, a primary repair is undertaken. If ankle instability is present or suspected following fibular harvest in children with significant remaining growth, consider distal tibiofibular fusion to prevent progressive valgus deformity at the ankle. In adults, postoperative muscle contractures in the lower extremity may require z-lengthening procedures.

# 72

# Halo Orthosis Application

*Kenneth C. Moghadam and R. John Hurlbert*

### Description

Proper halo application creates long-term immobilization of the cervical spine while ensuring patient safety and comfort.

### Key Principles

- Proper positioning of ring and screws
- Appropriate tightening of screws
- Snug-fitting vest
- Pin-site maintenance

### Expectations

Effective halo application and care should confer immobilization for complex unstable cervical spine conditions without producing pain, difficulty swallowing, or visual obscuration, while at the same time allowing patient mobility.

### Indications

For the nonsurgical management of cervical spine instability secondary to trauma, degenerative disease, infection, or as an adjunct to surgical reconstruction.

### Contraindications

- Frontal, temporal, or parietal skull fractures
- Scalp laceration at pin site
- Head injury necessitating craniotomy
- Major chest injury
- Life-threatening abdominal injury
- Pulmonary insufficiency

### Special Considerations

Skull pins should be retightened to 8 ft-lb at 24 to 36 hours postapplication. All other screws and straps should be checked and tensioned to their initial settings. The skin is cleansed in a circular fashion around each pin on a daily basis, utilizing sterilized cotton swabs soaked in normal saline. If crusts form on the skin at the pin sites, they should be moistened but not forcibly removed so as to prevent further skin breakdown. Mild irritation of the skin at the skull pins' site is common. However, reddened, shiny, elevated skin with purulent discharge indicates local infection. Cultures should be obtained and topical antibiotics applied in conjunction with oral antibiotics. Relocation of a pin at an infected site may be necessary if the infection persists or if the torque setting cannot be maintained at a minimum of 6 in-lb.

A well-fitted vest is essential to maintain spinal alignment. Follow-up visitation is required to ensure pin site health, vest position, and wear as well as patient compliance. Typically at the terminus of care, which may be 12 weeks or longer in duration, radiographic evidence is obtained to determine fusion of the affected region. The positioning rods may be removed to allow for flexion and extension films without removing the ring.

Removal of the halo is most easily accomplished with the patient sitting in a chair. The lock nuts securing the skull pins should be loosened first. If spinal integrity or muscle weakness is a concern, a cervical collar may be applied prior to halo ring and vest removal. To disassemble the vest, the rods are removed first and then the chest and shoulder straps loosened on one side. The patient leans forward slightly so that both vest plates can be removed in one step. After loosening the locking nuts, the anterior skull pins are loosened and backed away from the skin to at least 1 cm of clearance. An assistant may hold the ring firmly from behind the patient to reduce migration as the posterior pins are removed. It is important before removing the ring to ensure that all pins are backed away with sufficient clearance to prevent laceration to the skin. An antibiotic ointment is applied to reduce bone exposure to air at the pin sites. The antibiotic is reapplied 24 hours later. Normal skin closure occurs within 36 hours. Patients should avoid washing their hair until this time.

For cardiac emergencies, halo manufacturers either create a pre-creased area on the anterior vest to facilitate access to the chest for compression or electrostimulation, or they supply a box wrench to loosen the anterior rods allowing access to the chest. After the emergency, the vest may be reapplied, refastened, or replaced according to the manufacturer's specifications.

### Special Instructions, Position, and Anesthesia

The superstructure allowing connection to the halo ring is applied to both the anterior and posterior vest plates, composed of support rods and connectors. The anterior vest is applied to the anterior chest wall and secured to the halo ring. The patient is gently log rolled to one side using spinal precautions, and the posterior vest is slid into position. The patient is returned to a supine attitude, and the posterior vest is fastened to the ring with the remaining rods and connectors. Vest straps are applied to firm tension at the abdomen and shoulders. It may be necessary to reposition the head for best spinal alignment. Typically a neutral position is best; it is seen as an imaginary vertical line from the inferior lobe of the ear to the inferior tip of the nose. Radiographic evidence is required to confirm cervical alignment.

Positioning of the vest may require special attention in certain circumstances. Morbidly obese patients may require special accommodation of vest size and positioning, as it is important to ensure that the distal border of the anterior vest is superior to the diaphragm, leaving sufficient space for abdominal expansion for respirations. Emaciated patients require attention to potential pressure points to reduce risk of skin ulceration.

### Tips, Pearls, and Lessons Learned

Surgical bed adapters are commercially available to allow fixation of the halo ring to the operating table. Once positioned on the table and fixed in the adapter, the anterior or posterior vest may be removed easily without compromise to the cervical spinal alignment. If necessary, reapplication postoperatively is easily accomplished, with the adapter maintaining the head position.

### Imaging

Most halo orthoses are magnetic resonance imaging (MRI) compatible; however, the manufacturer's specifications should be examined to ensure compliance.

### Pediatric Applications

Selection of an appropriately sized ring is important. Measure the circumference of the head 1 cm above the ear and eyebrows and select the appropriate ring according to the halo manufacturer's sizing chart. In general, a closed ring is preferred to an open ring to accommodate the greater number of pin sites necessary due to immature development of the cranium. The number of pins placed into the skull and the degree to which they are tightened are age specific (**Table 72.1**).

**Table 72.1  Age Adjusted Pin Application**

| Patient Age | Number of Pins | Torque (in-lb) |
|---|---|---|
| <5 | 8–12 | 2–3 |
| 6–14 | 6–8 | 4–6 |
| 15 – 17 | 4–6 | 6–8 |
| Adult | 4 | 8 |

### Key Procedural Steps

#### Ring Type and Size

Halo rings are available in two styles, open-backed (horseshoe shaped) and closed-backed (ring shaped). The open-backed ring simplifies application because the patient's head can remain flat on the bed during positioning and pin insertion. It also leaves the posterior neck and occiput well exposed if posterior surgical management is required. The closed-backed ring allows for a greater number of pin placements. Different manufacturers provide rings of different sizes. A properly fitting ring should allow for about 1 to 2 cm of clearance circumferentially from the scalp, when positioned at or just below the equator of the skull.

#### Ring Application

The patient is positioned supine on the hospital bed. A positioning plate called a "spoon" is inserted underneath the patient in the midline of the spine so that it spans from the inferior border of the scapula to the posterior pole of the occiput. While gentle in-line traction is maintained, the patient and spoon are drawn up the bed to allow the head and neck to rest on the spoon, extending freely off the top of the bed. It is necessary to shave a 2.5-cm$^2$ area just behind and above the ear in preparation for the posterior (parietal) pins (**Fig. 72.1**). The frontal and parietal pin sites are prepared with Betadine, chlorhexidine, or alcohol sterilization.

The selected ring is placed around the skull with three positioning pins tightened finger tight against the skin (**Fig. 72.2**). When placing the positioning pins, it is best to utilize the most anterior hole to assist in midline orientation of the ring and also the first or second most posterior holes on the sides. This allows for the best positioning of the skull pins later. The ring should be at least 5 mm above the eyebrows and the superior helix of the ear. The positioning pins are tightened against the skin, ensuring that the anterior

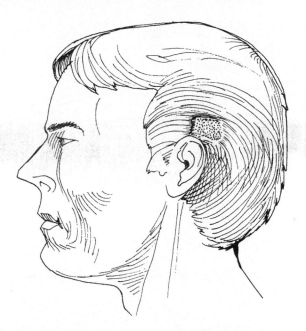

**Fig. 72.1** *A 2.5-cm² area is shaved just behind and above the pinna of the each ear to facilitate insertion of the posterior halo pins and to allow for optimum pin site care.*

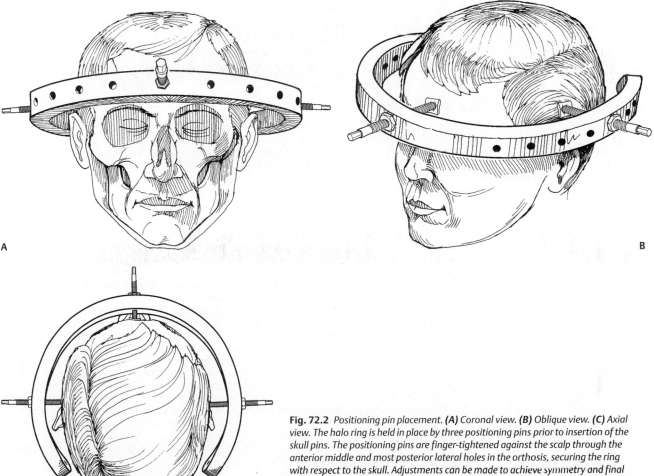

A

B

C

**Fig. 72.2** *Positioning pin placement. (A) Coronal view. (B) Oblique view. (C) Axial view. The halo ring is held in place by three positioning pins prior to insertion of the skull pins. The positioning pins are finger-tightened against the scalp through the anterior middle and most posterior lateral holes in the orthosis, securing the ring with respect to the skull. Adjustments can be made to achieve symmetry and final positioning with respect to: (1) the equator of the skull, (2) the eyebrows, and (3) the ears before the skull pins are inserted.*

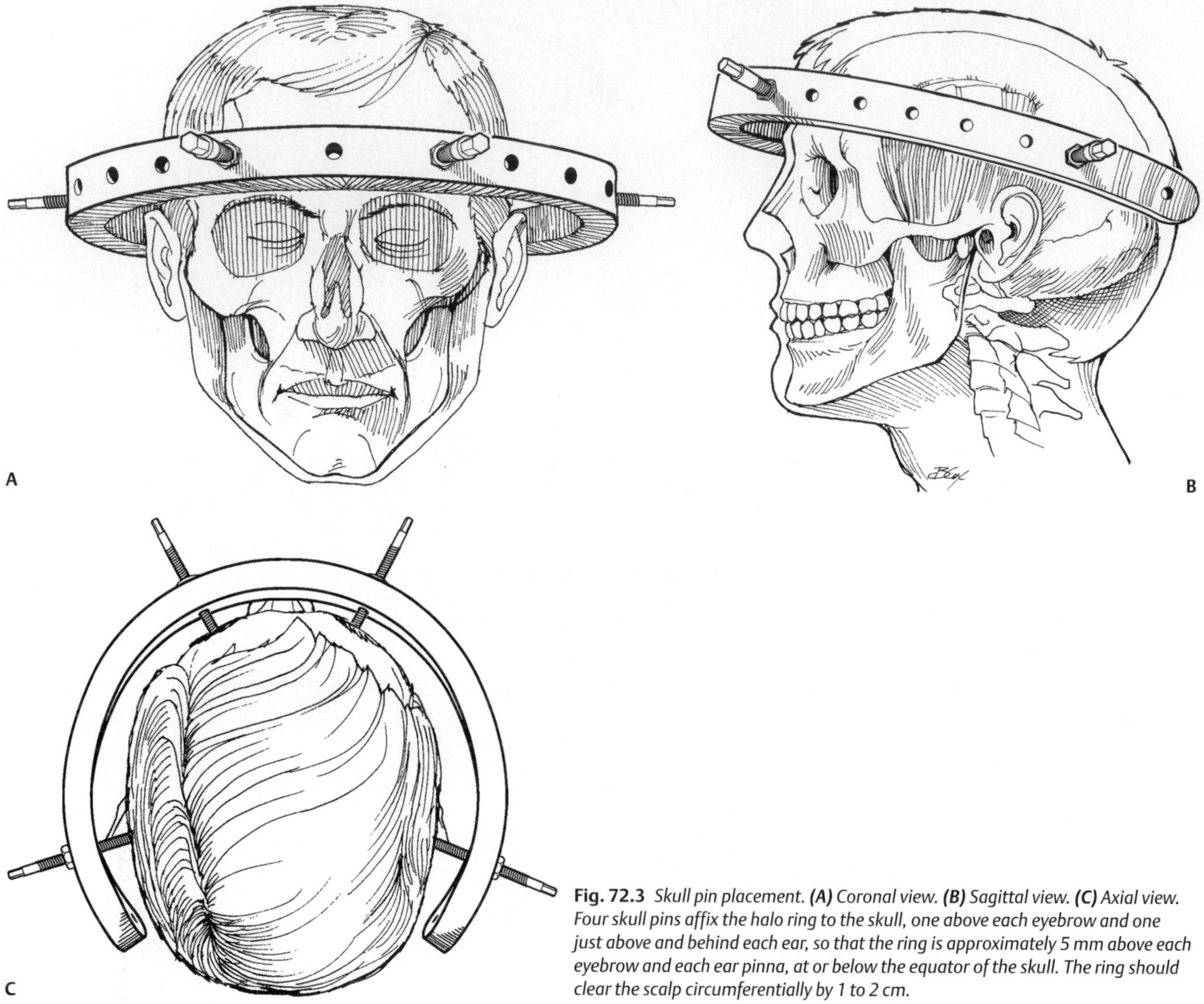

**Fig. 72.3** *Skull pin placement. (A) Coronal view. (B) Sagittal view. (C) Axial view. Four skull pins affix the halo ring to the skull, one above each eyebrow and one just above and behind each ear, so that the ring is approximately 5 mm above each eyebrow and each ear pinna, at or below the equator of the skull. The ring should clear the scalp circumferentially by 1 to 2 cm.*

pin is aligned with the midline of the forehead. Appropriate symmetry at this point aids in the alignment of the vest later. Adhesive tape placed underneath the mandible and attached to each side of the ring laterally is beneficial to prevent migration of the ring. Any touch-up to skin sterilization can be performed at this time.

Skull pins are placed just above the eyebrows, usually in the first or second ring holes lateral to the midline anterior positioning pin. Posterior skull pins are typically placed in the last available posterior hole of the open ring, adjacent to the posterior positioning pins (**Fig. 72.3**). The skull pins are advanced to within 1 mm of the skin in their selected positions, and the skin and periosteum are infiltrated with 2% Xylocaine. All pins are hand-tightened through the skin, allowing the person applying the halo to feel the solid purchase of each pin on the skull. Ensure that the patient's eyes are firmly closed during insertion of the anterior skull pins to prevent elevation of the eye brows and to allow the eyelids to completely cover the eye when the patient is at rest. A torque wrench set to 8 in-lb is utilized to complete the tightening on the skull pins in a "cross" (front-to-back and back-to-front) pattern advancing each one half to three quarters of a turn at a time until final torque is reached. Visual inspection is necessary during this procedure to ensure that the ring does not migrate. Once the skull pins are properly set, the lock nuts are applied to prevent pin loosening. The positioning pins and pads are removed, and the patient is lifted back down on the bed, with a physician controlling the head at all times.

Cranial defects or conditions such as osteogenesis imperfecta may necessitate default to a closed-backed ring and a pediatric (multiple) pin protocol.

# 73

# Closed Cervical Traction
# Reduction Techniques

*Gianluca Vadalà, Alexander R. Vaccaro, and Joon Yung Lee*

## Description
The graduated weighted reduction technique is commonly used for both traumatic and nontraumatic fractures and dislocation of the cervical spine. When performed under close supervision of an experienced surgeon, this is a safe and reliable method to achieve anatomic realignment.

## Key Principles
The anatomic abnormality is identified through use of various imaging modalities. Frequently, a lateral cervical spine x-ray is the quickest and most helpful screening modality to identify cervical malalignment. If a unilateral or bilateral facet dislocation of the cervical spine is identified, weighted-reduction techniques can be used to efficiently realign the spinal column and provide temporary stabilization. Computed tomography (CT) is also useful in identifying anatomic abnormalities in those cases where plain radiographs are inadequate or unrevealing. In the setting of a traumatic cervical dislocation, obtaining a magnetic resonance imaging (MRI) study prior to reduction is controversial. Some advocate obtaining MRI to confirm the presence or absence of a herniated disk at the site of dislocation to prevent further spinal cord damage during the reduction method. Others argue that as long as the patient is awake and alert, weighted reduction can be performed safely. If a herniated disk is identified anterior to the spinal cord prior to reduction, many surgeons proceed with an anterior decompression and stabilization procedure without performing a presurgical closed reduction.

Once the type of displacement is identified, the axis of traction needs to be determined. Frequently, in cases of unilateral or bilateral facet dislocations, the traction should be applied in the axis of flexion. It is not unusual to apply 30 to 45 degrees of flexion moment on the head through traction to begin the process of realigning the spine.

In cases of displaced odontoid fractures, bi-vector traction is often useful to obtain an efficient reduction. This technique combines both a longitudinal and flexion vector force to obtain a satisfactory realignment.

In patients with basilar invagination in the setting of rheumatoid arthritis, longitudinal low-weight traction (10 to 20 lb) often suffices.

Particular care must be taken in extension-type injuries. Frequently, injuries with extension mechanism are extremely unstable, and even a small degree of weight may result in excessive interspace distraction. In general, only a gentle graded flexion vector is used in extension-type injuries, or patients may be reduced in a halo vest with manual halo ring flexion.

## Expectations
The goal of the weighted traction reduction is to restore and maintain normal spinal alignment of the displaced cervical spine, providing temporary stabilization and indirect decompression of the spinal cord. This potentially allows for improved neurologic recovery and prevention of further neurologic injury. Traction is often a temporary measure, until more definitive management (usually surgical stabilization) is performed.

## Indications
The most common indications for closed traction reduction of the cervical spine are unilateral or bilateral dislocated facets. In these settings, higher weights on the order of 30 to 120 lb are frequently required to obtain a reduction. Lower weight traction (10 to 30 lb) is often used in the setting of displaced odontoid fractures, traumatic spondylolisthesis of the axis, rotatory atlantoaxial subluxation, basilar invagination, and cranial settling. Traction may also be used efficiently in other nontraumatic cervical spine conditions that result in instability or deformity such as tumor, infections, rheumatoid arthritis, and late posttraumatic kyphotic deformity or instability.

## Contraindications
Longitudinal traction in extension distraction injuries, and in patients who are not alert and cannot participate in their neurologic examination.

## Special Considerations
Physicians involved in the treatment of cervical spine injuries must be aware of the possibility of multiple noncontiguous levels of spinal injury before attempting reduction of any cervical fracture or dislocation.

This requires a thorough history and physical examination, as well as complete imaging of the entire spine in an orthogonal manner or with CT imaging. Good-quality x-rays (including a swimmer's view, if needed) or an entire spine CT is necessary. If a focal rotational deformity indicative of a unilateral facet joint dislocation is found on a lateral plain radiograph, it is useful prior to traction application to determine which facet is dislocated. This can be done clinically by observing head rotation, or through CT or MRI evaluation. On an anteroposterior plain x-ray, the more cephalic spinous process is rotated toward the side of the dislocated facet joint.

Following a successful or failed closed reduction and prior to an open reduction or in situ fusion procedure, MRI evaluation for the presence of a disk herniation or other space-occupying lesion should be done to determine the type of necessary surgical approach.

### Key Procedural Steps

Cranial tongs, head-halters, or halo rings can be used to hold weights for traction. We prefer the use of stainless-steel Gardner-Wells cranial tongs. The others have weight restrictions that are far less than what is sometimes necessary to achieve satisfactory reduction.

The position of the placement of the cranial tongs is crucial (**Fig. 73.1**). The pins are applied below the equator of the skull, approximately 1 cm superior of the pinna of the outer ear. Direct axial traction is applied with the tongs placed longitudinally in line with the external auditory meatus. Placement of the tongs more anteriorly or posteriorly applies an extension or flexion moment to the cervical spine, respectively.

A flexion moment is the most common vector required for a facet dislocation. In a unilateral or bilateral facet dislocation, up to 30 to 45 degrees of head flexion may be necessary to disengage or unlock the facets. This is achieved by elevating the traction pulley and positioning the cranial tongs posterior to the auditory meatus.

The bed is placed in a reverse Trendelenburg position. Initially 10 lb of weight is placed on the pulley, and the first lateral cervical spine x-ray is taken. The first radiograph must be scrutinized (1) for excessive distraction at the level of the injury; (2) for position of the head, to ensure that the vector of traction is correct; and (3) most importantly, to rule out cranial cervical junction injuries that may be missed. Only when all three of these factors are satisfactory can the reduction procedure proceed.

The weights are then added in 10-lb increments, and serial x-rays are taken. After the addition of each weight, the patient is examined to ensure that there is no adverse change in neurologic function. On review of each x-ray if there is any evidence of interspace overdistraction or if there is an adverse change in neurologic function, weight is expeditiously lessened and any change in head position is reversed. Traction is continued until there is radiographic evidence of facet perching. At this point the surgeon may proceed with a manual reduction maneuver (**Fig. 73.2**). In cases of bilateral facet dislocation, this involves standing behind the patient and cupping the posterior cervical spine with the treating physician's second

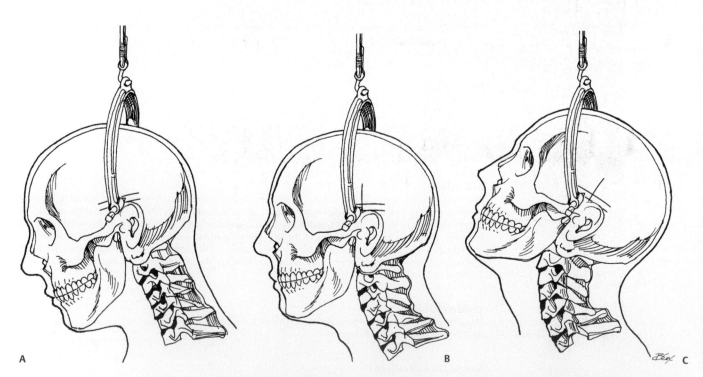

**Fig. 73.1** *Proper fixation points for Gardner-Wells tong application.* **(A)** *Posterior placement of tongs to produce flexion of head.* **(B)** *Normal placement of tongs to produce straight traction.* **(C)** *Anterior placement of tongs to produce hyperextension of head.*

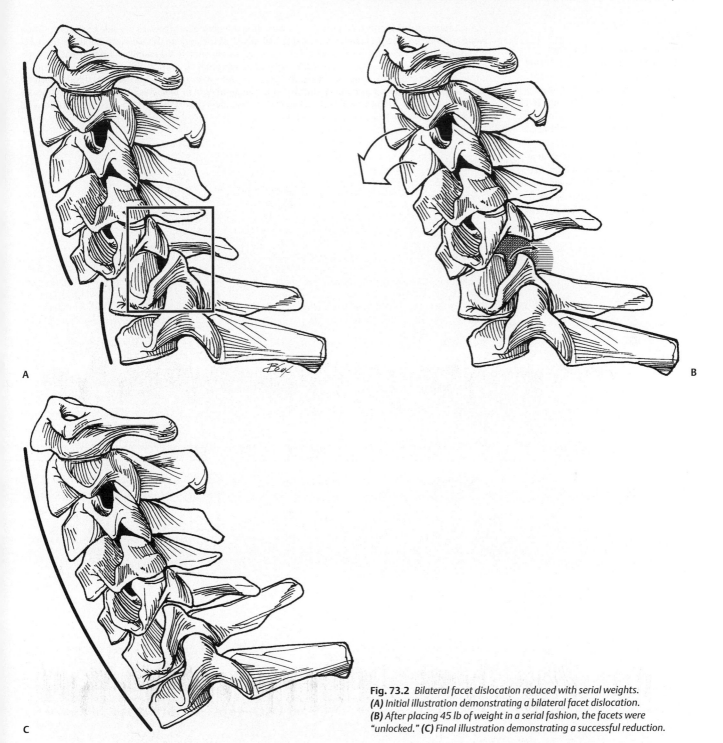

**Fig. 73.2** *Bilateral facet dislocation reduced with serial weights.*
*(A) Initial illustration demonstrating a bilateral facet dislocation.*
*(B) After placing 45 lb of weight in a serial fashion, the facets were*
*"unlocked." (C) Final illustration demonstrating a successful reduction.*

through fifth fingers on both sides of the neck, with the thumbs looped anteriorly over the traction pins. The thumbs are then used to gently extend the neck while the fingers are gently pressed anteriorly into the back of the neck at the estimated level of the dislocation. During this maneuver, assistants may gradually reduce the hanging weights to about 10 lb while the neck is gently lowered to a position in line with the axis of the body. Often a palpable click or clunk is felt or heard at the moment of reduction. The final position of the neck is in slight extension. Pillows are placed beneath the upper scapular to maintain this position. In the presence of a unilateral facet dislocation, the examiner positions his hands similar to that during a bilateral facet relocation and applies an axial load to the reduced side through the traction pin and gently distracts the dislocated side through the traction pin.

PITFALLS

• The treating physician should not attempt a manipulative reduction until the facets are perched, as this is often unsuccessful and may result in neurologic embarrassment or a facet fracture. Direct axial traction should not be performed in the setting of an unstable distraction extension injury. If there is evidence of neurologic worsening the reduction maneuver should be reversed and traction lessened. The patient should then be placed in a halo vest and proceed with a timely MRI of the cervical spine to search for significant spinal cord compression.

A rotational maneuver is then performed by rotating the neck gently toward the side of the dislocation while applying an anterior counterforce vector to the back of the neck on this side with the fingertips (second through fifth). During this maneuver the assistants slowly remove the weights, and the head is gently lowered to the level of the axis of the trunk. Again, at the time of facet relocation, a pop, click, or clunk is either heard or felt. Following this maneuver a careful physical examination is performed to confirm no adverse change in neurologic function. If the final plain radiograph indicates a successful reduction, all the weights except 10 lb are taken off. A halo vest is then applied with the neck in extension until surgical stabilization is performed.

# 74

# Nucleus Pulposus
# Replacement Techniques

*Jeff S. Silber and Jared F. Brandoff*

## Description

Techniques of selectively replacing the central nuclear portion of the diseased lumbar intervertebral disk with the goal of restoring as closely as possible the normal structural and functional properties of the native intervertebral disk have been described since the 1950s. Not until recently, however, have advances in biomaterials and mechanical testing techniques made selective nucleus replacement a feasible and viable technique.

In modern times, the gold standard of surgical management of end-stage degenerative disk disease is fusion of the diseased motion segment. To date, however, fusion procedures have yielded relatively unpredictable outcomes. Furthermore, fusion renders a patient potentially susceptible to various other morbidities, including posterior muscle atrophy, decreased motion and stiffness at the fused level, and transfer of loads leading to accelerated adjacent-level disease as well as morbidities at the bone-graft donor site associated with harvesting. Lehman et al have demonstrated that fusion leads to adjacent-level facet hypertrophy, spinal stenosis, and ultimately potential instability.

Moreover, in the case of disk herniation, partial diskectomy has been demonstrated to lead to gradual loss of disk space height over time. Removal of any significant portion of the nucleus pulposus changes the biomechanics of the remaining disk elements. In the normal intervertebral disk, axial loads are transferred through the viscoelastic nucleus pulposus to the surrounding anulus fibrosus. This leads to normal concordant out-bulging of both the inner and outer fibers of the anulus. Loss of nucleus material or loss of disk height from degenerated nucleus material leads to less efficient transfer of axial loads and discordant bulging of the inner and outer fibers of the anulus. The result is out-bulging of the outer fibers and in-bulging of the inner fibers. This disjointed bulging leads to increased exposure to shear forces within the anulus and ultimately decreased ability to resist compressive loads. In turn, this can lead to acceleration of the disk degenerative process as well as supraphysiologic transfer of loads to the facet joints posteriorly.

Conceptually, if the diseased or deficient nucleus material could be replenished with a material that exhibits the same biomechanical properties as nucleus pulposus material, then the physiologic biomechanics of the intervertebral disk could be restored. This is the goal of modern nucleus replacement technologies. These materials exhibit viscoelastic properties similar to native nucleus. They provide restoration of premorbid disk height and thus redistribution of forces during axial load. Current designs are biologically compatible, fatigue resistant (potentially withstanding 100 million cycles over a 40-year period), and resistant to the production of particulate debris. Several different designs are currently in different stages of preclinical and clinical testing. To date, however, all nucleus replacement materials and techniques are considered experimental. Significantly more research and clinical trials are required in this area.

## Expectations

In the setting of degenerative disk disease, it is theoretically desirable to remove the anterior portion of the disk nucleus, which has been described as a potential pain generator, and replace the diseased disk portion with a material that exhibits similar biomechanical properties to an undiseased or healthy disk. Specifically, it is expected that nucleus replacement will retain physiologic motion of the spinal segment while simultaneously retaining the inherent stability of that segment. This, in turn, should alleviate the transfer of stress to the posterior facet joints while simultaneously tensioning the anulus to minimize further irritation to the sinuvertebral nervous network. Ideally, this can be achieved through a minimally invasive approach, thus further preserving the surrounding soft tissue stabilizers and retaining stability at the segment. The implant should allow for stable motion similar to a healthy disk. Finally, the resulting restoration of disk height will decrease shear forces on the remaining anulus, facet joints, and stabilizing ligaments.

## Indications

Nucleus pulposus replacement techniques are indicated in patients with severe disability from lumbar degenerative disk disease who have failed at least 6 months of active, nonsurgical management. Imaging studies should demonstrate moderate disk degeneration with 10 to 50% loss of disk height. A lumbar provocative diskogram must demonstrate an intact anulus fibrosus, and pain provocation should be concordant with the patient's usual low back pain. Magnetic resonance imaging (MRI) findings should be limited to an early stage of degenerative changes, including a total disk height of greater than 5 mm, absent Schmorl's nodes, and mild facet arthrosis. Furthermore, this technique is indicated following a partial diskectomy for a disk herniation if the other aforementioned criteria are fulfilled, as a method of diminishing subsequent loss of disk height.

### Contraindications

Contraindications for this technique are associated with significant, end-stage degenerative disk disease. Specifically, significant fissuring of the anulus on the diskogram or advanced degenerative changes such as severe facet arthrosis or spondylolisthesis.

### Special Considerations

Available nucleus replacement implants today are either constrained or unconstrained. Constrained implants consist of an outer casing with a relatively fixed size and shape. This provides for less creep of the implant. Because of their predetermined size and shape, however, this design may not contact the entire surface of the adjacent vertebral end plates. This highlights the importance of having a compatible modulus between the implant and the end-plate bone. Incompatibility of modulus can lead to stress shielding, and, in accordance with Young's law, can lead to bone resorption at the end plates adjacent to the implant. This can predispose the implant to ultimate subsidence or extrusion. Unconstrained implants do not have a predetermined size or shape. They are injected and swell to fill the disk space, maximally providing the maximum surface area for stress distribution. This can lead to less implant motion and potentially fewer extrusions. Some hydrogel devices are made of a co-polymer of polyvinyl alcohol (PVA) and polyvinyl pyrrolidone (PVP). The Prosthetic Disc Nucleus (PDN) implants (Raymedica Inc., Bloomington/Minneapolis, MN) are composed of an internal hydrogel co-polymer pellet of polyacrylonitrile and polyacrylamide. It can be molded into sizes and shaped to the appropriate enucleated nucleus cavity formed following a diskectomy. The outer constraining cover is composed of a loosely woven high molecular weight polyethylene (HMWPE). The device can absorb water up to 80% of its dry weight to help provide force to elevate the disk space. However, unconstrained hydrogels require at least 5 mm of disk height for placement and expansion. These implants are ideally injected in a fluid phase and harden in vivo to the desired size and shape of the disk defect.

### Tips, Pearls, and Lessons Learned

Ideal patient selection for this technique is paramount. In patients undergoing a partial diskectomy either via a minimally invasive microdiskectomy approach with or without tubular retractor systems, placement of a nuclear replacement device may alter the natural history of continued degeneration. Technically, appropriate intervertebral preparation and proper placement of the device to avoid extrusion is key to optimizing long-term results.

### Key Procedural Steps

Specific procedural steps are outlined in the respective technique guides for each available implant type. Nearly all techniques employ a minimally invasive posterior approach that spares as much of the soft tissue sleeve as possible. It is recommended that laminar spreaders be used in an attempt to diminish the size of the laminotomy. The approach is similar to one performed for a microdiskectomy. A stab anulotomy is performed, and initially a smaller sized dilator is used followed by a larger one and rotated 90 degrees to stretch the outer anulus fibers. Pituitary rongeurs are used to remove the nucleus and attention is paid so as not to disrupt the anulus and vertebral end plates. A dural retractor is utilized to protect the neural elements. Once the appropriate amount of nucleus is removed, which can be checked with a probe, depth gauge, or intraoperative diskogram, the device is placed. The largest device size is chosen (constrained device), as measured with sizing instruments (**Fig. 74.1**). The device is placed with a flexible guide; the guide is placed into the nucleus cavity and a suture (No. 1 or 0 Vicryl) is sewn into the leading edge of the device (e.g., PDN device). The device is tamped in with an impactor following the flexible guide while pulling on the suture to help place the implant horizontally across the intervertebral disk space as best as possible (**Fig. 74.2**). Final positioning is confirmed with radiographic imaging (**Fig. 74.3**). If needed, a laminotomy and anulotomy may be performed on the opposite side to remove additional nucleus and aid in better device placement with the use of tamps and by pulling the suture attached to the leading device edge. Furthermore, when possible, it is desirable to employ anulus closing techniques, although presently none of the described techniques available today are completely satisfactory, to repair the requisite anulotomy after implant insertion. This should decrease the rate of implant extrusion. Finally, Bertagnoli has recently described a retroperitoneal trans-psoas approach that may be advantageous. It is generally advisable to avoid anterior approaches so that they may be retained for subsequent surgical intervention should the need arise.

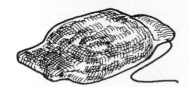

**Fig. 74.1** *The nuclear replacement device.*

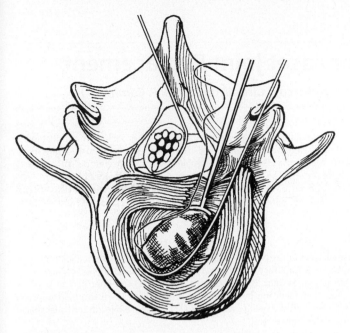

**Fig. 74.2** *Axial view showing the device being inserted with the use of a tamp, flexible guide, and pull suture.*

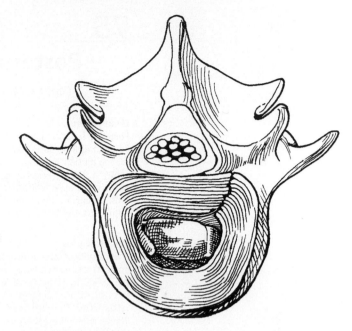

**Fig. 74.3** *Appropriate positioning of the device centered in the voided area after the nucleus pulposus is removed, leaving the anulus intact, except for the insertion anulotomy.*

PITFALLS

- Device extrusion has been the major problem with earlier devices. Proper surgical technique and better implant design has helped in decreasing extrusion rates. If this occurs with neurologic sequelae, emergent removal of the device is warranted. These devices should never be used in patients with extensive degeneration that may benefit more from a fusion procedure.

**Bailout, Rescue, Salvage Procedures**

There are two potential bailout/salvage techniques available if nucleus replacement fails. If the patient meets the indications for mechanical total disk replacement, it can be attempted; if the patient does not meet the indications, fusion of the spinal segment can be performed. Techniques that employ biologic, self-regenerating disk implants are currently being postulated, but to date no model exists for a usable implant.

# 75

# Posterior Facet Joint Replacement

*Seamus Morris, Federico P. Girardi, and Frank P. Cammisa, Jr.*

## Description

Posterior facet arthroplasty is an emerging technology aimed at addressing back pain and instability emanating from facet joint arthrosis, degenerative spondylolisthesis, and spinal stenosis, while maintaining motion. Facet arthroplasty may in the future also be combined with an anterior disk arthroplasty allowing 360 degrees of dynamic treatment of an arthritic motion segment. The incidence of adjacent-level disk degeneration may theoretically be decreased by the use of such technologies. Several devices are currently being developed and are undergoing clinical trials, though to date none has received Food and Drug Administration (FDA) approval.

## Key Principles

The majority of facet arthroplasty devices utilize pedicle-based fixation (TOPS Total Posterior Spine System, Impliant Inc., Ramat Poleg, Israel; TFAS Total Facet Arthroplasty System, Archus Orthopedics, Redmond, WA; AFRS Anatomic Facet Replacement System, Facet Solutions, Logan, UT) to either fully or partially reconstruct normal facet joint function following decompression. One device (Zyre Facet Arthroplasty System, Quantum Orthopedics, Carlsbad, CA) is being developed to act as a malleable intraarticular spacer device, augmenting the anatomy of the normal facet.

## Expectations

It is expected that facet arthroplasty devices will offer effective stabilization following posterior decompression and resection of pathologic bony and soft tissue elements. In vitro testing has confirmed that some of these systems (e.g., TOPS) maintain normal intradiskal pressures following laminectomy and facetectomy in addition to replicating a normal range of motion of the lumbar spine. Only limited clinical results are available from any of these systems.

## Indications

The TOPS system is intended for use in the treatment of facet arthrosis, grade I degenerative spondylolisthesis, and spinal stenosis at a single level from L3 to S1 in skeletally mature patients. Stabilization of an affected motion segment following wide decompression is therefore possible while still maintaining movement. It may also prove useful in "topping-off" multiple fused levels in a bid to prevent degeneration occurring at adjacent segments. In the future, facet arthroplasty systems may be combined with an anterior disk arthroplasty, in a hybrid construct, to comprise a total joint arthroplasty at a diseased motion segment.

## Contraindications

The contraindications are listed in **Table 75.1**.

**Table 75.1 Contraindications**

| Absolute | Relative |
|---|---|
| Primary diagnosis of discogenic back pain | More than one motion segment involved in the degenerative pathology to the extent that it justifies inclusion in a surgical procedure, unless a decompression alone can be done at that level without compromising stability |
| Previous total facetectomy or trauma at the index level | Prior surgery at any lumbar vertebral level except laminectomy, diskectomy, and foraminotomy; at least two thirds of the facets must be preserved if the patient has undergone prior surgery at the affected level |
| Lytic spondylolisthesis | Deformity of the spine that would compromise the implant, e.g., scoliosis of greater than 10 degrees |
| Clinically compromised vertebral bodies at the affected level(s) due to any traumatic, neoplastic, metabolic or infectious pathology | Morbid obesity defined as a body mass index >40 or a weight more than 100 lb over ideal body weight |
| Known allergy to the alloys or polymers that comprise the implant such as CoCr, titanium, poly-ether-ether-ketone (PEEK), polyester or polyurethane | Dual-energy x-ray absorptiometry (DEXA) bone density measured T score equal to or lower than −1.5 |
| Back or leg pain of unknown etiology | Paget's disease, osteomalacia, osteogenesis imperfecta, thyroid or parathyroid gland disorder, rheumatoid arthritis or other autoimmune or metabolic disease |
| Active infection: systemic or local | |

**Special Considerations**

Many of these devices are still in the investigational stage of development, and thus little information is available regarding their design. The TOPS system comprises a titanium "sandwich" with an interlocking polycarbonate urethane (PcU) construct, allowing for constrained axial rotation, and lateral bending, extension, and flexion movements in the affected segment (**Fig. 75.1**). This is achieved by the flexibility of the PcU element, which allows relative movement between the titanium plates (±1.5 degrees of axial rotation, ±5 degrees of lateral bending, 2 degrees of extension, and 8 degrees of flexion). The implant also blocks excessive posterior and anterior sagittal translation. Fixation is achieved using four hydroxyapatite-coated (HAC) polyaxial pedicle screws. The TOPS system is implanted via a posterior surgical approach, to both stabilize the affected vertebrae and to replace the skeletal elements such as the lamina and the facet joints that may be removed to achieve decompression.

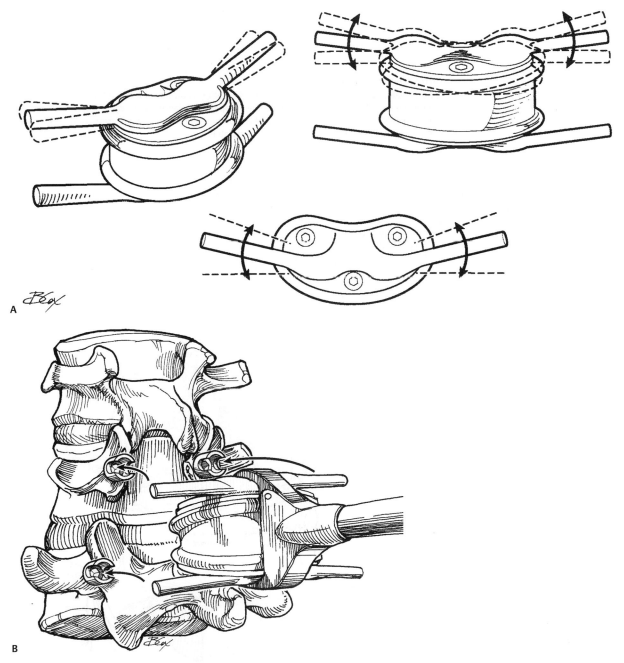

**Fig. 75.1** *(A)* The TOPS system is designed to partially constrain axial rotation, lateral bending, flexion and extension. *(B)* The TOPS device consists of a polycarbonate urethane (PcU) insert sandwiched between two titanium plates. The four arms extending from the device are inserted in tulip-head connections on pedicle screws.

# 76

# Posterior Interspinous Implant Placement

*Kern Singh and Frank M. Phillips*

## Description

Biomechanical studies have suggested that the restriction of segmental motion resulting from spinal fusion causes abnormal kinematics at adjacent mobile segments, potentially leading to instability and accelerated degeneration. In an attempt to eliminate problems innate to fusion surgery, the concept of dynamically stabilizing a diseased lumbar motion segment has been proposed.

## Key Principles

Theoretically, an interspinous process device should assist in the functioning of the diseased motion segment by providing stability while allowing motion and by load-sharing the forces transmitted through the posterior spinal elements.

## Expectations

The device for intervertebral assisted motion (DIAM) and the Wallis system are interspinous process "bumpers" designed to provide facet distraction, decrease intradiskal pressure, and reduce abnormal segmental motion and alignment.

## Indications

Indications for using interspinous prostheses remain poorly defined and largely reflect individual surgeon biases. The DIAM and Wallis devices have been used in the following situations:
- Disk herniation (with diskectomy)
- Spinal stenosis (with or without concomitant laminotomy)
- Facet syndrome
- Disk dysfunction or degenerative disk disease

## Contraindications

Isthmic spondylolysis, unstable spondylolisthesis (higher than grade I), neoplasia, fracture, and idiopathic scoliosis. Relative contraindications include osteoporotic bone and stable degenerative spondylolisthesis (grade I).

## Special Considerations

Preoperative imaging is essential to determine the etiologic and anatomic sites of neural compression. Plain radiographs, in addition to magnetic resonance imaging (MRI) or myelography and postmyelogram computed tomography (CT) imaging, are essential for identifying sites of neural compression and for identifying degenerative spinal pathologies.

## Special Instructions, Position, and Anesthesia

Traditional fusion procedures disrupt the normal segmental musculature and the inherent dynamic stabilization of the spine, likely degrading the surgical outcome. As such, the DIAM conforms to the interspinous anatomy and allows placement with minimal disturbance of the segmental muscles through a simple midline approach with preservation of the segmental anatomy. Patient is positioned in the standard prone position. These devices may be placed under local or general anesthesia.

## Tips, Pearls, and Lessons Learned

The most frequently involved anatomic level is L4-L5. The surgical approach is performed using a standard midline incision or a slightly lateral incision (10 mm lateral to the midline). A counterincision is necessary for insertion, preparation, and seating of the device. Care must be taken to maintain continuity of the supraspinous ligament by preserving a band at least 10 mm wide and as thick as possible. A window is created in the interspinous space using a scalpel that is ideally curved upward; the window is then enlarged with a curved Kerrison rongeur, taking care to preserve cortical bone (**Fig. 76.1**). At this stage, the interlaminar distractor can be inserted as far anteriorly as possible at the junction between the base of the spinous process and the laminae (**Fig. 76.2**). The appropriate trial (sizes available in 2-mm increments, from 8 to 14 mm) is positioned between the grooves of the distractor to determine the implant size (**Fig. 76.3**). Proper fit of the interspinous prosthesis should be based on re-tensioning of the supraspinous ligament and

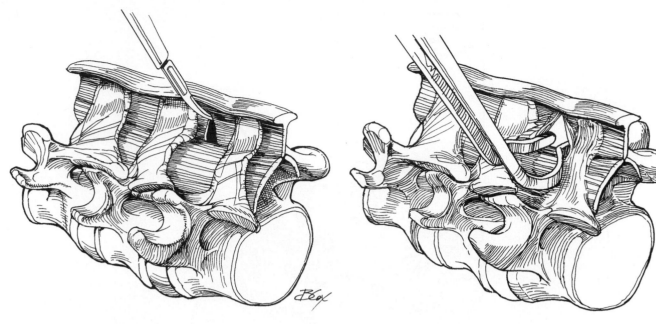

**Fig. 76.1** *Resection of the interspinous ligament down to the ligamentum flavum creating a window in the interspinous space.*

**Fig. 76.2** *Placement of the interspinous distractor.*

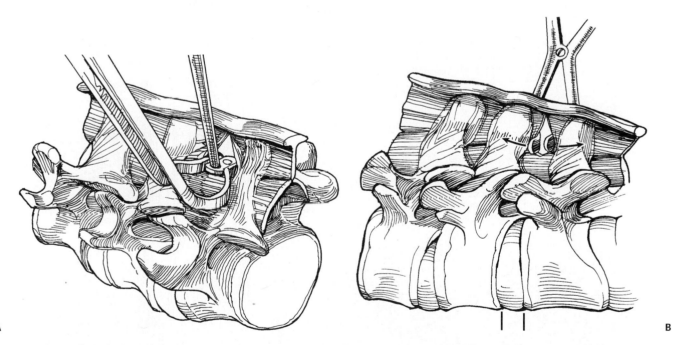

A

B

**Fig. 76.3** *Implant selection and prosthesis trial sizing. (A) A trial sizer is fitted between the spinous process. (B) Gentle distraction is applied between the spinous processes to appropriately tension the interspinous ligament.*

realignment of the facets and articular capsule (**Fig. 76.4**). Parallel alignment of the end plates can also be used as a reference for re-tensioning of the posterior longitudinal ligament. Pressing the trigger of the inserter both activates the claw and pulls back the arms of the inserter, allowing the wings to unfold, bringing them into contact with the spinous processes. The impactor is placed on top of the implant and the prosthesis is pushed down with gentle taps of the mallet. The posterior interspinous stabilizer is packaged with two independent ligaments that attach respectively to each adjacent spinous process (**Fig. 76.5**). The rivet is brought down to the loop, tensioned, and secured with the crimper. The rest of the ligament is cut off and removed.

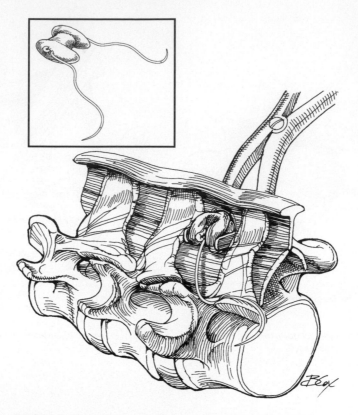

**Fig. 76.4** *Final positioning using the impactor. Inset figure shows inter-spinous device, which is inserted with the aid of gentle distraction.*

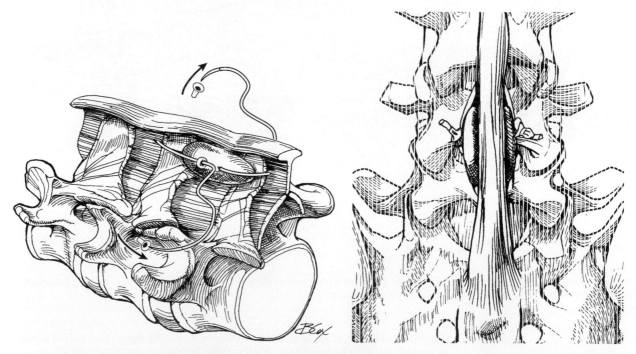

A

B

**Fig. 76.5** *Implant ligament fixation to the adjacent spinous processes. (A) The implant is inserted with the suturable ends passed through the inter-spinous ligament/around the spinous process. (B) The final position of the device with suturable ends appropriately tensioned and crimped.*

PITFALLS
- Care must be taken to maintain continuity of the supraspinous ligament by preserving a band at least 10 mm wide and as thick as possible. Excessive spinous process resection and undue force with the distractor may result in a fracture of the spinous process causing segmental spinal instability. Lastly, excessive distraction and oversized prosthetic implantation may result in creation of localized kyphosis and increased pressure on the disk accelerating spinal degeneration.

**Difficulties Encountered**

A window is created in the interspinous space using a scalpel that is ideally curved upward; the window is then enlarged with a curved Kerrison rongeur, taking care to preserve cortical bone. This step is critical and requires extreme caution. Using excessive force due to tissue entrapment may result in a fracture of the spinous process. In cases of overlapping and hypertrophic laminae (kissing laminae) or spinous processes, trimming is recommended.

**Key Procedural Steps**

1. Localizing lateral radiograph
2. Soft tissue dissection with preservation of the midline spinal structures
3. Counterincision necessary for insertion, preparation, and seating of the device
4. Neurologic decompression limited to sites of anatomic decompression identified on preoperative imaging studies
5. Resection of the interspinous ligament down to the ligamentum flavum, creating a window in the interspinous space (**Fig. 76.1**)
6. Placement of the interspinous distractor as far anteriorly as possible (**Fig. 76.2**)
7. Implant selection and prosthesis trial sizing (**Fig. 76.3**)
8. Final positioning using the impactor (**Fig. 76.4**)
9. Implant ligament fixation to the adjacent spinous processes (**Fig. 76.5**)

**Bailout, Rescue, Salvage Procedures**

Excessive interspinous ligament resection and spinous fracture may render the interspinous implant unusable. A standard decompression should be performed with spinal fusion implemented if the motion segment is deemed to be unstable.

# 77

# Cervical Disk Replacement

*Rick C. Sasso and Ben J. Garrido*

## Description

Anterior cervical diskectomy and fusion has historically been the gold standard treatment for patients experiencing cervical radiculopathy or myelopathy refractory to nonoperative measures. The safety and effectiveness of this procedure have been established and demonstrated in the literature; however, limitations have evolved, and subsequently alternatives such as disk replacement are being investigated. Such innovative technology has addressed kinematic and biomechanical factors in cervical spine motion. Intervertebral disk replacement is designed to preserve motion, both at the affected and adjacent levels, and avoid limitations of fusion. Hilibrand et al have described adjacent level degeneration in patients having undergone cervical fusion at a rate of 2.9% of patients per annum. Such new-onset degenerative changes and possible recurring neurologic symptoms may be deferred or eliminated with cervical disk replacement. In addition, potential complications related to fusion such as pseudarthrosis, anterior plate problems, and morbidity associated with bone graft harvest may be avoided. Cervical disk arthroplasty is designed to provide physiologic motion and eliminate abnormal loading stresses at adjacent levels that lead to accelerated degeneration.

## Expectations

Disk arthroplasty results may be highly subject to procedural technique. Preoperative planning with magnetic resonance imaging (MRI) or computed tomography (CT) myelogram is essential to determine neural compressive lesions. Appropriate disk sizing and assessment of excessive osteophytes is performed with preoperative CT scans. Disk height should be relatively normal without profound collapse, facet joints must not be extremely degenerated, and reasonably normal motion must be present. Intraoperative patient positioning is supine, with the spine stabilized in neutral position without hyperextension. It is important to perform adequate decompression of both the spinal canal and the bilateral neuroforamen. With motion-sparing techniques, it is extremely important to adequately decompress the asymptomatic side as well as the target site. Appropriate end-plate preparation is critical to allow for bony ingrowth into the prosthetic shell while maintaining the strong subchondral end plate. Undersizing the base-plate area may result in end-plate damage and implant subsidence. Prosthetic disk placement is confirmed under fluoroscopy. Postoperative immobilization is not required.

## Indications

Intervertebral disk replacement is indicated for cervical radiculopathy due to a herniated disk or osteophyte complex at a single level between C3 and C7. These patients must have failed aggressive nonoperative treatment modalities and be skeletally mature with relatively normal segmental motion.

## Contraindications

Cervical disk replacement surgery should not be performed in patients with sagittal plane abnormalities, spondylolisthesis, retrolisthesis, spondylolysis, or any evidence of segmental instability. Poor surgical candidates and those with active systemic or operative site infection should be excluded. Those patients who have a history of previous cervical surgery, metabolic bone disease, progressive neuromuscular disease, or significant osteoporosis, or are on corticosteroid therapy, should not be considered for this procedure. In addition, radiographically confirmed ankylosis, ossification of the posterior longitudinal ligament (OPLL), fixed kyphosis, and incompetent end-plate or severe facet joint arthritic changes should also be excluded. Cervical myelopathy secondary to factors other than a soft disk herniation at the level to be treated via an anterior diskectomy decompression should be avoided.

## Special Considerations

There are several disk arthroplasty systems for which early data has been reported but long-term outcomes are still pending. Wigfield et al recently reported favorable results after 2 years with the Prestige I disk design (Medtronic Sofamor Danek, Memphis, TN). They concluded that motion was successfully preserved without sacrificing device stability. No devices dislocated, and procedural complications were limited to two cases of transient hoarseness, which resolved demonstrating procedural safety. Goffin et al also reported early excellent results for the Bryan disk (Medtronic Sofamor Danek) placed at a single level in 60 patients. Sasso et al compared the initial functional outcome results on the Bryan disk replacement with anterior cervical fusion. This study used multiple outcome measures, also demonstrating favorable results for disk replacement compared with anterior cervical arthrodesis. Significant more motion at 3, 6, and 12 months was retained in the disk replacement group (**Fig. 77.1**). The clinical benefits of maintaining motion and providing symptom relief are postulated to delay or avoid adjacent level degeneration. These

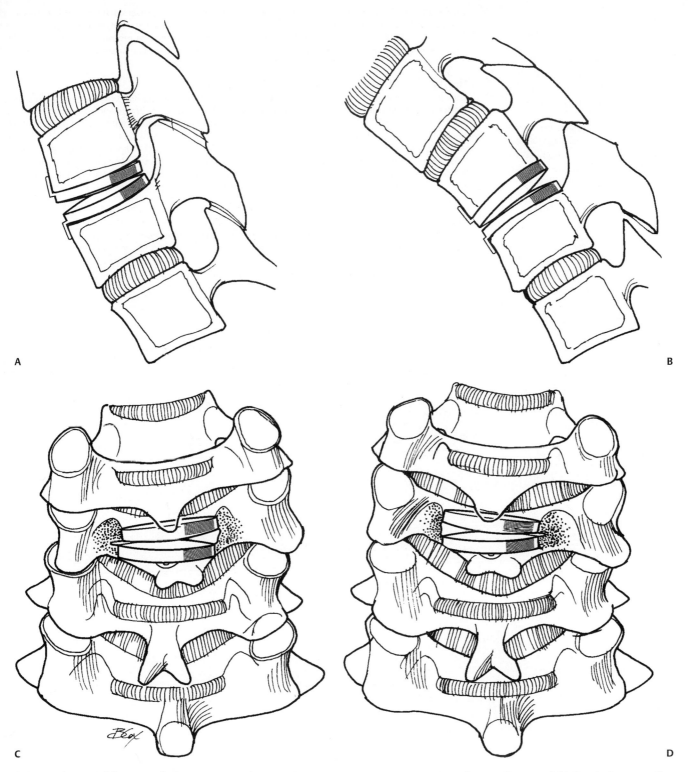

**Fig. 77.1** *Three-year follow-up on the first patient to undergo cervical artificial disk replacement in the United States. This Bryan disk is functioning very well as demonstrated by these illustrations in extension **(A)**, flexion **(B)**, and left **(C)** and right **(D)** side-bending.*

PITFALLS

• Malplacement of the artificial disk implant can result in a neurologic deficit or later malfunction of the disk. It is imperative that the cervical disk replacement implant be well positioned. This is much more critical than positioning of a bone graft for fusion.

• Early postoperative pitfalls include recurrent laryngeal nerve palsy, dysphagia, and implant migration. Late pitfalls may include heterotopic ossification, implant loosening, and juxtalevel changes.

promising results suggest that artificial cervical disk replacement is comparable, if not superior, to fusion at least in the short term. Although not the current standard, wide acceptance will depend on long-term outcome studies. Current success with artificial cervical disk replacement has demonstrated that the intended effects are being achieved, sparing cervical motion and decreasing future fusion associated morbidity.

**Tips, Pearls, and Lessons Learned**

Important considerations for a good outcome include adhering to strict patient selection, complete preoperative preparation, and meticulous surgical technique. One of the most important lessons learned is the importance of careful and complete neural decompression when motion-sparing devices are implanted. Neural tissue is protected in a fused nonmobile setting; however, neural tissue is placed at risk in a mobile segment, especially if the motion is increased and residual compressive disk tissue or osteophyte remains. This can be troublesome if relative stenosis is present on the asymptomatic side and meticulous attention has not been paid to this side during decompression of the symptomatic side. Radicular symptoms may begin postoperatively on the initial asymptomatic side as increased motion commences.

**Key Procedural Steps**

1. Intraoperative positioning in physiologic alignment, not hyperextension
2. Complete diskectomy with neural decompression
3. Verification of midline
4. Preparation of end plates
5. Insertion of device
6. Radiographic verification of position

**Bailout, Rescue, Salvage Procedures**

Most cervical disk replacements can be repositioned intraoperatively if acceptable placement is not initially achieved. Those devices that achieve initial stability with a keel that is cut into the vertebral body may be difficult to realign. The ultimate bailout, rescue, and salvage procedure for a cervical disk replacement is a standard anterior cervical fusion with instrumentation.

# 78

# Lumbar Spinal Arthroplasty

*Scott L. Blumenthal*

## Description

Spine fusion for degenerative disk disease has been regarded as the gold standard, but this has not produced excellent results, with pseudarthrosis being an all-too-common occurrence, as well as patients who achieve a solid fusion but who do not have a favorable clinical outcome. Spine fusion surgery has also given rise to the phenomenon of adjacent segment disease related to the relatively rigid fusion segment being adjacent to a previously normal segment. These concerns have highlighted the need for a surgical treatment that spares spinal motion, allowing motion to be closer to that of pre-illness levels and to allow a more rapid return to work and other activities without having to rely on a solid fusion first taking place.

## Key Principles

It is essential first to identify the cause of the low back pain. Disk replacement should not be considered in patients with fracture, infection, spondylolisthesis, spinal stenosis, sacroiliac problems, or facet-related pain. These diagnoses should be ruled out as the primary pain source. History and physical examination followed by anteroposterior (AP) and lateral flexion and extension radiographs should be performed. Magnetic resonance imaging (MRI) is a helpful study to evaluate the intervertebral disks, spinal canal, and neural foramen. One must be cautious in assuming that every degenerated "black disk" found on MRI is a source of pain. We have found it helpful to perform a diskography to evaluate intradiskal pressure and volume, disk morphology, and most importantly, reproduction of the patient's usual pain during disk injection. Pain intensity during injection can be assessed on a 0 to 10 visual analogue scale (VAS) at each level. The patients should be awake and blinded to the level being tested. Facet pain may be ruled out by history and physical examination. If in doubt, a facet injection may be performed. Bone densitometry should be obtained on all patients being worked up for a spinal arthroplasty procedure, especially if there is any concern about patients' bone quality or if their history indicates a high risk of osteoporosis.

## Expectations

Pain arising from degenerative disk disease at one or more lumbar levels not responding to nonoperative measures is the primary indication for spinal arthroplasty. The goals of spinal arthroplasty are to maintain motion, relieve pain, preserve disk space height, maintain neural foraminal height, and preserve the facet joints. It is important to have longevity of any implant through millions of cycles and to aim for avoidance of revision surgery. This requires excellent wear characteristics of any spacer, excellent shock absorbing capacity, and a solid interface between the device and the host bone without sacrificing revision options. The expectation of the surgical procedure is that patients experience significant relief of their back pain complaints and are able to resume activities of daily living as well as some recreational activities or a preinjury occupation. It is hoped that the long-term potential of symptomatic adjacent level disease is minimized with the placement of a motion-sparing device rather than a spinal fusion.

## Indications

Infection and instability must be ruled out as well as low bone density, typically defined as a density value one standard deviation below the normal population mean. Typically, patients may be no older than 60 years of age. Facet arthrosis at the level being considered may be present but should not be severe.

The presence of radicular pain in addition to axial pain is acceptable if there is no severe canal stenosis and it is thought that the radicular pain is mostly from foraminal stenosis secondary to loss of disk height at that level. This may be corrected with the distraction that is performed during insertion of the artificial disk.

## Contraindications

The presence of infection or disruption of posterior structures or any instability from a pars defect or pedicle fracture should be regarded as absolute contraindications. The presence of a rigid deformity is a contraindication. Bending films may be obtained to differentiate sciatic scoliosis from other rigid forms such as degenerative or idiopathic.

## Special Considerations

Most artificial disk devices consist of a metal end plate that anchors into the vertebral endplate (**Fig. 78.1**). These metal end plates articulate with a spacer (**Fig. 78.2**), which allows motion at the segment (**Fig. 78.3**). The metal end plates are available in different cross-sectional sizes and lordotic angles, and come with or

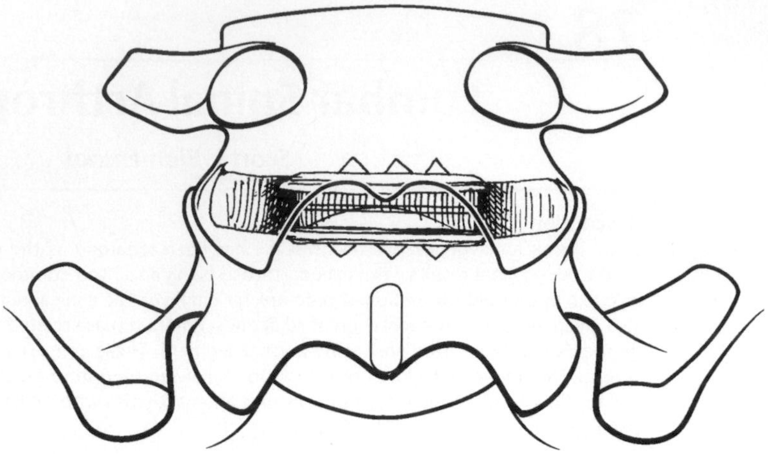

**Fig. 78.1** *The implant as it should be positioned at the midline of the vertebral body.*

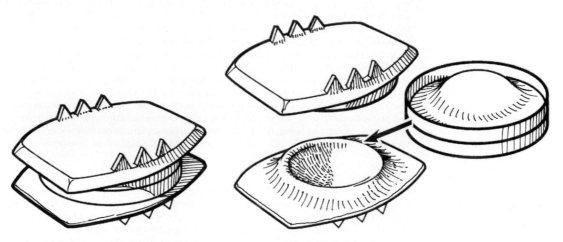

**A**

**B**

**Fig. 78.2** *(A) The fully assembled prosthesis as it would sit in vivo. (B) Exploded view of the prosthesis showing its three components (from top to bottom): vertebral body side of upper metal end plate showing spikes for bone anchoring; polyethylene spacer; and lower end plate showing smooth concave inner side for contact and motion with spacer.*

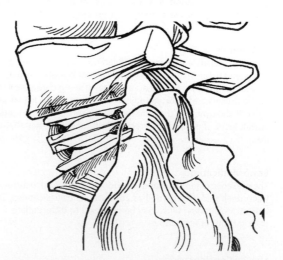

**Fig. 78.3** *A properly positioned implant. Note the posterior placement, but with no penetration of the canal at the posterior aspect of the superior end plate of S1.*

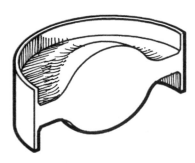

**Fig. 78.4** *Cross section of a polyethylene spacer.*

without a porous coating and have either teeth or keels to gain stability into the bony vertebral end plate. The spacers come in various thicknesses and consist of either metal or polyethylene (**Fig. 78.4**). The total disk replacement (TDR) devices have varying levels of constraint.

### Special Instructions, Position, and Anesthesia
The help of an access surgeon is strongly advised. A rolled towel may be placed under the patient's lumbar spine to help local lordosis and assist in disk tissue removal and implantation of the device. The towel may later be removed on device insertion. Similarly, the table can be re-flexed and flexed to open up the disk space when desired.

### Tips, Pearls, and Lessons Learned
Recently, results of the multicenter Food and Drug Administration (FDA)-regulated trial conducted to assess the safety and effectiveness of the Charité artificial disk were published. The study involved 304 patients and included 24-month follow-up. Patients were randomized to TDR or anterior interbody fusion using cages. Although patients in both groups improved, the TDR group experienced improvement more quickly and were significantly more satisfied. Complications in the two groups were similar.

Long-term follow-up of TDR patients has been published from Europe where TDR has been performed since the mid-1980s. A study with a minimum 10-year follow-up for 100 patients found that 62% of patients had an excellent outcome, with an additional 28% indicating a good outcome. The return to work rate was 91%. Five patients (5%) required a secondary posterior fusion. There was no indication of significant problems with the durability of the devices long-term.

### Difficulties Encountered
Because an anterior approach is required, the presence of vessel calcification, which may be seen on lateral radiographs, should be evaluated with a CT scan. If circumferential calcification is present, it is inadvisable to proceed except at the L5-S1 level, where the vessels need minimal retraction. A vascular opinion can be sought in cases of uncertainty.

### Key Procedural Steps
A direct anterior approach is used with a transverse incision for a one-level replacement or vertical incision for multilevel procedures. A retroperitoneal approach is preferred but a transperitoneal may also be used. Care must be taken to preserve sympathetic and parasympathetic nerves to avoid erectile dysfunction and retrograde ejaculation in the male patient. It is also important to avoid lymphatic structures and to protect all vascular structures at all times.

It is important to obtain wide exposure of the disk space and perform a total diskectomy, while being careful to avoid damaging the end plates. Intact end plates are important for obtaining good fixation and avoiding subsidence. To avoid lateral tilt, care must be taken to restore the appropriate lordosis and obtain adequate end-plate coverage. The spacer insert must be of the appropriate thickness to allow a snug fit without overdistracting the disk space. When working above the L5-S1 level, it may be necessary to allow the vessels to relax from time to time to allow some blood flow into the left leg. The vessels and distal pulses should be palpated at the end of the surgery to ensure no vascular insult.

It is important to place the device as close to the true midline as possible and as far posterior as possible without breaching the spinal canal.

### Postoperative Protocol
All patients may be weight bearing immediately after surgery and are encouraged to stand and ambulate with a therapist the day of surgery. Standing x-rays are obtained the morning after surgery to document the position and rule out migration in the weight-bearing position. Patient-controlled analgesia is used on the first postoperative night for pain control. Compression stockings and sequential foot or leg pumps are also used on the first postoperative night. Most single-level patients go home the following morning. Patients are advised to avoid extension, stooping, excessive twisting, or any heavy lifting the first 6 weeks, and may then gradually resume normal activities. Participation in extreme or contact sports is not encouraged.

### Bailout, Rescue, Salvage Procedures
Revision options include avoiding the entire anterior implantation area completely and performing a posterior fusion. If removal of the device is indicated, it may be replaced with either a new TDR, or an anterior fusion may be performed with or without a supplemental posterior construct. The approach for removing the primary TDR prosthesis may be done through a repeat direct anterior approach or through a lateral approach, avoiding the area of scar tissue.

---

**PITFALLS**
Potential complications of disk replacement include:
- Subsidence
- Device dislocation and migration
- Radicular pain, weakness, dysesthesia
- Infection
- Polyethylene wear, osteolysis, and loosening
- Metal debris and oncogenic potential (no clinical cases identified)
- Acceleration of facet joint arthrosis
- Instability (too thin of a spacer)
- Postoperative scoliosis (poor device positioning)

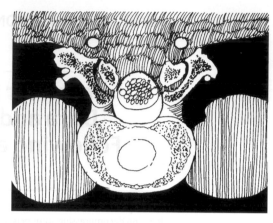

**Fig. 79.1** *The position of the rods and facets in relation to the dura. These structures may be used as landmarks in estimating the depth of epidural scar resection.*

• Intraoperative blood loss tends to be increased in revision surgeries due to distortion of the normal tissue planes. During decompression, achievement of adequate hemostasis may be difficult, and bipolar cautery, thrombin-soaked patties, Gelfoam, and Floseal are all useful modalities for coagulating or tamponading epidural venous bleeding. Bone wax may also be utilized to minimize bleeding from exposed cancellous surfaces. Prior to wound closure, routine placement of a subfascial drain is recommended. Wounds should be irrigated copiously with antibiotic containing normal saline solutions due to longer operative times and higher incidence of infection in revision cases. Appropriate redosing of prophylactic intravenous antibiotics intraoperatively is also recommended. Postoperative management should include close neurologic monitoring for any deterioration that may be indicative of an epidural hematoma. Drains typically are left in place longer compared with nonrevision procedures because of continued wound bleeding or extravascular fluid accumulation. Serial monitoring of the coagulation panel, complete blood count, and electrolytes is recommended for several days postoperatively for procedures with intraoperative blood losses in excess of 1 L.

aid in differentiating scar from other pathologies. MRI is also helpful in identifying the presence of a pseudomeningocele and arachnoiditis. Pseudomeningocele may sometimes be confused with a seroma. Arachnoiditis typically appears as irregular nerve roots that are thickened or clumped together. MRI may have limited utility, however, due to excessive postoperative scar formation or the presence of metal instrumentation, which produces artifact. The mainstay of postoperative imaging is postmyelography CT.

A CT myelogram is useful in evaluating the bony anatomy. Pars interarticularis defects may easily be identified as well as the presence of bridging laminar bone that may still be present if the previous procedure was a limited type of decompression. These bony structures serve as important landmarks. Another crucial observation is the level of the pars with respect to the dura. With the exception of L5-S1, the pars is usually posterior to the most superficial portion of the dura, making this a critical landmark for safely resecting epidural scar tissue (**Fig. 79.1**). At L5-S1 the dura is often above the level of the pars, however, and scar resection must be carefully performed at this level to avoid an inadvertent durotomy. Pseudomeningocele identified on MRI is also important to confirm on CT myelogram.

### Special Instructions, Position, and Anesthesia

To reduce epidural bleeding, a Jackson or Andrews table is used to allow the abdomen to hang free, reducing intraabdominal pressure and the resultant intravenous pressure and engorgement of the epidural veins. Anticipated blood loss and anesthesia duration are somewhat more unpredictable in revision surgery. One should consider the use of arterial line monitoring of blood pressure, pay close attention to ensuring that all bony prominences are well padded, and take extreme care to avoid external ocular pressure during the prone positioning of the patient.

### Difficulties Encountered

Dural injury is among the most common complications of revision decompression surgery. Durotomy closure may be facilitated with the use of a microscope and microsurgical instruments with monofilament suture (e.g., 6-0 Prolene). Closure may be reinforced with commercially available adjuvant products such as a DuraGen (Integra Life Sciences Corp., Plainsboro, NJ) patch or a fibrin glue product. Valsalva maneuver performed by the anesthesiologist helps to assess the adequacy of the closure. If a durotomy is repaired, patients will typically be on bed rest for 48 hours with the head of the bed flat. Caffeine intake may also be encouraged to treat severe headaches that do not resolve spontaneously.

### Key Procedural Steps

The previous incision may be used, but is often extended in the cranial and caudal direction to enhance exposure. The previous scar is often excised to enhance cosmesis. After the fascia is incised in the midline, aggressive epidural scar removal is advocated. To assess the depth of safe scar removal, several landmarks may be utilized. The position of the dura with respect to the pars should be evaluated on CT myelogram. Usually, scar tissue can be safely removed in the midline to the level of the pars bilaterally. An exception may be at L5-S1 where the dura is often superficial to the pars. A sharp Cobb elevator is the instrument of choice for removing scar tissue safely. Bovie cautery may also be used, but care must be taken to avoid thermal injury to the dura. The Cobb provides tactile feedback once the pars had been reached on each side of the canal. The epidural scar may then be removed to the depth of the pars using a Cobb elevator or Leksell rongeur. The lamina above and below the laminectomy defect should also be identified, as well as any bridging bone, to aid in determining the desired depth of scar resection.

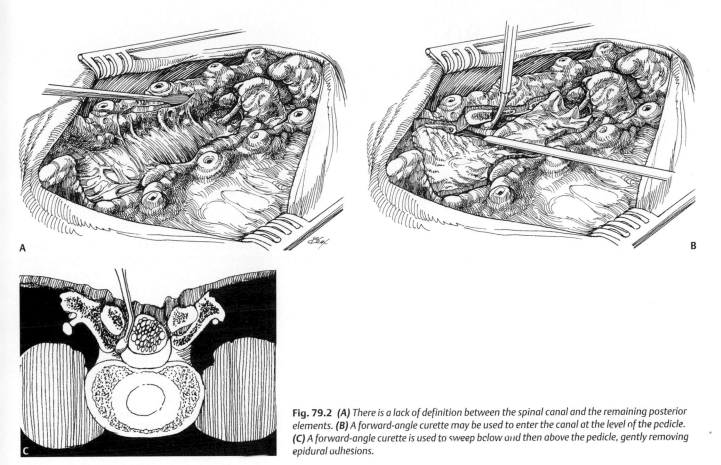

**Fig. 79.2** *(A) There is a lack of definition between the spinal canal and the remaining posterior elements. (B) A forward-angle curette may be used to enter the canal at the level of the pedicle. (C) A forward-angle curette is used to sweep below and then above the pedicle, gently removing epidural adhesions.*

Once the excessive epidural scar has been removed and self-retaining retractors are placed, a microscope may be brought into the field (under sterile conditions) to safely enter the spinal canal. The next objective is to define the interface between the pars and epidural scar at the lateral edge of the canal. A sharp Cobb is usually the best instrument to remove scar tissue at this interface. The high-speed burr is also a safe instrument to define this interface because it is fairly resistant to cutting through scar tissue. Bovie cautery is sometimes used, but again may risk thermal injury to the dura.

Once the edge of the canal is defined, a forward-angle Karlin curette may be used to enter the canal at the level of the pedicle. Staying adjacent to the bone of the pedicle can avoid injury to the dura or nerve roots, and the scar can be safely elevated away from the side wall of the canal. Sweep below the pedicle and then above, gently removing epidural scar adhesions. Next, move to the adjacent pedicle and perform the same maneuver. Connecting adjacent levels may be safely accomplished once the nerve roots have been identified at the level of each pedicle (**Fig. 79.2**).

The high-speed burr is useful in safely widening the bone resection of previous laminotomies or laminectomy defects. Once the bone has been resected, areas devoid of epidural scar may be used to enter the canal and define a plane to release the scar tissue. A thin shell of bone may be created at the interface between bone and scar that may be safely removed using a forward angle curette.

### Bailout, Rescue, Salvage Procedures

Revision decompression surgery is challenging, but adherence to a routine set of management guidelines and operative techniques helps ensure optimal outcomes. Indirect decompression may also be utilized as an accessory tool in revision decompression cases. Indirect techniques include anterior lumbar interbody fusion to restore disk height as well as the use of pedicle screw distraction (unilateral or bilateral). Indirect decompression techniques increase the foraminal area without direct nerve root manipulation and neurolysis. Overdistraction should be avoided due to the risk of stretch nerve root palsies and nerve irritation.

# Dural Repair and Patch Techniques: Anterior and Posterior

*Milan G. Mody and Laurence D. Rhines*

### Description
Incidental or inadvertent durotomies are infrequent (4 to 14% incidence) but serious complications in spinal surgery. Several intra- and postoperative surgical strategies are available for proper and timely management of cerebrospinal fluid (CSF) leaks.

### Key Principles
Timely effective strategies for controlling CSF leaks can lead to good clinical outcomes and avoid serious sequelae such as postural headaches, pseudomeningocele, meningitis, durocutaneous fistulas, epidural abscess, and persistent neuropathy.

### Expectations
These techniques can provide stable control of CSF egress from incidental durotomy.

### Indications
The gold standard for treatment of all CSF leaks is primary repair of the dural defect with 5-0 or 6-0 Prolene or Neurilon. There are certain pathologic situations and intraspinal locations for which primary repair may be technically formidable or impossible and require patch techniques (**Fig. 80.1**). This includes a durotomy in the setting of anterior cervical or lumbar diskectomy, en bloc removal of tumor with adherent dura, resection of an intradural tumor, microdiskectomy with adherent nerve root sleeve, adherent stenotic ossification of the posterior longitudinal ligament (OPLL) or ligamentum flavum, and traumatic bony laceration of dura.

### Contraindications
Do not attempt primary dural repair if under tension secondary to a large defect or constraining adhesions. Pinhole high-pressure leaks are better treated with enlargement and primary suture closure. A patch repair cannot be performed if a dural edge cannot be circumferentially exposed. Management of durotomy in the setting of an acute infection is a challenge.

### Special Considerations
There is a published association of dural tears with smoking, diabetes, more than three epidural steroid injections 6 months prior to surgery, trauma, and revision surgery. Preoperative planning enables the surgeon to be prepared for dural repair with a choice of graft. Patients must be informed of the nature, purpose, risks, benefits, and alternatives of autograft (fascia lata, lumbodorsal fascia, or fat), allograft (cadaveric dura or pericardium), xenograft (bovine pericardium), or synthetic (Gore-Tex or DuraGen [Integra Life Sciences Corp., Plainsboro, NJ] collagen matrix suture or sutureless) patch grafts.

### Special Instructions, Position, and Anesthesia
A surgical microscope or loupes can enhance the evaluation and repair of durotomies. The availability of specialized instruments such a watchmaker's or knot-tying forceps, microscissors, microneedle holder, and knot-pusher can mitigate the technical difficulty of a small workspace.

If autograft fascia lata is to be used for patch repair, then the patient's lateral thigh should be available, prepped, and draped at the start of the procedure. Anesthesia personnel will have to perform Valsalva maneuver to test the repair or sometimes identify the pinhole tear.

### Tips, Pearls, and Lessons Learned
Local erector spinae fascia or fat is readily available without increased risks. Collagen matrix onlay can be successful with limited technical or time demands but adds to material costs. Autograft fascia lata has the best handling characteristics and does not pose the risk of disease transmission but requires separate incision with associated morbidity including possible weakness of leg abduction.

Placement of an intradural lumbar drain for 3 to 5 days reduces CSF pressure on the repair; however, the surgical and nursing staff must be extremely diligent in monitoring the flow (<10 cc/hr) and position (ear or shoulder level). Remember to continue prophylactic antibiotics until the drain is discontinued. If CSF appears cloudy or turbid, then fluid should be sent for Gram stain and cultures. We recommend placing a skin stitch upon drain removal to minimize leakage. If there is persistent drain-site leakage, then place a pressure dressing and institute bed rest for 2 to 3 more days.

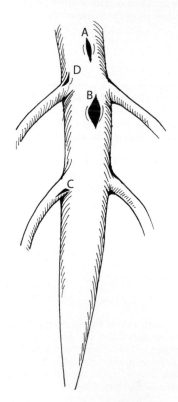

**Fig. 80.1** *Type A tear can be repaired primarily, whereas type B opening requires patch technique. Types C and D tears should be considered for fat, fibrin glue, or collagen matrix onlay bailout.*

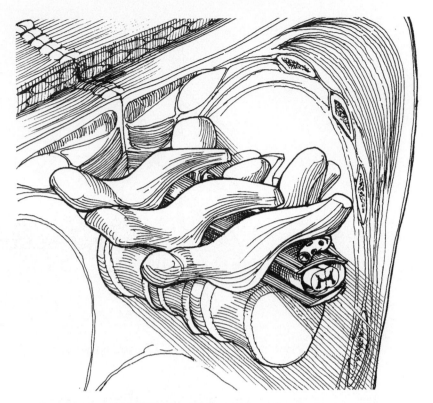

**Fig. 80.2** *With a collagen matrix onlay graft, the recommended subfascial drain will remove any residual fluid and transient CSF effusion, especially when the patient is mobilized. Drains can also help obliterate dead space.*

Strategies to reduce perioperative intrathecal pressure include decreasing central venous pressure if a central line is present, smooth reversal of anesthesia to decrease tracheal irritation and coughing, Foley catheter for 2 to 5 days to facilitate bed rest, curbing narcotic use or providing stool softeners or laxatives to decrease constipation, antitussives, and locking the head of bed to <30 to 45 degrees. One should also avoid postoperative steroids if possible to promote physiologic augmentation of the primary or patch dural repair.

Some authors have wisely advised that we label these events as "intraoperative dural openings" and drop the medicolegal-laden terms such as "inadvertent or incidental durotomy or dural tears."

### Difficulties Encountered
If using DuraGen collagen matrix onlay (sutureless) technique, then a local drain is required (**Fig. 80.2**). With other techniques, however, local drains may pose the risk of repair breakdown or encourage formation of CSF fistula. If a local drain is preferred, then we recommend draining off the suction. Although a Gore-Tex synthetic graft is readily available, it is relatively stiff and requires special needles and suture, which makes it challenging in a narrow workspace. Patch suturing does leave pinholes from the suture needle that can be sealed with fibrin glue.

### Key Procedural Steps
Expose the entire dural defect and debride the frayed edges. This may require additional bony decompression or exposure than originally intended; however, one must maintain osteoligamentous stability. It is necessary to have at least 2 mm of dura exposed beyond the tear to suture a patch. Template the patch with cottonoid, glove-tip, or calipers.

A watertight primary closure with 5-0 or 6-0 nylon, Prolene, or Neurilon is highly recommended if possible rather than simple fibrin glue application or packing with Gelfoam. Fibrin glue can be applied to augment a repair. If a dural tear cannot be repaired primarily, then these steps must be taken: patch and seal the tear, achieve a watertight wound closure, and decrease perioperative intrathecal pressure with the provided strategies.

Local fascia is easily obtained with electrocautery and prepared on the back table by removing fat or muscle bluntly. A fat graft can also be applied if only a small defect is present. Fascia lata is harvested through a linear incision on the lateral thigh. It is always wise to harvest a larger graft than needed, as the size can

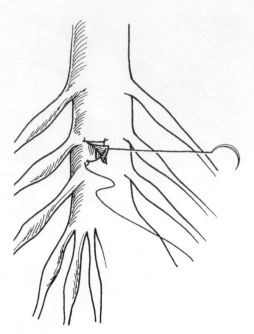

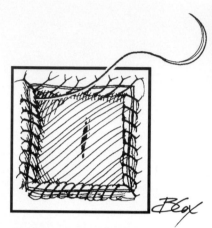

**Fig. 80.3** *Tack graft in place with stay sutures in all corners.*

**Fig. 80.4** *Complete repair with interrupted or running sutures.*

always be made smaller. If allograft, xenograft, or synthetic graft is to be used, then follow the thawing and preparation directions, which may require some time, so plan accordingly. At minimum, the patch material must be pliable and able to take needle passage when the patch repair is begun.

Stay sutures are placed at all corners of the graft and a running stitch is used to complete the repair (**Figs. 80.3** and **80.4**). Sewing from the graft to the dura is an easier and safer technique. Anterior patch repair may not allow working room for suturing, and therefore collagen matrix onlay may be necessary (**Figs. 80.5** and **80.6**). Fibrin glue can reinforce the suture line, especially the pinholes from needle entry. Anesthesia-induced Valsalva maneuver at a pressure of 40 mm $H_2O$ in the reverse Trendelenburg position

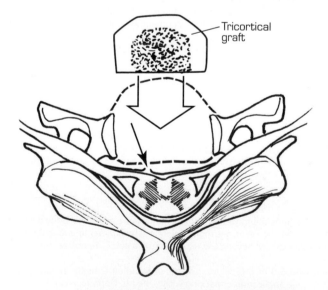

Tricortical graft

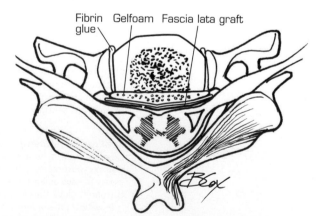

Fibrin glue    Gelfoam    Fascia lata graft

**Fig. 80.5** *A small dural defect (arrow) during an anterior cervical diskectomy or corpectomy may be difficult to widely expose for repair. Black arrow shows the small dural defect. Large arrow shows the tricortical graft placement.*

**Fig. 80.6** *Autologous fascia or fat or collagen matrix is laid gently over the defect and held in place with a piece of Gelfoam. Fibrin glue is added to secure the fascial graft, and a tricortical graft is placed in the usual fashion. It is important to measure the depth of the corpectomy defect to avoid iatrogenic spinal cord compression. Once the graft is in place, more fibrin glue can be added in the lateral gutters.*

PITFALLS

- Placing the patient in the Trendelenburg position to minimize CSF accumulation in the wound can lead to blood entry into the dural defect and can cause intradural hematoma neural compression. The dura mater where an inadvertent durotomy occurs is often fragile and may easily tear further when suturing. Therefore, great care must be taken to maintain only gentle traction on the suture at all times. Placement of a local wound drain is necessary when using DuraGen collagen matrix onlay (sutureless) technique. Otherwise, a local wound drain is the surgeon's choice because recent published reports dispute the increased risk of durocutaneous fistula from local drains.

- If a primary or patch dural repair is performed in the setting of an anterior thoracic corpectomy or approach, then attention must be paid to completely isolate the repair and spinal compartment from the pulmonary compartment and the inherent inspiratory negative pressure. The pulmonary effect can exacerbate CSF egress. Therefore, monitor the chest tube output for quantity and quality because this complication could be life-threatening with uncal herniation.

should be performed to test the primary or patch repair. If the repair is not watertight, then use fibrin glue rather than repeating the repair due to the fragility of the dura.

If the durotomy was large, repair was tenuous, or a patch technique was used, then percutaneously place a lumbar CSF drain proximal to the repair for 3 to 5 days. Postoperative management of drain and CSF pressure has been previously discussed. Closure of the wound should also be watertight with minimal dead space. Removing the spinous processes if possible will facilitate this closure. If posterolateral hardware is in place, then bilateral relaxing fascial incisions will allow the muscle and fascia to come together at the midline.

### Bailout, Rescue, Salvage Procedures

If a tear cannot be completely repaired, reinforcement with Gelfoam or fibrin glue can be performed. In anterior cervical or lumbar diskectomy cases, direct repair may be technically impossible and therefore requires onlay of Gelfoam, autogenous fascia or fat, or collagen matrix sealed with fibrin glue (**Figs. 80.5** and **80.6**).

A watertight wound closure over bony and neural elements by relaxing fascial incisions can also salvage an incomplete or difficult dural repair. You may need to utilize any and all strategies discussed here to ensure cessation of CSF egress from an incidental durotomy. The reported failure rate of durotomy repairs is about 5%, and failure often requires reoperation.

Postoperative discovery of an unknown incidental durotomy based on a patient's symptoms requires observation and 2 to 3 days of bed rest. If symptoms are progressive or persistent, then identify the problem with magnetic resonance imaging (MRI) or computed tomography (CT) myelogram. Treatment with epidural blood patch, CT-guided fibrin glue therapy, or lumbar CSF drain is reasonable and supported by the literature. If there is suspicious wound drainage but patient remains asymptomatic, then $\beta_2$-transferrin assay of the fluid will identify if this is a CSF leak. Early intervention is emphasized because delayed management can prolong symptoms and may lead to formation of a fistula, pseudomeningocele, or increased scar tissue.

# 81

# Wound Vacuum Assisted Closures (VAC) Management for Spinal or Bone Graft Wound Infections

*John M. Beiner and Linda Mascolo*

### Description

Traditional management of postoperative spinal (or bone graft donor site) wound infections, consisting of repeated operative debridement or bedside dressing changes, has largely been supplanted by the use of closed-system suction devices known as wound Vacuum Assisted Closures (VACs). This system consists of a specifically designed sponge that is placed into the infected wound bed, covered by an adhesive, occlusive drape, with suction applied via a vacuum device to promote wound healing, decrease wound size, help remove interstitial fluid allowing tissue decompression, improve perfusion, and assist in the removal of infectious materials (**Fig. 81.1**).

### Key Principles

Generalized wound treatment principles should be emphasized. Necrotic tissue and purulent fluid must be removed, and an abscess cannot be treated with anything other than operative debridement. Once the gross bacterial load has been reduced, the wound can begin to form granulation tissue. Adequate nutrition (prealbumin above 15 mg/dL) must be stressed. The wound VAC (KCI, San Antonio, TX) can speed closure of an infected spinal or bone graft site wound.

### Expectations

The wound VAC is expected to shorten time to healing, encourage granulation tissue formation, and reduce the need for repeat trips to the operating room with their attendant risks, (anesthesia, nutritional depletion, and blood loss) as well as decrease hospital length of stay. Once all gross purulence and necrotic tissue have been removed, the VAC should be applied and changed every 48 hours. The expected outcomes of this therapy are to promote an environment for healthy granulation tissue growth, decrease bacterial colonization, and improve time to wound closure or graft.

### Indications

Postoperative posterior spinal wound infections, iliac crest wound infections, or de novo spinal infections, once adequate debridement has been performed. The wound VAC also has clinical applications throughout the surgical arena for soft tissue loss and infections.

### Contraindications

Active CSF leak. The wound VAC in this setting can contribute to the formation of a pseudomeningocele.

#### Relative Contraindications

- History of dural tear or CSF leak that has been repaired
- Long-term steroid use with fragile skin

### Special Considerations

Some animal studies have shown that exposed bone should be decorticated to encourage granulation tissue to form. If exposed dura is present, suction may be decreased to 75 to 100 mm Hg; any radicular sensation may indicate excessive suction causing neural irritation. VAC vers-foam, a dense hydrophilic foam (white in color) is a nonadherent material that helps protect delicate structures and should be placed deep to the fascia on top of the dura. Granufoam, a reticulated hydrophobic foam (the black sponge) may then be placed superficial to this to allow a relative gradient in suction to protect the dura.

### Special Instructions, Position, and Anesthesia

Wounds below the fascial level may necessitate conscious sedation for removal and changing of the sponge. This decreases apprehension in patients who may already be frustrated with their infection, and allows a better debridement of tissue. This may be arranged in the operating room, the recovery room, or an intensive care unit. Alternatively, saline may be used to moisten the sponge to allow it to be removed more easily. Lidocaine can also be injected into the sponge prior to removal, as a topical anesthetic to

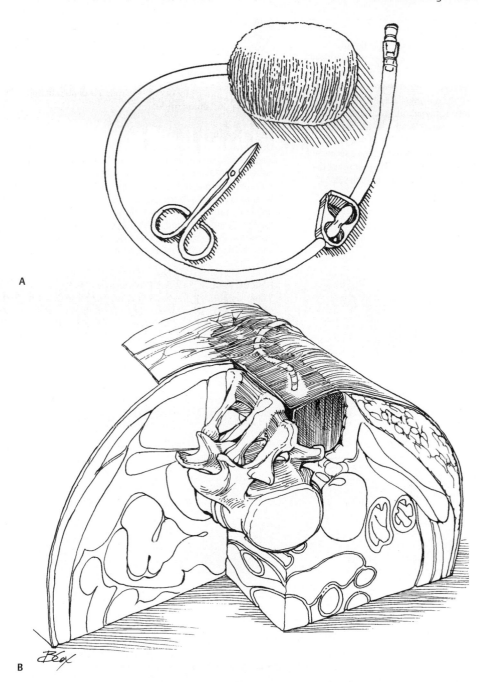

**Fig. 81.1** *(A)* *Typical components of the wound vacuum assisted closure packs: black sponge, tubing, and scissors.* *(B)* *Close-up of a wound with the component layers in place (from inside out): sponge, suction tubing, and occlusive layer.*

improve pain control during the dressing change. With wounds superficial to the fascia, bedside changes are often well tolerated.

### Tips, Pearls, and Lessons Learned
The VAC should be placed only into a relatively clean wound; it will not draw interstitial fluid and bacteria away from necrosis or purulence. It is important that the foam dressing be placed in the wound covering the entire wound base and sides, tunnels, and undermining; packing only superficially will encourage the fascia to close prematurely and may cause the treatment to fail. If purulent material is noted with the packing change, the surgeon should resort to repeated operative debridement or saline gauze wet to dry dressing changes until the wound is clean prior to reapplication of the VAC.

## PITFALLS

- If diskitis is present, a posterior application of the wound VAC will likely fail. The disk and any anterior phlegmon must be debrided before the posterior wound will granulate and heal without abscess formation. Brace wear may be uncomfortable with the suction tubing in place. The final closure of a wound can be expedited by performing a secondary closure in the operating room once the wound is approximately 80 to 90% granulated.

### Difficulties Encountered

Staff members may be reluctant to fully pack the sponge into the cavity. The sponge should be cut to the contour of the soft tissue deficit, but not packed into compression. Because this often generates significant pain in subfascial wounds, the resident, nurse, or physician's assistant is often reluctant to pack deep enough. A responsible care provider should personally supervise most VAC dressing changes, preferably with the skin/wound care nurse who is available at many hospitals, to ensure that healing is progressing from inside out, with no pockets forming.

### Key Procedural Steps

Operative debridement should occur until the wound is clean. The sponge is then contoured and placed into the soft tissue defect (often at the time of the last operative debridement), followed by an occlusive adherent dressing. A hole is then cut into the middle of this dressing, allowing placement of the suction/therapeutic regulated accurate care (TRAC) (KCI, San Antonio, TX) pad over this hole. The tubing may then be supported with more sponge and adhesive dressing to secure it to the skin in a convenient position to prevent pain from "laying on the tubing" and to allow improved patient mobilization. The wound edges may be "window-paned" with a hydrocolloid dressing (Duoderm) to protect the skin from shear stress. Suction is then applied: 125 mm Hg for most cases, but see above for exceptions. The dressing should be changed and assessed every 48 hours.

### Bailout, Rescue, Salvage Procedures

Saline wet to dry dressing changes, "feed me–drain me" irrigation systems, or silver-impregnated VAC sponges can be used for resistant infections. Hardware removal is rarely necessary.

# Index

Note: Page numbers followed by *f* indicate figures.